Basil C. Tarlatzis and Serdar E. Bulun, Editors

Proceedings of The IFFS 21st World Congress on Fertility and Sterility 2013

Transforming Reproductive Medicine Worldwide

Proceedings of

The International Federation of Fertility Societies

21st World Congress on Fertility and Sterility

and

The 69th Annual Meeting of the

American Society for Reproductive Medicine

Boston, Massachusetts, 2013

Basil C. Tarlatzis and Serdar E. Bulun, Editors

Delivered by:
Craftsman Printing, Inc.
120 Citation Court
Birmingham, Al 35209
1-205-945-4155
Email: gbevis@craftsmanprintinginc.com
Internet: www.craftsmanprintinginc.com

Library of Congress Cataloging-in-Publication Data

Library of Congress Control Number: 2013946613
Published by Craftsman Printing, Inc. located in Birmingham, Alabama

ISBN: 978-0-615-85253-9

Table of Contents

Preface

The 21st World Congress of the International Federation of Fertility Societies was organized in conjunction with the 69th Annual Meeting of the American Society for Reproductive Medicine (Boston, 12-17 October 2013). The editors of these Proceedings are proud to present this compendium of summaries of the IFFS trilogies given at the meeting.

The IFFS Scientific Committee worked diligently to identify topics of great relevance to clinicians and scientists working in the area of reproductive medicine and biology. Renowned experts from around the world were recruited to provide global perspectives on the pathophysiology, diagnosis, and treatment of diseases of the reproductive system. Each topic is addressed from three points of view, hence the name "trilogy": basic science, translational science, and clinical medicine. The trilogies are designed to update clinicians on the most current therapies and also provide them with a view to the future of emerging technologies.

The 15 trilogies provide gynecologists, urologists, endocrinologists, internists, and family practitioners with insights into the treatment of endometriosis, infertility, premature ovarian insufficiency, fibroids, polycystic ovary syndrome, and exposure to environmental toxicants. In addition, specialists in assisted reproductive technologies, embryology, and andrology learn the latest procedures for fertility preservation, ART in the developing world, optimizing endometrial receptivity and ART outcomes, preimplantation genetic diagnosis, and minimizing the occurrence of multiple pregnancy. Finally, the trilogy program includes discussions of global contraceptive efforts and the impact of obesity on reproduction.

The Editors are grateful to all of the trilogy authors for their generous contributions to the program and to this volume.

Basil C. Tarlatzis, M.D., Ph.D.
Serdar E. Bulun, M.D.

Trilogy 1. David Healy, M.D., Ph.D., Memorial Trilogy: Endometriosis

Genetics and epigenetics of endometriosis

Grant W. Montgomery
Queensland Institute of Medical Research, Brisbane, Australia

Introduction

Endometriosis is a common, chronic gynecological disorder defined by the presence of lesions containing endometrial glands and stroma outside the uterus. The lesions occur at multiple sites on the peritoneum, on the ovaries, in the rectovaginal septum, and occasionally at other sites outside the pelvis. Endometriosis causes pelvic pain, dysmenorrhea, and subfertility (1, 2). Endometriosis affects 6%-10% of women of reproductive age with a 6-8-fold higher risk in infertile women with a normal cycle whose partner has normal sperm (3). Diagnosis is usually made on visual inspection of the pelvis by laparoscopy and the average time from first symptoms to diagnosis is 8 years (2). Medical treatment options are limited and surgical intervention may not prevent recurrence (1, 4).

Genetic contributions to endometriosis

Endometriosis is a complex trait and risk of disease is influenced by both genetic and environmental factors. Higher rates of endometriosis are found among the relatives of endometriosis cases in both hospital (5, 6) and population-based (7) samples. Genetic effects on endometriosis risk have been reported in studies with twins (8-10) and in non-human primates (11). The best estimate for the heritability of endometriosis comes from a study in Australian twins with a reported heritability of 51% (10).

Genetic mapping studies

A major goal of research in endometriosis is to better define the genes and pathways contributing to disease risk and use this knowledge to develop more effective methods of diagnosis and treatment. Genetic studies provide one important approach to define pathways influencing endometriosis, and the number of studies has increased as the role of genetic factors has become more widely accepted. The basic requirements to map genes for a given disease are: (1) evidence for a genetic contribution to disease risk; (2) samples from either case/control or family-based studies; (3) genotype data on large sample sets with sufficient power to detect effects; and (4) replication in an independent sample. Approaches to gene mapping include candidate gene studies, linkage mapping, and genome-wide association studies.

Candidate gene and linkage mapping

Candidate gene studies have reported association between endometriosis and markers in many genes and have been the subject of several reviews (12, 13). Despite a large number of reported associations, results have generally not been replicated in subsequent studies (12-14). Lack of replication is likely due to issues with study design including the lack of power in small-scale studies that detect only variants with large effect, failure to adequately correct for multiple testing, publication bias, differences in disease definitions, and case/control population sampling issues (15). Linkage mapping studies are designed to search for disease-causing variants in families with a high prevalence of disease. For complex diseases like endometriosis, the most common approach is to study families with sister pairs who both have surgically confirmed disease and genotype highly polymorphic markers (16). Markers were typically microsatellite markers with many alleles, although current designs could include multiple single nucleotide polymorphism (SNP) markers. A linkage scan conducted by the International EndoGene Consortium in sister pair families identified a region of significant linkage on chromosome 10q26 (16). There was no evidence for association with potential candidate genes implicated in endometriosis and/or endometrial cancer immediately under the linkage peak (17). Extensive fine-mapping under the linkage peak identified evidence for association with SNPs in the region of the cytochrome P450 subfamily C (CYP2C19) gene and the signal replicated in an independent sample (18). CYP2C19 is a plausible candidate for endometriosis since it is involved in the metabolism of drugs and estrogen (18).

Subsequent analysis in a subset of 248 families with 3 or more affected family members identified a second region on chromosome 7p13-15 suggesting one or more rare variants following near-Mendelian patterns of inheritance contribute to disease risk in this region (15). Follow-up studies have included sequencing of potential candidate genes in the region (INHBA, SFRP4, and HOXA10). Results show that novel variants in the coding regions of these genes do not account for the linkage signal (13).

Genome-wide association studies

Genome-wide association studies (GWAS) have transformed gene mapping studies in complex traits. Four studies on endometriosis cases report at least nine gene regions with robust evidence for association with endometriosis risk (Table 1) (19-22). A study by Uno and others included 1,423 Japanese cases and 1,318 controls in the discovery sample with a mixture of surgically confirmed and clinically diagnosed cases and identified association with rs10965235 on chromosome 9p21.3 (22). The sentinel SNP (SNP with the lowest P value) rs10965235 is located in intron 6 of the cyclin-dependent kinase inhibitor 2B antisense RNA (CDKN2BAS), a region implicated in a range of complex diseases. A GWAS conducted by the International EndoGene Study included 3,194 surgically confirmed endometriosis cases and 7,060 controls from Australia and the United Kingdom in the discovery sample (21). Following replication of the top 70 SNPs in an independent dataset comprising 2,392 self-reported cases and 2,271 controls from the Nurses' Health Study I and II, the study reported significant association to an intergenic region on 7p15.2 (21). The International EndoGene Study also replicated a result from the Japanese study for association with rs7521902 on 1p36.12 (close to WNT4) (21).

Two recent studies genotyped top SNPs from the GWAS to attempt to replicate results. Four variants were genotyped in a small study of 305 surgically confirmed endometriosis cases in Italy and results compared with 2,710 population controls (23). This included a SNP rs1250248 close to FN1 on chromosome 2q35 that was genome-wide significant in the International EndoGene discovery sample ($P = 3.2 \times 10^{-8}$), but did not replicate in the Nurses' Health Study sample (21). SNPs close to CDKN2BAS, WNT4, and FN1 showed evidence of association with disease in this independent sample. A second study found nominal evidence for association with rs1250248 close to FN1 (24). The other variants did not show significant association, but the directions of effects were the same as for the large GWAS samples.

A meta-analysis of 4,604 endometriosis cases and 9,393 controls from the European and Japanese GWA datasets (21, 22) demonstrated that the top hit on chromosome 7p15.2 for SNP rs12700667 in Europeans did replicate in Japanese cases with strong evidence of association for this SNP ($P = 9.55 \times 10^{-10}$, odds ratio (OR) = 1.22) (14). Meta-analysis confirmed association with rs7521902 in the region of WNT4 ($P = 4.88 \times 10^{-8}$, OR = 1.18) and replicated association with rs13394619 in the gene growth regulation by estrogen in breast cancer 1 (GREB1) on chromosome 2p25.1 ($P = 2.14 \times 10^{-5}$, OR = 1.12), previously reported to be associated ($P = 3.80 \times 10^{-5}$, OR = 1.35) in a small independent Japanese GWA study (14, 19). The analysis also identified association with rs10859871 at 12q22 near the VEZT gene (OR = 1.18, 95% confidence interval (CI) = 1.12–1.25; $P = 5.5 \times 10^{-9}$).

Additional meta-analyses, excluding endometriosis cases with known minimal (Stage A) endometriosis (rAFS stage I or II disease) (25) from the Australian and Oxford samples, implicated a novel locus on 6p22.3 (rs7739264; $P = 5.82 \times 10^{-8}$, OR = 1.21) close to ID4 and an independent intergenic SNP on 9p21.3 approximately 55 kb from rs10965235 and 49 kb from the 3' end of CDKN2BAS (rs1537377; $P = 1.11 \times 10^{-8}$, OR = 1.21).

A recent GWAS analysis in 2,019 endometriosis cases with surgically confirmed disease from a Caucasian sample in Utah (20) provided strong replication for association in the region of LINC00339-WNT4 on chromosome 1p36. They also reported evidence for novel associations with rs1519761 and rs6757804 on 2q23.3 between RND3 and RBM43 ($P = 4.70 \times 10^{-8}$, OR = 1.20 and $P = 4.05 \times 10^{-8}$, OR = 1.20, respectively) in combined analysis of the discovery and replication sample. They also reported suggestive association with two regions; RNF144B-ID4 on chromosome 6p22.3 (rs6907340; $P = 2.19 \times 10^{-7}$, OR = 1.20) and HNRNPA3P1-LOC100130539 on chromosome 10q11.21 (rs10508881; $P = 4.08 \times 10^{-7}$, OR = 1.19).

Additional applications of genome-wide marker data

Association results must pass stringent thresholds for significance and be replicated in independent studies before evidence for association with disease risk is accepted. Only a few of the top signals in GWAS meet these criteria. Many other variants with signals just below the significance threshold will be "truly" associated with disease, although these cannot be distinguished from the false-positive signals. Methods can be applied to data from genome scans to use the predictive information from markers at the top of the distribution including many "true" signals to evaluate the genetic contribution to disease subtypes and genetic comorbidity with other diseases. Estimates from genome-wide marker data from the International EndoGene Study show common genetic variants contribute substantially to genetic risk for endometriosis (21, 26). The results show stronger genetic loading for moderate to severe endometriosis (Stage B disease; rAFS stage III or IV) compared to minimal endometriosis (Stage A disease; rAFS stage I or II) (21). The meta-analysis of European and Japanese samples (14) also demonstrated a significant overlap in polygenic risk for endometriosis between the European and Japanese GWA cohorts, peaking in SNPs nominally associated with $P < 0.1$ ($P = 8.81 \times 10^{-11}$). These results show many common genetic variants nominally associated with endometriosis risk ($P < 0.1$) represent true endometriosis risk loci. Moreover, similar mechanisms underlie disease risk on the European and Japanese populations and targeted disease therapy and risk prediction can be transferred across these populations.

Epigenetics

Epigenetics refers to stable changes in gene function and cell phenotype that can be transmitted through mitosis and/or meiosis without a change in the sequence of DNA (27, 28). Epigenetic modifications include addition of several types of "marks" to either DNA or chromatin that cause transient or persistent changes in gene transcription through DNA methylation and histone modification. The epigenetic state for each individual can be partly inherited and partly generated during development and continues to be altered during adult life (27).

Epigenetic changes can act at the level of the cell, tissue, or organism and could lead to alterations in cell fate affecting risk or progression of endometriosis. Evidence for epigenetic alterations in endometriosis (reviewed in Guo et al., 2009) includes hypermethylation of the promoter for homeobox A10 gene (HOXA10) and isoform B of the progesterone receptor (PGR-B), hypomethylation of steroidogenic factor 1 (SF-1) and estrogen receptor 2 (ESR2), and alterations in the expression of DNA methyltransferases. Promoter hypermethylation is usually associated with gene silencing and both HOXA10 and PGR-B are down-regulated in endometriosis. Similarly SF-1 and ESR2 are over-expressed in endometriosis.

Endometriosis is generally considered a benign disease, but it is associated with an increased risk of clear-cell, low-grade serous, and endometrioid invasive ovarian cancers (29). There is evidence of a monoclonal origin of some endometrial lesions associated with the development of ovarian cancers, and epigenetic alterations may play a role in progression of disease including possible links with ovarian cancer (30, 31). Genetic polymorphisms that predispose to endometriosis could act through alterations in histone modification or DNA methylation leading to altered gene expression in specific tissues or at critical times during development. Additional studies with greater numbers of relevant clinical samples using newer methods in genomics will be required to help define the role of epigenetics in molecular pathways that lead to endometriosis and predispose to ovarian cancer.

Future studies

The GWAS results represent the first convincing evidence for gene regions associated with endometriosis. Evidence from many complex diseases show that the number of variants discovered is strongly correlated with experimental sample size (32). Above a given threshold for each disease, doubling study size doubles the number of genes or regions identified. GWAS have been successful in endometriosis despite modest sample sizes when compared with many other disease studies. The associated variants all have small effects, explain only a very small proportion of disease prevalence, and are not useful as diagnostic markers. However, the data provide a valuable starting point to define the underlying pathways contributing to the disease and help in the development of better diagnostic tests and future treatments. Future studies should include larger samples with detailed phenotypic data to increase the number of markers and gene regions associated with disease risk and better define different aspects of endometriosis. Functional studies must be carried out to define the specific genes in each region contributing to disease risk to realize the potential for translation of these results.

Chromosome	SNP	P value	OR	95% CI	Gene	Reference
1p36.12	rs7521902*	7.6×10^{-13}	1.19	1.13–1.25	WNT4	Nyholt et al., (2012)
2p14	rs4141819*	4.1×10^{-8}	1.15	1.09-1.21	-	Nyholt et al., (2012)
2p25.1	rs13394619	6.1×10^{-9}	1.15	1.09-1.20	GREB1	Nyholt et al., (2012)
2q23.3	rs6757804	6.4×10^{-8}	1.20	1.13–1.29	RND3	Albertsen et al., (2013)
2q35	rs1250248*	3.9×10^{-9}	1.29	1.19-1.40	FN1	Pagliardini et al., (2013)
6p22.3	rs7739264*	2.1×10^{-10}	1.17	1.11-1.23	ID4	Nyholt et al., (2012)
7p15.2	rs12700667*	1.1×10^{-9}	1.18	1.11–1.25	-	Nyholt et al., (2012)
9p21.3	rs10965235	5.6×10^{-12}	1.44	1.30–1.59	CDKN2BAS	Uno et al., (2010)
9p21.3	rs1537377*	5.8×10^{-12}	1.15	1.10-1.21	CDKN2BAS	Nyholt et al., (2012)
12q22	rs10859871	5.1×10^{-13}	1.20	1.14-1.26	VEZT	Nyholt et al., (2012)

Table 1: Gene regions associated with endometriosis risk with P values for association for the sentinel SNP together with reported odds ratio (OR), 95% confidence intervals (95% CI) and nearest gene where this is less than 100 kb from the sentinel SNP. For SNPs marked with an asterisk, the evidence for association was stronger for more severe cases and results are reported for moderate-severe cases.

References

1. Giudice LC. (2010) Clinical practice. Endometriosis. N Engl J Med 362, 2389-2398.
2. Treloar S, Hadfield R, Montgomery G, Lambert A, Wicks J, Barlow DH, O'Connor DT, Kennedy S and Group, I.E.S. (2002) The International Endogene Study: a collection of families for genetic research in endometriosis. Fertil Steril 78, 679-685.
3. Meuleman C, Vandenabeele B, Fieuws S, Spiessens C, Timmerman D, D'Hooghe T. (2009) High prevalence of endometriosis in infertile women with normal ovulation and normospermic partners. Fertil Steril 92, 68-74.
4. Rogers PA, D'Hooghe TM, Fazleabas A, Gargett CE, Giudice LC, Montgomery GW, Rombauts L, Salamonsen LA, Zondervan KT. (2009) Priorities for endometriosis research: recommendations from an international consensus workshop. Reprod Sci 16, 335-346.
5. Kennedy S, Mardon H, Barlow D. (1995) Familial endometriosis. J Assist Reprod Genet 12, 32-34.
6. Simpson JL, Bischoff FZ. (2002) Heritability and molecular genetic studies of endometriosis. Annals of the New York Academy of Sciences 955, 239-251.
7. Stefansson H, Geirsson RT, Steinthorsdottir V, Jonsson H, Manolescu A, Kong A, Ingadottir G, Gulcher J, Stefansson K. (2002) Genetic factors contribute to the risk of developing endometriosis. Hum Reprod 17, 555-559.

8. Hadfield RM, Mardon HJ, Barlow DH, Kennedy SH. (1997) Endometriosis in monozygotic twins. Fertil Steril 68, 941-942.
9. Moen MH. (1994) Endometriosis in monozygotic twins. Acta Obstet Gynecol Scand 73, 59-62.
10. Treloar SA, O'Connor DT, O'Connor VM, Martin NG. (1999) Genetic influences on endometriosis in an Australian twin sample. Fertil Steril 71, 701-710.
11. Zondervan KT, Weeks DE, Colman R, Cardon L, Hadfield RH, Scheffler J, Trainor AG, Coe CL, Kemnitz JW, Kennedy SH. (2004) Familial aggregation of endometriosis in a large pedigree of rhesus macaques. Hum Reprod (in press).
12. Montgomery GW, Nyholt DR, Zhao ZZ, Treloar SA, Painter JN, Missmer SA, Kennedy SH, Zondervan KT. (2008) The search for genes contributing to endometriosis risk. Hum Reprod Update 14, 447-457.
13. Rahmioglu N, Missmer SA, Montgomery GW, Zondervan KT. (2012) Insights into Assessing the Genetics of Endometriosis. Curr Obstet Gynecol Rep 1, 124-137.
14. Nyholt DR, Low SK, Anderson CA, Painter JN, Uno S, Morris AP, MacGregor S, Gordon SD, Henders AK, Martin NG, et al. (2012) Genome-wide association meta-analysis identifies new endometriosis risk loci. Nat Genet 44, 1355-1359.
15. Zondervan KT, Treloar SA, Lin J, Weeks DE, Nyholt DR, Mangion J, MacKay IJ, Cardon LR, Martin NG, Kennedy SH, et al. (2007) Significant evidence of one or more susceptibility loci for endometriosis with near-Mendelian inheritance on chromosome 7p13-15. Hum Reprod 22, 717-728.
16. Treloar SA, Wicks J, Nyholt DR, Montgomery GW, Bahlo M, Smith V, Dawson G, Mackay IJ, Weeks DE, Bennett ST, et al. (2005) Genomewide linkage study in 1,176 affected sister pair families identifies a significant susceptibility locus for endometriosis on chromosome 10q26. Amer J Human Genet 77, 365-376.
17. Treloar SA, Zhao ZZ, Le L, Zondervan KT, Martin NG, Kennedy S, Nyholt DR, Montgomery GW. (2007) Variants in EMX2 and PTEN do not contribute to risk of endometriosis. Mol Hum Reprod 13, 587-594.
18. Painter JN, Nyholt DR, Morris A, Zhao ZZ, Henders AK, Lambert A, Wallace L, Martin NG, Kennedy SH, Treloar SA. et al. (2011) High-density fine-mapping of a chromosome 10q26 linkage peak suggests association between endometriosis and variants close to CYP2C19. Fertil Steril 95, 2236-2240.
19. Adachi, S., Tajima, A., Quan, J., Haino, K., Yoshihara, K., Masuzaki, H., Katabuchi, H., Ikuma, K., Suginami, H., Nishida, N. et al. (2010) Meta-analysis of genome-wide association scans for genetic susceptibility to endometriosis in Japanese population. J Hum Genet, 55, 816-821.
20. Albertsen, H.M., Chettier, R., Farrington, P. and Ward, K. (2013) Genome-wide association study link novel Loci to endometriosis. PLoS One, 8, e58257.
21. Painter, J.N., Anderson, C.A., Nyholt, D.R., Macgregor, S., Lin, J., Lee, S.H., Lambert, A., Zhao, Z.Z., Roseman, F., Guo, Q. et al. (2011) Genome-wide association study identifies a locus at 7p15.2 associated with endometriosis. Nat Genet, 43, 51-54.
22. Uno, S., Zembutsu, H., Hirasawa, A., Takahashi, A., Kubo, M., Akahane, T., Aoki, D., Kamatani, N., Hirata, K. and Nakamura, Y. (2010) A genome-wide association study identifies genetic variants in the CDKN2BAS locus associated with endometriosis in Japanese. Nat Genet, 42, 707-710.
23. Pagliardini, L., Gentilini, D., Vigano, P., Panina-Bordignon, P., Busacca, M., Candiani, M. and Di Blasio, A.M. (2013) An Italian association study and meta-analysis with previous GWAS confirm WNT4, CDKN2BAS and FN1 as the first identified susceptibility loci for endometriosis. J Med Genet, 50, 43-46.

24. Sundqvist, J., Xu, H., Vodolazkaia, A., Fassbender, A., Kyama, C., Bokor, A., Gemzell-Danielsson, K., D'Hooghe, T.M. and Falconer, H. (2013) Replication of endometriosis-associated single-nucleotide polymorphisms from genome-wide association studies in a Caucasian population. Hum Reprod, 28, 835-839.
25. Society, T.A.F. (1985) Revised American Fertility Society classification of endometriosis: 1985. Fertil Steril, 43, 351-352.
26. Lee, S.H., Harold, D., Nyholt, D.R., Goddard, M.E., Zondervan, K.T., Williams, J., Montgomery, G.W., Wray, N.R. and Visscher, P.M. (2013) Estimation and partitioning of polygenic variation captured by common SNPs for Alzheimer's disease, multiple sclerosis and endometriosis. Hum Mol Genet, 22, 832-841.
27. Fleisch, A.F., Wright, R.O. and Baccarelli, A.A. (2012) Environmental epigenetics: a role in endocrine disease? J Mol Endocrinol, 49, R61-67.
28. Guo, S.W. (2009) Epigenetics of endometriosis. Mol Hum Reprod, 15, 587-607.
29. Pearce, C.L., Templeman, C., Rossing, M.A., Lee, A., Near, A.M., Webb, P.M., Nagle, C.M., Doherty, J.A., Cushing-Haugen, K.L., Wicklund, K.G. et al. (2012) Association between endometriosis and risk of histological subtypes of ovarian cancer: a pooled analysis of case-control studies. Lancet Oncol, 13, 385-394.
30. Peltomaki, P. and Butzow, R. (2011) Endometriosis as an epigenetic disease. Epigenomics, 3, 690-691.
31. Peltomaki, P. and Butzow, R. (2011) Pathogenesis of endometriosis and its relationship to gynecological cancers. Epigenomics, 3, 689-690.
32. Visscher, P.M., Brown, M.A., McCarthy, M.I. and Yang, J. (2012) Five years of GWAS discovery. Am J Hum Genet, 90, 7-24.

Clinical applications of stem cells

Hugh S. Taylor and Levent Mutlu

Yale University, New Haven, United States

Introduction

Despite years of research, a definition of the term 'stem cell' remains elusive. The 'stem cell' does not designate a specific cell type, but is rather a heterogeneous group of cells capable of differentiating into a variety of mature cell types. While some can generate an entire organism, others are capable only of differentiating into a single mature cell type. Despite their diversity in differentiation potential, stem cells have two properties in common: self-renewal and differentiation. Self-renewal ensures the constancy of stem cells after cellular division. Differentiation, on the other hand, is the process through which the stem cells produce progeny that successfully incorporate into the tissue and maintain homeostasis. Taken together, stem cells play a vital role in maintaining tissue homeostasis in physiological as well as pathological conditions such as tissue injury. Stem cells in tissues like gut, epithelium, and endometrium display a quite remarkable regeneration capability, whereas stem cells in brain and cardiac tissue have only a limited ability to regenerate the organ. When the extent of tissue injury exceeds the ability of self-repair, commonly seen endpoints are cellular death and subsequent functional loss. Intuitively, this mechanism – at least partly – contributes to the massive burden of chronic diseases related to cardiovascular, central nervous system, and other tissues that have limited regeneration capacity. The rationale of stem cell therapy is to replace cells in organs that were damaged beyond their ability for self-repair.[1]

General aspects of stem cell therapies

Embryonic stem cells (ESCs) are pluripotent, derived from inner cell mass of the preimplantation blastocyst. ESCs are able to form all three germ layers and subsequently differentiate to every cell type found in the body. ESCs can self-replicate endlessly. There are a limited number of ESC lines available today and increasing data suggest that they tend to develop karyotypic abnormalities due to prolonged culture times. Despite their high differentiation potential, their use is limited by concerns issuing from ethical/moral constraints and the immunological mismatch between currently available ESC lines and the candidate recipients as well as the risk of teratoma formation after transplantation. Consequently, we are led to seek alternatives to ESCs.

Introduction of induced pluripotent stem cells (iPS) to regenerative medicine was a major step in stem cell research. Transfection of mouse fibroblasts with Oct3/4, Sox2, Klf4, and c-MYC resulted in reprogramming of fibroblastic cells into a pluripotent state.[2] As far as can be determined, there is no major difference in the differentiation potential between iPS and ESCs. iPS cells seem superior in some ways, as they circumvent the ethical issues related to ESCs. Additionally, they can be produced from any patient and therefore the risk of immune rejection is eliminated. Similar to ESCs, transfer of undifferentiated iPS cells may result in teratoma formation.

Organ-specific multipotent stem cells are widely distributed and can be isolated from adult tissues. They are somewhat differentiated compared to ESCs and iPS cells and have a more restricted cell fate. Hematopoietic stem cells (HSCs) and mesenchymal stem cells (MSCs) are examples of multipotent stem cells. As in the case of HSC transplantation, they can be easily harvested and cultured in vitro. They can be transferred back to the patient without immune rejection risk. Like HSCs, MSCs are easily cultured, although they may be more difficult to collect.

Since they have a more restricted differentiation potential compared to ESCs, multipotent stem cells were classically accepted to be lineage-restricted cells. However, studies within the last decade questioned this belief and suggested that multipotent stem cells may show remarkable plasticity and could 'jump' across lineage barriers (transdifferentiation). HSCs are well-studied examples of this phenomenon and neuron-like, hepatocyte-like, cardiomyocyte-like differentiation has been demonstrated. Similar to HSCs, MSCs exhibit remarkable transdifferentiation capability. Additionally, MSCs secrete immunosuppressive cytokines and trophic factors and actively regulate the microenvironment promoting tissue regeneration.3 These features make adult stem cells an attractive source for stem cell therapy.

There are multiple ways to administer stem cells for cell replacement purposes. They can be injected into the blood stream or can be applied into the damaged tissue. Cytokines like SDF and HIF as well as the local microenvironment in the injured tissue regulate stem cell chemotaxis and differentiation. Alternatively, stem cells can be differentiated in vitro, and the differentiated cells may be administered. The decision regarding the type of stem cells and the route of administration should be tailored to the patient and disease.

Endometrial stem/progenitor cells

Human endometrium undergoes approximately 400 menstrual cycles during the reproductive age period. This level of tissue regeneration is comparable to other highly regenerative tissues such as epidermis, gut epithelium, and bone marrow. One would expect that endometrium houses a rich stem/progenitor cell population.

Note, however, that the majority of studies constituting our current knowledge on endometrial stem/progenitor cells were published within the last decade. In 2004, Gargett found that 0.22% of epithelial and 1.25% of stromal cells exhibited clonogenicity and suggested the presence of stem/progenitor cells in endometrium.[4] Others have suggested that the progenitor cells are c-kit and CD34 expressing cells in the basalis layer of endometrium.[5] These cells may constitute the progenitor cells that give rise to endometrium in each menstrual cycle.

In the same year, we showed that bone marrow contributes to endometrium. Two percent to 52 percent of uterine stroma and epithelium was donor derived in women who had undergone single HLA mismatched bone marrow transplantation.[6]

We have further studied bone marrow's contribution to uterine endometrium in murine model. After bone marrow transplantation from male mice, Y chromosome$^+$ cells were observed in the endometrium of the recipient mice. One out of 5,000 cells was Y chromosome positive in uterine epithelium. The extent of contribution to uterine stroma was nearly twice that of epithelium.[7]

In the following years, studies mainly focused on finding potential markers for endometrial stem/progenitor cells. Sorting PDGF-β^+CD146$^+$ cells resulted in 8- to 10-fold enrichment for MSC-like cell compared to unfractionated endometrium.[8] Therefore, PDGF-β+CD146+ double positivity was suggested as a marker for endometrial MSC-like cells. In vitro assays showed that these cells are able to differentiate to adipocytes, chondrocytes, and osteocytes.[8,9] Recently, W5C5 was introduced as an alternative single marker to purify the same PDGF-β^+CD146$^+$ endometrial stem/progenitor cell population.[10]

The following studies on endometrial stem/progenitor cells utilized Hoechst 33342 dye exclusion assays to identify stem cell activity. Hoechst 33342 excluding Side Population (SP) cells express ATP Binding Cassette-G2 (ABCG2) on their cytoplasmic membrane, which pumps a DNA-binding dye (Hoechst 33342) out of the cell, hence giving these cells the name 'side population' in flow cytometric analysis. In a study published in 2010, Masuda et al. found that SP cells preferentially expressed endothelial cell markers. When cultured in vitro, SP cells differentiated to epithelial, stromal, and endothelial cells, whereas the main population cells differentiated only to stromal cells.[11] SP cells' differentiation potential and quiescent nature rendered them a possible candidate for stem cells.

Endometrial regeneration with bone marrow-derived stem cells

Asherman's syndrome is associated with infertility due to destruction of the basal layer of endometrium and intrauterine synechiae. Treatment of Asherman's syndrome aims to break up the synechiae and restore the uterine cavity. Since the endometrial stem/progenitor cells residing in basalis layer can be damaged or lost, endometrial growth in women with Asherman's syndrome is inconsistent. Recently, we created a murine model of Asherman's syndrome to test bone marrow-derived cells' (BMDCs) contribution to uterine regeneration after endometrial injury. After uterine horn injury, mice were randomized to receive bone marrow (BM) or sham transplantation. Three months after transplantation, BMDCs were observed in both uterine horns of the transplant recipients. There was no difference between the numbers of bone marrow-derived Y chromosome+ cells between each horn in the BM-transplanted group. Notably, the BM-transplanted mice showed substantially higher pregnancy rates compared to the PBS-transplanted mice ($P=0.02$). Our findings suggest that BMDCs play a functional role in endometrial regeneration (article in review).

Endometrial stem cells in regenerative medicine

As discussed above, multipotent stem cells have emerged as an alternative source for cell replacement therapies. Bone marrow-derived stem cells have been long used for cell replacement therapies with varying degrees of success. We have recently concentrated on endometrium, which is a readily accessible stem cell source obtained by the minimally invasive endometrial biopsy. Actually, endometrium is the only source where adult mesenchymal stem cells can be obtained without the need for analgesia. Finally, as a patient's own stem cells are used, immune rejection is not an issue.

HEDSC to neuron-like cells

A promising therapeutic role example of endometrial MSC transdifferentiation came from our laboratory in 2010. We differentiated human endometrium stem cells (HESCs) to neuron-like cells in vitro. Differentiated cells exhibited neurite-like processes and expressed several neuronal markers, including tyrosine hydroxylase, the enzyme that catalyzes the rate limiting step in dopamine production. In vitro electrophysiologic studies using patch clamp showed that the differentiated cells expressed barium sensitive potassium inward rectifying channels as seen in central neurons. Differentiation was also tested in an MPTP-treated Parkinson's disease (PD) mouse model. Undifferentiated human endometrial-derived stem cells (HEDSCs) were transplanted into the striatum of the recipient mice. These stem cells migrated to substantia nigra, increased nestin expression, and adopted a neuron-like morphology in vivo. Additionally, dopamine and its metabolite, DOPAC, concentrations were significantly higher in the HEDSC-transplanted mice compared to the sham transplant.

Although higher levels of dopamine and its metabolite observed in the transplanted mice might be explained – at least partially – by the protective effect of stem cell transplantation itself on neuronal death, transplanted cells clearly recapitulated normal cellular allocation and expressed the rate-limiting enzyme (tyrosine hydroxylase) in dopamine synthesis. Therefore, the dramatic difference between the sham and the HEDSC-transplanted mice cannot be solely explained by the protective mechanism of the transplantation itself, but also by the active contribution of differentiated HEDSC to dopamine production.[12]

HESC differentiated into insulin-producing cells

In a separate study, we differentiated HESCs into pancreatic beta-like cells. After incubation for one week in differentiation media, HESC expressed early pancreatic developmental genes NGN3 and PDX1. After three weeks a fraction of HESCs formed clusters with islet-like morphology in cell culture. Furthermore, mature beta cell markers like GLUT2 and insulin were expressed in HEDSC-derived pancreatic beta-like cells. Beta-like cells were responsive to the glucose concentrations in vitro and increased insulin secretion when glucose concentration in the media was increased. To assess the therapeutic potential of HESC-derived beta-like cells in type-1 diabetes, beta-like cells or endometrial stromal cells were transplanted under the kidney capsule of mice treated with streptozocin to induce diabetes. Mice that were transplanted with endometrial stromal cells developed more severe hyperglycemia compared to the mice that had been transplanted with pancreatic beta-like cells. Notably, transplantation of pancreatic beta-like cells prevented worsening of hyperglycemia in the recipient mice, whereas stromal cell transplantation failed to do so. Although beta-like cell transplantation did not normalize glucose levels, it prevented/slowed down the development of diabetes-associated complications such as dehydration, weight loss, and cataracts.[13]

Li et al.[14] used a different approach to differentiate human endometrial mesenchymal stem-like cells (EMSCs) to pancreatic beta-like cells. In this study, EMSCs were cultured in a specific differentiation medium and finally formed spheroid bodies (SBs) that secreted insulin. After transplantation, SB-EMSC normalized glucose levels in the streptozocin-treated diabetic mice. Interestingly, SB-EMSC showed resistance to oxidative stress and prolonged survival in the recipient mice.

HEDSC to cardiac precursor-like cells

Heart disease is the most common cause of hospitalization and death in adults. Not surprisingly, cell-based therapies to replenish the lost cardiomyocytes have generated great interest. Embryonic stem cells, bone marrow-derived mesenchymal stem cells, endothelial progenitor cells have been employed as a stem cell source in murine cardiac infraction models. Nevertheless, many investigators speculated that the improved cardiac functions observed were due to increased angiogenesis after myocardial infarction.

A novel source of cardiac precursor-like cells was proposed in 2008. Hida et al.[15] successfully differentiated human menstrual blood-derived mesenchymal stem cells (MMCs) or endometrial regenerative cells (ERCs) to spontaneously beating cardiomyocyte-like cells. These cells are easily collectible in menses and were shown to retain their transdifferentiation potential for approximately 28 generations in vitro. After culturing with murine cardiac cells, human MMC-derived cells exhibited strong contractility. Additionally, mRNA expression of human genes encoding cardiac proteins was increased in the MMCs that were co-cultured with murine cardiomyocytes, whereas a similar trend was not observed in the control group.

Electrophysiologic studies on differentiated cells showed pacemaker potentials and action potentials that are characteristic for cardiomyocytes. The transdifferentiation potential of MMCs was also tested in murine models. Two weeks after ligation of left coronary artery and resultant left ventricular infarction, either MMC or bone marrow-derived mesenchymal stem cells (BM-MSC) were injected in the infarct zone. Notably, left ventricular systolic functions were superior in MMC compared to BM-MSC recipients. Additionally, as the transplantation was done after myocardial necrosis had been completed, improved cardiac function was not merely due to MMC-induced angiogenesis. These findings suggest that MMCs have a substantial capacity to transdifferentiate into cardiomyocyte-like cells.

Limitations

Regardless of the stem cell source, generating large numbers of differentiated stem cells is necessary for successful therapeutic applications. Differentiation in current studies is still in need of optimization.

Another hurdle to overcome is sorting and transplanting a pure population of differentiated cells to minimize the risk of tumor formation or proliferation of inappropriate cell types. As discussed above, ESCs and iPS cells have remarkable proliferation and differentiation capacity; however, transplantation of single undifferentiated cell might result in teratoma formation.

Validity of the HSC or MSC plasticity has been questioned in the past decade. Some researchers argue that the transplanted stem cells do not transdifferentiate into other tissues, but merely fuse with endogenous mature cells. Similarly, these cells often fail to undergo clonal expansion in order to replace or regenerate damaged tissue. Trophic factors secreted from stem cells may play a large role in the therapeutic effects seen in some studies described above. Identification of these trophic factors would allow for their direct use, perhaps eliminating the need for cellular delivery. Alternatively, the role of direct cell contact and active ongoing signaling between cells may necessitate the use of intact stem cells.

Conclusions

Stem cell therapy has a tremendous potential but it is still in its infancy. Improvements in identification, purification, differentiation, and transplantation of stem cells will likely increase the availability and success of cell replacement therapies. Adult stem cells and iPS cells both hold great promise and will continue to be an active area of research in the near future.

There is a growing body of evidence that the adult endometrial stem cells show a high level of differentiation potential and could be used for stem cell therapies. Endometrial-derived stem cells have produced functional improvements in animal models of Asherman's syndrome. Similarly, endometrium-derived stem cells can be successfully differentiated into neuron-like, pancreatic beta-like, and cardiomyocyte-like cells. We are only beginning to understand the potential of endometrial stem/progenitor cells. Endometrium, due to its versatility and ready availability, may be the optimal source of stem cells for future regenerative therapies.

References

1. Sahni V, Kessler JA. Stem cell therapies for spinal cord injury. Nature reviews Neurology 2010;6:363-72.
2. Yamanaka S, Takahashi K. [Induction of pluripotent stem cells from mouse fibroblast cultures]. Tanpakushitsu kakusan koso Protein, nucleic acid, enzyme 2006;51:2346-51.
3. Caplan AI. Adult mesenchymal stem cells for tissue engineering versus regenerative medicine. Journal of cellular physiology 2007;213:341-7.
4. Chan RW, Schwab KE, Gargett CE. Clonogenicity of human endometrial epithelial and stromal cells. Biology of reproduction 2004;70:1738-50.
5. Cho NH, Park YK, Kim YT, Yang H, Kim SK. Lifetime expression of stem cell markers in the uterine endometrium. Fertility and sterility 2004;81:403-7.
6. Taylor HS. Endometrial cells derived from donor stem cells in bone marrow transplant recipients. JAMA : the journal of the American Medical Association 2004;292:81-5.
7. Du H, Taylor HS. Contribution of bone marrow-derived stem cells to endometrium and endometriosis. Stem Cells 2007;25:2082-6.

8. Schwab KE, Gargett CE. Co-expression of two perivascular cell markers isolates mesenchymal stem-like cells from human endometrium. Hum Reprod 2007;22:2903-11.
9. Wolff EF, Wolff AB, Hongling D, Taylor HS. Demonstration of multipotent stem cells in the adult human endometrium by in vitro chondrogenesis. Reprod Sci 2007;14:524-33.
10. Masuda H, Anwar SS, Buhring HJ, Rao JR, Gargett CE. A novel marker of human endometrial mesenchymal stem-like cells. Cell transplantation 2012;21:2201-14.
11. Masuda H, Matsuzaki Y, Hiratsu E, et al. Stem cell-like properties of the endometrial side population: implication in endometrial regeneration. PloS one 2010;5:e10387.
12. Wolff EF, Gao XB, Yao KV, et al. Endometrial stem cell transplantation restores dopamine production in a Parkinson's disease model. Journal of cellular and molecular medicine 2011;15:747-55.
13. Santamaria X, Massasa EE, Feng Y, Wolff E, Taylor HS. Derivation of insulin producing cells from human endometrial stromal stem cells and use in the treatment of murine diabetes. Molecular therapy : the journal of the American Society of Gene Therapy 2011;19:2065-71.
14. Li HY, Chen YJ, Chen SJ, et al. Induction of insulin-producing cells derived from endometrial mesenchymal stem-like cells. The Journal of pharmacology and experimental therapeutics 2010;335:817-29.
15. Hida N, Nishiyama N, Miyoshi S, et al. Novel cardiac precursor-like cells from human menstrual blood-derived mesenchymal cells. Stem Cells 2008;26:1695-704.

The management of pelvic pain with infertility

Mauricio S. Abrão

São Paulo University, São Paulo, Brazil

Introduction

Endometriosis is a common disease that affects 10% to 15% of women of reproductive age. It is known to be an important cause of pelvic pain and infertility (Giudice, 2010). In the last few years, our understanding of endometriosis underwent major modifications because of recent findings involved in the diagnosis and treatment of this disease. Following the definition of deep endometriosis, as described in 1989 (Cornillie et al., 1990), and the subsequent finding that endometriosis affecting the ovary, peritoneum, and rectovaginal septum should be considered three separate conditions (Nisolle and Donnez, 1997), specific attention has been paid to the diagnostic and therapeutic aspects of the disease affecting each of these three sites for patients with pain and infertility. Deep endometriosis was, for the first time, recognized as a separate entity requiring special consideration.

The diagnosis

The main symptoms of endometriosis are dysmenorrhea, deep dyspareunia, non-cyclic pelvic pain, and bowel and urinary tract alterations during menses and infertility. Evaluation of patients includes a thorough physical examination, looking for lesions involving the vaginal mucosa, and a digital examination, detecting areas of thickening or enlargement of the adnexae and nodules in the uterosacral ligaments, retrocervical region, vaginal fornix, and/or the rectovaginal septum (Abrão et al., 2007; Bazot et al., 2009). For lesions of the vaginal pouch itself, which consist of nodules in the posterior vaginal fornix and rectovaginal septum, digital examination may provide greater certainty of diagnosis.

In the case of patients whose clinical status and physical examination are both suggestive of a diagnosis of endometriosis, an imaging method can be helpful to map the pelvis. Transvaginal ultrasonography with simple bowel preparation prior to the exam is the method of choice for this purpose. It permits adequate visualization of the internal pelvic organs and their interface with the urinary and intestinal tracts allowing for detection of lesions of deep and ovarian endometriosis with a high degree of accuracy. Bowel preparation consists of the use of a mild oral laxative on the eve of the exam and a rectal enema consisting of 120 mL of dibasic sodium phosphate approximately one hour prior to initiation of the exam. Bowel preparation is performed in order to eliminate any fecal residue and gases present in the rectosigmoid (Abrão et al., 2008; Gonçalves et al., 2009; Gonçalves et al., 2010).

Magnetic resonance imaging (MRI) also is a good method for evaluating endometriosis, although it has the limitation of not being as widely available as ultrasonography. Furthermore, it is more expensive and patients who are unable to tolerate the exam have to be sedated (Chamie et al., 2009). In a study comparing these imaging methods, our group reported sensitivity of 98.1% in cases of rectal endometriosis and 95.1% in retrocervical endometriosis with the use of transvaginal ultrasonography with prior bowel preparation, whereas sensitivity with MRI was 83.3% and 76% for rectal and retrocervical endometriosis, respectively (Abrão et al., 2007).

Management of endometriosis

The treatment of endometriosis can be clinical or surgical and should also depend on symptoms of pain and/or infertility. In the case of infertility, the clinical treatment options include the induction of the ovulation, insemination, or in vitro fertilization. In the presence of pain and two previously failed in vitro fertilization (IVF) treatments, the best option is for surgical resection of the lesions, depending on the organ that is compromised. The concept of endometriosis as three distinct diseases (peritoneal, ovarian, and deep disease) allows us to consider the therapeutic options according to these different sites of the disease:

Peritoneal endometriosis

The best modality of treating peritoneal disease is controversial. For infertile patients, in 1997, the Canadian Collaborative Group on Endometriosis published an important study suggesting advantages for the surgical treatment in comparison to conservative treatment, but after two years, the Gruppo Italiano per lo Studio dell'Endometriosi showed no advantage for the surgical treatment versus conservative treatment.

Ovarian endometriosis

Patients with ovarian endometriomas may be asymptomatic or may have symptoms such as pain and/or infertility. The decision regarding therapy depends on the patient's age, her symptoms, the preoperative diagnosis, and her desire for future fertility.

Reasons for recommending surgical treatment of endometriomas are:

- Pain relief (dysmenorrhea, acyclic pain, and dyspareunia) (Hart et al., 2005);
- Treatment of infertility (Donnez et al., 1995);
- Lower probability of recurrence with surgical treatment compared to medical treatment (Donnez et al., 1995);
- Possibility of malignant transformation (Nishida et al., 2000).

The Guidelines of the European Society of Human Reproduction and Embryology (ESHRE) state that histologic confirmation should be obtained from cysts > 3 cm in diameter with characteristics of endometriomas (Kennedy et al., 2005).

Laparoscopy is the method of choice for the treatment of endometriomas. Compared to laparotomy, this method results in shorter duration of hospitalization, lower costs, reduced postoperative pain intensity, and a lower incidence of postoperative adhesions. Cumulative pregnancy rates following surgery and recurrence rates of cysts are comparable whether laparoscopy or laparotomy is used for surgical access (Hart et al., 2005).

Management of deep endometriosis

The treatment of deep endometriosis compromising the retrocervical region and the bladder for patients with pain consists on the excision of the lesions by laparoscopy.

Bowel involvement may be present in 3%-37% of all cases of endometriosis (Zwas et al., 1991), affecting the rectosigmoid in 90%, and, less frequently, other bowel segments such as the cecum, appendix, terminal ileum, and jejunum.

Evaluating the symptoms of 70 patients with bowel endometriosis undergoing laparoscopic treatment, Abrão et al. (2003) reported complaints of dysmenorrhea in all cases, and in 38.8% the severity of the pain prevented them from carrying out their routine activities. Deep dyspareunia, likely caused by local lesions, was present in 72.2% of cases and acyclic pelvic pain in 66.7%. Cyclical bowel symptoms were present in 88.9% and were significantly related to bowel endometriosis. Cyclical bowel symptoms were the principal complaint in 50% of patients (n=35) and included pelvic pain at evacuation and/or diarrhea during menstruation and, more characteristically, blood in the feces during menstrual periods. Physical examination was suggestive of deep endometriosis in 73.3% of cases. In view of this observation, the value of the physical examination should not be underestimated; this exam should be carried out systematically as it may result in identification of areas of thickness and nodules in the anterior and posterior cul-de-sac and in the uterosacral ligaments as well as in the rectovaginal septum.

The medical treatment of deep endometriosis and endometriosis of the rectovaginal septum remains controversial. Fedele et al. (2000) reported an important improvement in pain during six months of treatment with GnRH analogues; however, there was early recurrence after discontinuing treatment. The discrete but significant reduction in the size of the endometriotic lesions during therapy disappeared 6 months after treatment with GnRH. Guidelines published by the European Society of Reproductive Medicine (ESHRE) offer recommendations with respect to this subject: In cases of deep endometriosis there is no evidence that hormonal suppression of ovarian function is effective for the treatment of infertility. Furthermore, the patient is unable to achieve pregnancy during treatment and thereafter until normal ovulatory function is re-established.

In regard to deep endometriosis associated primarily with pain, there appears to be a consensus in the literature that the treatment of choice is surgical (Jerby et al., 1999; Redwine et al., 2001; Varol et al., 2000; Minelli et al., 2003). Surgical access may be achieved by laparotomy or laparoscopy depending on the surgeon's experience and the extent of the disease.

In regard to infertility patients with deep endometriosis, there are no randomized controlled studies or meta-analyses to support that surgical treatment is preferable.

Abrão et al. (2008) evaluated cases of bowel endometriosis and observed that endometriosis lesions that compromise the rectum deeper than the inner muscularis layer have more than 40% of the circumference of the rectum affected by the disease. On the other hand, when the superficial or serous layer of the bowel wall is affected, these same authors recommend resection of the nodule only.

Considerations in management of infertile patients with endometriosis with pain

Considering the absence of consensus on many aspects of the treatment of patients with pain and infertility, we consider the following aspects before deciding to pursue surgery and/or clinical treatment (i.e., induction of ovulation or IVF):

- Age of the patient (less or more than 35 years old)
- Ovarian reserve (follicle-stimulating hormone [FSH] and antimüllerian hormone levels)
- Intensity of pain (less or more than 7 according to the visual analogic scale)
- The site of the disease (peritoneal, ovarian, or deep disease)
- Concerns about cancer
- Tubal patency

For young patients (less than 30 years old) with good ovarian reserve, surgery may be a good option followed by the infertility treatment (induction of ovulation for patients with normal tubal patency or IVF for patients with tubal obstruction). For older patients, or those with low ovarian reserve, IVF must be considered, and in most of these cases, cryopreservation of oocytes or embryos before surgery must be offered to the patients.

Conclusion

In summary, our approach to endometriosis has changed significantly with greater understanding of the three different types of endometriosis. Many treatment options are currently available for patients with infertility and should be made only after consideration of multiple critical factors.

References

1. Abrao MS, Dias JA, Jr., Bellelis P, Podgaec S, Bautzer CR, Gromatsky C. Endometriosis of the ureter and bladder are not associated diseases. Fertil Steril. 2009 May;91(5):1662-7.
2. Abrao MS, Goncalves MO, Dias JA, Jr., Podgaec S, Chamie LP, Blasbalg R. Comparison between clinical examination, transvaginal sonography and magnetic resonance imaging for the diagnosis of deep endometriosis. Hum Reprod. 2007 Dec;22(12):3092-7.
3. Abrao MS, Neme RM, Averbach M. Rectovaginal septum endometriosis: a disease with specific diagnosis and treatment. Arq Gastroenterol 2003;40(3):192-7.
4. Abrao MS, Podgaec S, Dias JA, Jr., Averbach M, Silva LF, Marino de Carvalho F. Endometriosis lesions that compromise the rectum deeper than the inner muscularis layer have more than 40% of the circumference of the rectum affected by the disease. J Minim Invasive Gynecol. 2008 May-Jun;15(3):280-5.
5. Bazot M, Lafont C, Rouzier R, Roseau G, Thomassin-Naggara I, Darai E. Diagnostic accuracy of physical examination, transvaginal sonography, rectal endoscopic sonography, and magnetic resonance imaging to diagnose deep infiltrating endometriosis. Fertil Steril. 2009 Dec;92(6):1825-33.
6. Chamie LP, Blasbalg R, Goncalves MO, Carvalho FM, Abrao MS, de Oliveira IS. Accuracy of magnetic resonance imaging for diagnosis and preoperative assessment of deeply infiltrating endometriosis. Int J Gynaecol Obstet. 2009 Sep;106(3):198-201.
7. Chapron C, Barakat H, Fritel X, Dubuisson JB, Breart G, Fauconnier A. Presurgical diagnosis of posterior deep infiltrating endometriosis based on a standardized questionnaire. Hum Reprod. 2005 Feb;20(2):507-13.
8. Cornillie FJ, Oosterlynck D, Lauweryns JM, et al. Deeply infiltrating pelvic endometriosis: histology and clinical significance. Fertil Steril 1990;53(6):978-83.
9. Donnez J, Nisolle M, Squifflet J. Ureteral endometriosis: a complication of rectovaginal endometriotic (adenomyotic) nodules. Fertil Steril. 2002 Jan;77(1):32-7.
10. Fedele L, Bianchi S, Zanconato G, et al. Gonadotropin-releasing hormone agonist treatment for endometriosis of the rectovaginal septum. Am J Obstet Gynecol 2000;183(6):1462-7.
11. Giudice, L.C. Endometriosis. N Engl J Med 2010; 24:362:2389-98.
12. Goncalves MO, Dias JA, Jr., Podgaec S, Averbach M, Abrao MS. Transvaginal ultrasound for diagnosis of deeply infiltrating endometriosis. Int J Gynaecol Obstet. 2009 Feb;104(2):156-60.
13. Goncalves MO, Podgaec S, Dias JA, Jr., Gonzalez M, Abrao MS. Transvaginal ultrasonography with bowel preparation is able to predict the number of lesions and rectosigmoid layers affected in cases of deep endometriosis, defining surgical strategy. Hum Reprod. 2010 Mar;25(3):665-71.
14. Hart R, Hickey M, Maouris P, et al. Excisional surgery versus ablative surgery for ovarian endometriomata: a Cochrane Review. Hum Reprod 2005;20(11)3000-7.
15. Kennedy S, Bergqvist A, Chapron C, et al. ESHRE guideline for the diagnosis and treatment of endometriosis. Hum Reprod 2005;20(10):2698-704.

16. Jerby BL, Kessler H, Falcone T, et al. Laparoscopic management of colorectal endometriosis. Surg Endosc 1999;13(11):1125-8.
17. Marcoux S, Maheux R, Bérubé S. Laparoscopic surgery in infertile women with minimal or mild endometriosis. Canadian Collaborative Group on Endometriosis. N Engl J Med. 1997 Jul 24;337(4):217-22.
18. Minelli L, Barbieri F, Fiaccavento A, et al. Complete laparoscopic removal of endometriosis for the management of pain symptomatology. J Am Assoc Gynecol Laparosc 2003;10(S):11.
19. Nishida M, Watanabe K, Sato N, et al. Malignant transformation of ovarian endometriosis. Gynecol Obstet Invest 2000;50 Suppl 1:18-25.
20. Nisolle M, Donnez J. Peritoneal endometriosis, ovarian endometriosis and adenomyotic nodules of the rectovaginal septum are three different entities. Fertil Steril. 1997; 68:585-96.
21. Parazzini F. Ablation of lesions or no treatment in minimal-mild endometriosis in infertile women: a randomized trial. Gruppo Italiano per lo Studio dell'Endometriosi. Hum Reprod. 1999 May;14(5):1332-4.
22. Varol N, Maher P, Woods R. Laparoscopic management of intestinal endometriosis. J Am Assoc Gynecol Laparosc 2000;7(3):405-9.
23. Zwas FR, Lyon DT. Endometriosis. An important condition in clinical gastroenterology. Dig Dis Sci 1991;36(3):353-64.

Trilogy 2. Female fertility preservation

Fundamentals of cryobiology

Claus Yding Andersen and Christina Hnida

University Hospital Copenhagen, Copenhagen, Denmark

Introduction

The outlook for using cryopreservation today in a number of areas related to fertility preservation and assisted reproduction techniques is imminent. This especially includes cryopreservation of ovarian tissue and/or oocytes to safeguard the fertility of girls and young woman with a cancer disease as well as many other aspects of modern assisted reproduction treatment of infertile couples (1, 2). Thus, understanding the fundamentals of cryobiology has turned into an issue of utmost importance, which is essential to establishing and running effective cryopreservation programs in fertility clinics and in centers dealing with fertility preservation. This review focuses on the fundamentals of cryopreservation with special emphasis of oocytes and ovarian tissue in the context of the two most-used methods, slow-freezing or vitrification.

Rationale for an increased use of cryotechnology in fertility treatment and in fertility preservation

Rationale for using cryotechnology in cancer treatment

The 5-year survival rate after many, especially childhood, cancers has improved significantly during the last two decades and now reaches or exceeds 80% in many instances (3, 4). This remarkable success is based mainly on the development of modern aggressive chemotherapy regimens and targeted radiotherapy treatment. The wanted destruction of cancer cells on one side may, however, lead to unwanted side effects such as the elimination of ovarian function on the other side, which reflects that all the ovarian follicles may be destroyed. The growing cohort of cancer survivors, especially girls and young women, has led to a great desire to preserve fertility and has created great motivation to develop effective fertility preservation methods. Thus, the incorporation of fertility preservation into the clinical practice has been a long-term goal of many practitioners, especially during the last 10 to 20 years. At the center of this new development are new effective methods to store mature oocytes, embryos, and now also ovarian tissue, all of which are based on cryopreservation (5, 6).

Rationale for using cryotechnology in assisted reproductive technology (ART)

A challenge in modern in vitro fertilization (IVF) treatment is to balance the number of embryos transferred per cycle relative to embryo quality, chance of conception, and risk of multiple pregnancies. Obstetrical complications, including significant health risks for both the mother and her babies, as the result of multiple pregnancies are very well known and documented (7). The continuous effort to optimize IVF protocols, including refining embryo culture systems/strategies as well as embryo quality assessment, has resulted in generally improved clinical pregnancy rates and increased number of surplus, top-quality embryos, highlighting the necessity for effective cryoprotocols. This is especially so because implantation rates of frozen/

thawed embryos replaced in the natural cycle appear to be considerably improved compared to that of the fresh cycles (8). Furthermore, single embryo transfer is increasingly used to prevent multiple pregnancies, resulting in cryopreserving the remaining top-quality embryos for later potential treatment cycles (2, 7, 9).

Oocyte freezing in oocyte donation regimes

Oocyte cryopreservation can be used as an effective strategy in oocyte-donation programs to overcome synchronization issues between recipient and donor (10). Furthermore, oocyte cryopreservation allows a quarantine period of the donated oocytes to minimize the risk of disease transmission (9). However, the biological competence of the frozen/thawed oocytes should be comparable to fresh oocytes to legitimize cryopreservation in oocyte donation programs (2, 10).

Oocyte freezing to "rescue" IVF cycles

Cryopreservation of mature oocytes immediately after oocyte aspiration can be a successful strategy when there is an imminent risk of ovarian hyperstimulation or no sperm cells could be collected on the day of oocyte retrieval or if the endometrium has responded suboptimally (9).

Oocyte/ovarian tissue banking for social reasons

In modern society, elective delayed childbearing is becoming an increasingly important issue. Storing good-quality oocytes in a woman's younger years may secure fertility later on in life. Furthermore, cryopreservation techniques may in the future also complement assisted reproduction in some fertile woman who may want to use the endocrinological features of their ovarian tissue to postpone menopause by having some ovarian tissue excised and cryostored in their young years (9, 11, 12).

Rationale for using cryotechnology in studying development of diseases

There is a growing interest in studying development of diseases by evaluating the appearance of specific disease markers from before a specific person became sick until symptoms become manifest in the same individual. So, studies on the development of disease with time require large biobanks with both cells/tissue and body fluids that obviously need to be cryopreserved in a way that allows sufficient quality in the measurements of the relevant comparisons.

Fundamentals of cryobiology

The purpose of freezing cells and tissues is to maintain long-term viability after long-term storage. In order to accomplish this, all biological activities within the cells need to be brought to a halt and into a state of suspended animation representing a condition from which they may recover and resume viability. Liquid nitrogen, at a temperature of minus 196°C, is the preferred environment for long-term storage. At this temperature all biological activity has stopped. Although the threshold temperature that allows long-term storage probably is higher, liquid nitrogen is convenient to use and allows certain flexibility when handling samples. Human cells can probably be stored in liquid nitrogen for a very long time, and it has been demonstrated that sperm cells after 25 years and human ovarian tissue after 10 years in liquid nitrogen, respectively, remain functional. These time spans are sufficient for most practical purposes, and cells and tissue can be considered safely stored in liquid nitrogen. Thus, it is therefore important to realize that damage to cells and tissue in connection with long-term storage takes place during the transition processes of freezing and/or thawing/warming.

In order to accomplish cryopreservation, cells and tissues are exposed to numerous stress factors that include mechanical, thermal, and chemical factors (13, 14), which may compromise cell function and cause cell death. The establishment of a successful cryopreservation program that will allow cells and tissue to resume their original activity following thawing/warming is therefore dependent on controlling these stress factors as they may affect one or several of all the complex intracellular organelles and processes that are necessary for normal cell function. Damage may, therefore, be variable and cause transient disturbances from the normal state or sublethal or permanent and lethal injuries.

Substances with cryoprotective properties

Reducing damage to cells and tissue during cryopreservation can be accomplished by substituting water molecules with water soluble organic molecules that don't expand in size in the crystalline state at subzero temperatures and that help to avoid intracellular ice crystal formation. Usually two types of cryoprotectants are used: those that penetrate cells and those that remain in the extracellular space but reduce water activity within the cell, usually termed the permeating and nonpermeating cryoprotectants.

Permeating cryoprotectants

Permeating cryoprotectants are small organic molecules that easily permeate the cell membrane, either by simple diffusion or through membrane channels (9, 11). The most commonly used permeating cryoprotectants are propylene glycol (PROH), ethylene glycol, glycol, and dimethylsulfoxide (DMSO). In principle they prevent ice crystallization by forming hydrogen bonds with water molecules.

At low concentrations they lower the freezing temperature of both the intra- and extracellular solution. The toxicity at low concentrations is relatively low. However, their ability to prevent ice formation is limited. At high concentrations they occupy so much cellular space that it makes it difficult for water molecules to form organized crystals. This results in the formation of a non-crystalline (glassy) state, where water is solidified (9, 11).

However, increasing concentrations of the permeable cryoprotectants significantly increase their toxic effect on cellular functions. Thus, exposure time as well as cooling/warming rate has to be adjusted. Usually, higher concentrations of permeable cryoprotectants mandate a shorter exposure time, and faster cooling rate is necessary (9, 11).

Nonpermeating cryoprotectants

Nonpermeating cryoprotectants are molecules not able to permeate into the cell (sucrose and other disaccharides are commonly used), therefore increasing the extracellular osmotic pressure and assisting the dehydrating process of the cell.

When used together with permeating cryoprotectants, the net concentration of intracellular permeable cryoprotectant concentration is increased, resulting in further decreased freezing temperature, which helps in preventing ice crystal formation. However, their most critical function may be during thawing, preventing osmotic stress. As the extracellular ice is melting, the extracellular osmotic pressure is decreasing rapidly in the absence of nonpermeating cryoprotectants. The intracellular permeable cryoprotectants may not be able to defuse out of the cell as rapidly as water is diffusing into the cell. The result will be swelling or even rupture of the cell (9, 11).

Biological challenges that need to be overcome in connection with cryopreservation

In order to maintain a functional cellular machinery following cryopreservation, there are three main stress factors that need to be managed and avoided as much as possible during the transition from 37°C to liquid nitrogen and back again:

- Ice crystal formation
- Solution effects
- Osmotic shock

This is normally accomplished by the use of various combinations of cryoprotectants as mentioned above, which, however, may act as stress factors themselves, while they also facilitate the transition to a solid state. However, as the commonly used cryoprotectants have potential toxic effects, the following critical parameters need to be considered to maintain their toxicity at a minimum.

- The time that cells are exposed to the liquid cryoprotectants
- The concentration of cryoprotectants used
- The temperature at which the cells and tissues are exposed to the cryoprotectants (metabolism is reduced by 50% for every 10°C decrease)
- The freezing method used to reach the liquid nitrogen state

Ice crystal formation

When water in a solution transitions from liquid to ice, all solutes present in the liquid are excluded from the ice crystals and the ice crystals are pure water. Formation of ice is introduced when a small crystal spontaneously forms (i.e., nucleation) that rapidly grows. If the initial crystal formation takes place within a cell/tissue, the entire biological material may almost immediately become a crystalline solid that has expanded and caused damage. Thus, intracellular nucleation is a very critical event that has to be avoided when cryopreserving biological material (11, 15).

Ice crystal formation often starts outside the cells/tissue, resulting in an increased concentration of other solutes in the non-crystallized surroundings, as ice crystals solely consist of water molecules. Thus, due to lower solute concentration within the cell, the permeable solutes will diffuse across the plasma membrane into the cells in order to reach osmotic equilibrium. Simultaneously, water within the cell will diffuse out as the water activity in the surroundings is reduced due to the ice crystal formation.

Cryoprotectants (permeable or nonpermeable) are solutes changing the intra- and/or extracellular osmotic concentrations, thereby affecting the osmolarity of fluid within the cell, thus determining the direction and amount of water flux across the cell membrane. The following cellular factors affect the ability of the cell to adjust its osmolarity when introduced to cryoprotectants:

1. Membrane permeability for given cryoprotectants
2. Membrane permeability for water
3. Membrane surface area to cell water volume (surface/volume ratio)
4. Temperature (9)

However, these cellular factors are cell and/or cell-stage specific. As an example, oocytes have been shown to have lower permeability to cryoprotectants than early embryos and blastocysts (16) and oocytes have the lowest surface/volume ratio. Thus, oocytes are less efficient to decrease water content and to take up cryoprotectants than embryos. Furthermore, the diffusion rate of cryoprotectants and water across the oocyte membrane is relatively low. Collectively, this explains the relatively long exposure times needed to equilibrate oocytes to cryoprotectants and makes oocytes more vulnerable to suboptimal conditions with the risk of intracellular ice formation.

In general, the exposure time needed to remove water from the cell and to load it with sufficient concentrations of cryoprotectants is longer in larger cells than in smaller cells (9, 16, 17). Thus, ice crystallization in extracellular space introduces a concentration gradient forcing toward an equilibrium balanced by the temperature, concentration, and composition of the solutes and the degree of ice crystal formation.

Solution effects

Cryopreservation processes reduce the intracellular water activity to avoid ice crystal formation while ice proliferates in extracellular space. This leads to high intracellular concentrations of cryoprotectants in which the levels of electrolytes can be very high (11). High levels of electrolytes may denature intracellular proteins and in this way cause cell stress and damage.

Osmotic shock

In living cells osmosis describes the net movement of water through the semipermeable cell membrane from a region of lower solute concentration into a region of higher solute concentration. The osmotic pressure is defined as the pressure required for maintaining equilibrium, with no net movement of water. Osmotic shock/stress, however, is a result of sudden significant extra- or intracellular change in the solute concentration, causing a rapid change in the movement of water across the cell membrane. Sudden low extracellular solute concentrations, which may be a result of thawing, will result in a large net influx of water into the cell, resulting in cell stress like swelling or even rupture and/or apoptosis. Cells have regulatory mechanisms to recover from and tolerate osmotic stress as calcium dependent efflux of osmolytes. However, when freezing or thawing cells, significant changes of solute concentrations, caused by exposure to cryoprotectants and/or as a result of ice crystal formation or melting, may introduce more or less reversible cell injuries.

Principles of cryopreservation techniques

Slow freeze

Slow freezing is based on the principle of cellular equilibrium. Using a refined balance between cryoprotectant concentrations and cooling rate, cells and tissue can be cooled slowly to low temperatures, while minimizing intracellular stress like ice formation, solutions effects, and osmotic trauma (9, 11). Slow freezing protocols use relatively low concentrations of permeable cryoprotectant (usually 1.5 mol/L) with equilibration starting at room temperature, where cellular metabolism still is significant. At these low concentrations, however, the cytotoxicity of permeating cryoprotectants is low. The concentration of the cryoprotectants will, as temperature drops, increase in parallel with the growth of extracellular ice crystal formation as only pure water will be integrated in the ice crystals. As metabolism decreases around 50% for every 10°C, toxicity imposed by higher concentrations of cryoprotectants are only observed at lower subzero temperatures. In connection with slow freezing protocols, a small extracellular crystal is normally formed by the so-called seeding procedure at a temperature of around -6 to -9°C from which the ice crystal will enlarge as the temperature drops. After a short equilibration period, the temperature is lowered very slowly (approximately 0.3ºC/minute) allowing further diffusion of permeable cryoprotectants into the cells while maintaining equilibrium with the extracellular space. The growing extracellular ice formation assisted by nonpermeable cryoprotectants results in further dehydration of the cells. At a temperature of about -30 to -40°C (still well above the freezing temperature of the commonly used permeable cryoprotectants), the intracellular concentrations of cryoprotectants reach levels similar to those used in connection with vitrification, and the cells/tissue can be plunged directly into liquid nitrogen during which the remaining solution rapidly is vitrified to a solid, glassy state. During thawing, temperature is quickly raised to reach the liquid state in order to prevent recrystallization to occur, which potentially may result in stress and cause cell damage. To avoid osmotic stress, relatively high concentrations of nonpermeable cryoprotectants are normally used in this step to avoid a rapid influx of pure water released from melting ice crystals into the cells (9, 11).

Vitrification

Vitrification is achieved by very rapid cooling. Exposure to very high concentrations of cryoprotectants results in extremely viscous intra- and extracellular solutions that can be supercooled forming a solid, glassy state while maintaining the molecular distribution of the original liquid phase. Thus, no ice crystal formation and no spatial expansion occur. The very high cooling rate is a critical factor that has to be balanced in relation to concentration, toxicity, and exposure time of the cryoprotectants. However, once successfully supercooled below the glass transition temperature, a stabile state is reached (5, 9, 11, 15).

Due to exposure to the cryoprotectants at room temperature, water exchange occurs quickly (i.e., a high osmotic velocity), and the cells immediately shrink. However, as the permeable cryoprotectants diffuse into the cells, the cells equilibrate to normal volume. Depending on the temperature, kind of biological material, and membrane permeability of the used cryoprotectants, this equilibration time is normally achieved between 3-15 minutes.

The final step before fast cooling is exposure to the vitrification medium, which contains both permeable and nonpermeable cryoprotectants in high concentrations (i.e., 6 mol/L). In order to minimize toxicity at room temperature of the vitrification medium, the exposure time should be no longer than 30-90 seconds, depending on media composition, exact temperature, and physiological properties of the cells (9). Vitrification is done by loading cells/tissue on a suitable carrier device and the subsequent plunging into liquid nitrogen. These steps determine the cooling rate that has to be ultra rapid. The use of open carrier systems (for example Cryotop® or Cryoleaf™), where the biological material is in direct contact with the liquid nitrogen, results in higher cooling rates (about 20,000°C/minute) than using closed systems (<1,500°C/minute) as CryoTip® or Rapid-i™, which have a space of air between the biological material and nitrogen (9).

Furthermore, loading the biological material on a minimum volume (e.g., 0.5 – 1.0 μL) is an additional factor to optimize the cooling rate. However, the equilibration time, cryoprotectant composition, and cooling rate need optimization for each given type of biological material. Rapid cooling rates have to be complemented by rapid warming rates to prevent ice recrystallization or devitrification. Successful thawing requires, therefore, a refined balance of the critical factors that corresponds to the previous cooling protocol (11, 15).

Conclusions

Each type of cell, and especially each type of tissue, where different types of cells are present simultaneously, often requires a unique set of conditions to obtain optimal results in connection with cryopreservation. The penetration rate and the time to obtain equilibration of the cryoprotectants are dependent of the temperature, their viscosity and water solubility, and of the properties of membrane permeability. Toxicity of cryoprotectants depends on different factors, such as temperature, the specific biochemical properties, and their concentrations within the cells. In general, an optimized setup, supporting the cell survival after freezing and thawing, is commonly achieved experimentally based on an understanding of the fundamental rules of cryobiology and cryotechnology. The differences between slow freezing and vitrification are outlined in the table below.

	Slow freezing	**Vitrification**
CPA concentration	**1.5 mol/L**	**≈ 5 – 6 mol/L**
Volume	**0.3 – 1.0 mL**	**≤ 1 µL**
Contact between cell and N2	**No**	**Yes – in most techniques**
Freezing	**Slow**	**Ultra-rapid**
Cooling rate	**≈ 0.3°C/minute**	**≈ 20.000°C/minute**
Thawing/warming	**Slow**	**Rapid**
Time required	**180 – 240 minutes**	**≈ 10 minutes**
Risk of osmotic injury	**Low**	**High**
Ice crystal formation	**Yes**	**No**
Seeding	**Yes**	**No**
Device (cost)	**High (initial)**	**High (running)**

Table. Comparison of slow-freezing and vitrification methods for cryopreservation of cells/tissues.

References

1. Schmidt KTL, Larsen EC, Yding Andersen C, Nyboe Andersen A: Risk of ovarian failure and fertility preserving methods in girls and adolescents with a malignant disease. British J Obstet. Gynaecol. 2010;117:163-74.
2. Roque M, Lattes K, Serra S, Sola I, Geber S, Carreras R, Checa MA. Fresh embryo transfer versus frozen embryo transfer in in vitro fertilization cycles: a systemic review and meta-analysis. Fertil Steril 2013; 99 (1): 156-162.
3. Gatta G, Capocaccia R, Coleman MP, Ries LAG, Berrino F. Childhood cancer survival in Europe and the United States. Cancer 2002;95:1767–72.
4. Edgar AB, Morris EMM, Kelnar CJK, Wallace WHB. Long-term follow-up of survivors of childhood cancer. Endocr Dev 2009;15:159–80.
5. Smith GD, Motta EE, Serafini P. Theoretical and experimental basis of oocyte vitrification. Reproductive BioMedicine Online 2011;23:298–306.
6. Rosendahl M, Schmidt KT, Ernst E, Rasmussen PE, Loft A, Byskov AG, Andersen AN, Andersen CY. Cryopreservation of ovarian tissue for a decade in Denmark: a view of the technique. Reprod Biomed Online 2012;25:146-167.
7. Roberts SA, McGowan L, Hirst WM, Vail A, Rutherford A, Lieberman BA, Brison DR and the toward SET collaboration. Reducing the incidence of twins from IVF treatments: predictive modeling from a retrospective cohort. Hum Reprod 2011;26(3):569-575.
8. Shapiro BS, Daneshmand ST, Garner FC, Aguirre M, Hudson C, Thomas S. Evidence of impaired endometrial receptivity after ovarian stimulation for in vitro fertilization: a prospective randomized trial comparing fresh and frozen-thawed embryo transfer in normal responders. Fertil Steril. 2011;96:344-348.
9. Alpha Scientists in Reproductive Medicine. The Alpha consensus meeting on cryopreservation key performance indicators and benchmarks: proceedings of an expert meeting. Reprod Biomed Online 2012; 25: 146-167.
10. Cobo Cabal A, Carrido N, Castello D, Meseguer M, Pellicer A, Remohi A. Evaluation of four years experience of an ovum donation (OD) program using cryo-banked oocytes. Hum Reprod 2011;26(Suppl 1), i33.
11. Jain JK, Paulson RJ. Oocyte cryopreservation. Fertil Steril 2006;86 (Suppl 3):1037-1046.
12. Andersen CY, Silber SJ, Berghold SH, Jorgensen JS, Ernst E. Long-term duration of function of ovarian tissue transplants: case reports. Reprod Biomed Online. 2012;25:128-32.
13. Mazur, P., Leibo, S., Chu, E., 1972. A two-factor hypothesis of freezing injury: evidence from Chinese hamster tissue-culture cells. Exp. Cell Res. 71, 345–355.
14. Meryman, H., 1971. Cryoprotective agents. Cryobiology 8, 173–183.
15. Yavin S, Arav A. Measurement of essential physical properties of vitrification solutions. Theriogenology 2006; 67:81-89.
16. Pedro P, Yokoyama E, Zhu S, Yoshida N, Valdez D, Tanaka M, Edashige K, Kasai M. J. Permeability of mouse oocytes and embryos at various developmental stages to five cryoprotectants. Reprod Dev 2005;51:235-246.
17. Maneiro E, Ron-Corzo A, Julve J, Goyanes VJ. Surface area/volume ratio and growth equation of the human early embryo. Int. J. Dev. Biol.1991;35:139-143.

Clinical application of fertility preservation

Mitchell P. Rosen

University of California, San Francisco, United States

Introduction

Loss of reproductive potential after cancer treatment negatively impacts quality of life (QOL) in young survivors.[1,2] Recent studies have indicated that the potential iatrogenic loss of fertility has a profound impact on young women and, at times, may be more stressful than the cancer diagnosis itself.[3,4] Loss of fertility represents a large-scale survivorship issue according to 2006 Surveillance, Epidemiology and End Results (SEER) statistics: Approximately 120,000 women aged <50 years develop cancer each year in the United States.[5] And although counseling and fertility preservation rates have improved over the last decade, a significant unmet need remains among cancer patients who desire the opportunity to undergo fertility preservation.[6] Oncologists have cited many reasons for the lack of such discussions with patients, including lack of knowledge, insufficient time to discuss the issue, and perceptions that patients cannot delay treatment.[7]

Multiple strategies have emerged to preserve fertility in females with different types of malignancies. These include oocyte and embryo cryopreservation, cortical and whole ovary cryopreservation, ovarian transplantation, ovarian transposition, and use of gonadotropin-releasing hormone (GnRH) agonist.[8] The indications for ovarian transposition or treatment that does not involve controlled ovarian stimulation (COS) are limited to cases of pelvic radiation or those with stringent short-term time constraints, respectively.

Currently, embryo and mature oocyte cryopreservation with COS are the only techniques endorsed by the American Society for Reproductive Medicine (ASRM), while the other methods are still considered investigational.[9,10] The purpose of COS is to maximize the number of embryos and oocytes cryopreserved. This is critically important for those undergoing treatment that is potentially gonadotoxic, not only because the patient likely only has a single cycle opportunity, but also to increase the chances for future pregnancy(ies). However, when stimulating cancer patients, several unique issues are important to consider:

1. Avoidance of delays for cancer treatment. Time delays can create increased stress for both the patient and the oncologist. Thus, a potential delay may mean the patient may not be able to go through treatment to preserve fertility.
2. Consideration of additional safety issues. It is important to avoid a high estrogenic state with cancers that are positive for estrogen receptors (i.e., breast, uterine). Additionally, it is important to understand the co-morbid conditions as they may precipitate sequelae from COS and/or the oocyte retrieval procedure.

1) Avoidance of potential delays

The choice of the specific COS protocol is generally determined based upon preferences of each in vitro fertilization (IVF) center and influenced by the time available until the initiation of radio/chemotherapy. Although multiple different COS protocols are being used, the majority of the patients are treated with a GnRH antagonist-based protocol because they significantly decrease the interval from patient presentation to embryo/oocyte cryopreservation.[11]

Conventionally, regardless of the protocol, COS is initiated at the beginning of the follicular phase with the idea that this would optimize clinical outcomes. As a result, depending on the women's menstrual cycle phase at presentation, 2 to 6 weeks may be required to complete a cycle for fertility preservation. Adhering to this convention may result in either significant delay of cancer treatments or forgoing fertility preservation due to time constraints. Therefore, a modification from conventional early follicular phase start was necessary.

For patients presenting in the luteal phase, GnRH antagonists were used to initiate luteolysis as a first attempt to shorten the luteal phase and minimize potential delays for cancer treatment.[12,13] Several case series have shown with the administration of a GnRH antagonist (e.g., single dose of cetrorelix 1g subcutaneously) during the mid-luteal phase, menses ensued a few days later[12-15] (Figure 1B).[16] Ovarian stimulation then began immediately following menses and a synchronized cohort of follicles developed with oocyte number and fertilization rates similar to what would be expected with a standard follicular phase start. These studies suggested that by initiating luteolysis the luteal phase can be shortened, decreasing the potential delay to cancer treatment. However, this approach still required a follicular phase start of gonadotropins.

For a more rapid start, and potentially a shorter delay for patients who present in the luteal phase, random start stimulation with simultaneous luteolysis regression was then proposed. In a small prospective multi-center study (n=40), ovarian stimulation during the luteal phase was described in a cohort of cancer patients.[17] GnRH antagonists to eliminate luteinizing hormone (LH) secretion and initiate luteolysis were started simultaneously with recombinant follicle-stimulating hormone (FSH), thus avoiding exogenous LH activity, which might prevent luteolysis. Compared with cancer patients stimulated during the follicular phase (n=28) with either a short "flare-up" protocol or an antagonist protocol, the luteal phase group (n=12) had a similar number of aspirated oocytes, number of metaphase II oocytes,

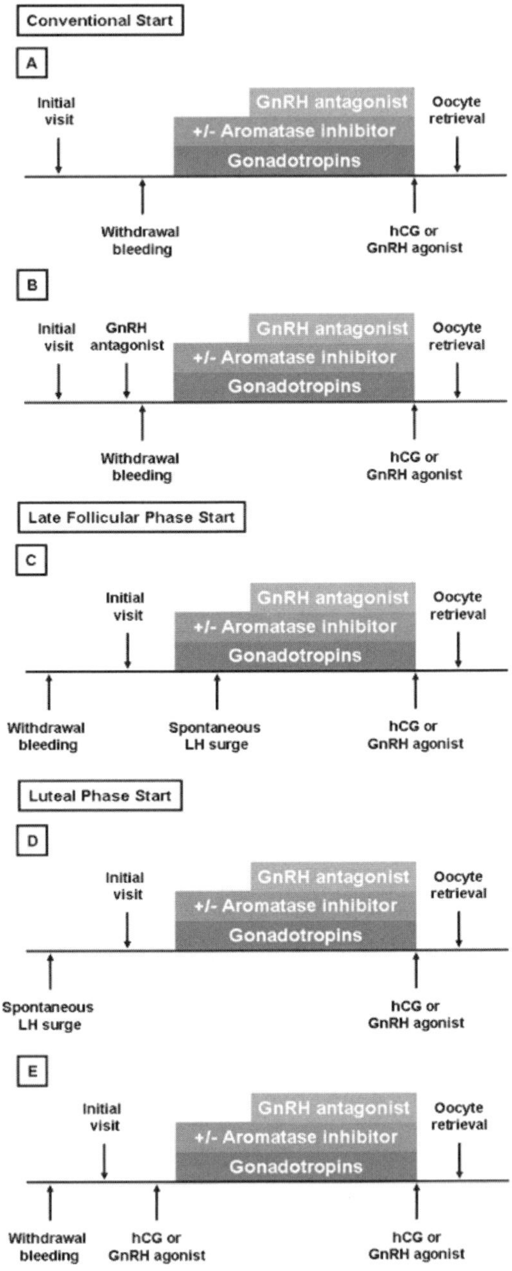

Figure 1. Conventional and random-start antagonist IVF protocols for cancer patients undergoing fertility preservation

Reference: Cakmak H, Rosen MP. Ovarian stimulation in cancer patients. Fertility and sterility. In press.

and fertilization rate.[17] Interestingly, several of the patients in this study were also stimulated late in the follicular phase, raising the potential that patients can be stimulated at any point in the cycle.

Two case studies evaluated the effectiveness of initiating ovarian stimulation at the time of patient presentation (menstrual cycle day 11, 14, and 17) rather than waiting for spontaneous menses.[18,19] GnRH antagonist was started to prevent premature LH surge when the lead follicle measured over 13 mm. In the 2 patients who presented in the luteal phase, gonadotropins were administered without simultaneous GnRH antagonist. The results showed similar cycle length and a reasonable ovarian response with 7–10 embryos cryopreserved per patient.[18] These case studies supported the idea that it is possible to start a COS at any time in the menstrual cycle (random start).

At the University of California, San Francisco, we compared the outcomes of random start ovarian stimulation to conventional start with the same protocol over the same time period.[20] The protocol that was administered to the patient was dependent on the menstrual phase at presentation.

If the patient did not present near the first day of menses, the phase of menstrual cycle was evaluated by the onset of the last menstrual period, by ultrasound and/or by progesterone concentrations. The late follicular phase was defined as after menstrual cycle day 7 with emergence of a dominant follicle (larger than 13 mm) and a progesterone level lower than 2 ng/mL. The luteal phase was determined by progesterone level higher than 3 ng/mL.

If the cancer patient presented in the late follicular phase, we preceded with one of the following treatment plans:

a) Ovarian stimulation was started at the time of presentation. If the follicle cohort following the lead follicle was smaller than 12 mm and continued to be smaller than 12 mm before spontaneous LH surge, no GnRH antagonist was started (Figure 1B).[16] After the spontaneous LH surge, GnRH antagonist was added when the secondary follicle cohort reached 12 mm to prevent secondary LH surge prior to human chorionic gonadotropin (hCG) trigger (Figure 1B).[16] If the follicle cohort following the lead follicle reached 12 mm before the spontaneous LH surge, pituitary suppression with GnRH antagonist was initiated and continued until triggering final oocyte maturation with hCG or GnRH agonist (Figure 1C).[16]
b) Ovulation was induced when the dominant follicle reached 18 mm in diameter with hCG or GnRH agonist, and ovarian stimulation was started in 2-3 days in luteal phase (Figure 1E).[16]

If the cancer patient presented in the luteal phase or the ovulation was induced, ovarian stimulation was started without GnRH antagonist (Figure 1D and E).[16] Similar to conventional COS, to prevent premature secondary LH surge, GnRH antagonist administration was initiated later in the cycle when the follicle cohort reached 12 mm and was continued until the hCG or GnRH agonist trigger.

Table 1 shows comparisons between random start and conventional start. The number of total and mature oocytes retrieved, oocyte yield (i.e., number of metaphase II [MII] oocytes/antral follicle count [AFC]), and fertilization rates were similar between groups. However, the length of ovarian stimulation was about 2 days longer, and therefore, the total dose of gonadotropin used was significantly higher in late follicular and luteal phase start groups compared to conventional start group. Ongoing data on late follicular and luteal starts have been collected and compared to conventional start and continue to show similar outcomes with no differences between late follicular or luteal starts (data not shown).

	Conventional Start (n=87; 101 cycles)	Random Start (n=24; 24 cycles)	P value
Age (years)	33.9 ± 5.2	34.6 ± 5.0	NS
AFC	13 (9-19)	11.5 (6-16)	NS
Days of ovarian stimulation	9 (8-10)	11 (10-12)	<0.001
Total dose of gonadotropins (IU)	3386 ± 1085	4201 ± 1147	0.001
Follicles ≥ 13 mm	12 (6-17)	10 (8-15.5)	NS
Oocytes retrieved	15 (9-23)	12.5 (9-20.5)	NS
Mature oocytes (MII) retrieved	11 (6-16)	9 (5-14.5)	NS
Oocyte/AFC ratio	1.1 (0.8-1.7)	1.2 (0.9-1.7)	NS
Mature oocyte/AFC ratio	0.8 (0.5-1.1)	0.8 (0.6-1.2)	NS
Fertilization rate after ICSI (2PN/MII)	0.77 ± 0.22	0.87 ± 0.15	NS

Table 1. Comparison of characteristics and outcomes of conventional and random start antagonist IVF cycles in cancer patients. Data are presented as mean ± SD or median (interquartile range 25%-75%) (19). AFC: Antral follicle count, NS: Not significant; ICSI: intracytoplasmic sperm injection; PN: pronuclear.

Overall, this approach provides a significant advantage by decreasing total time for the IVF cycle, and in emergent settings, ovarian stimulation can be started at a random cycle time for the purpose of fertility preservation without compromising oocyte yield and maturity. This is consistent with a newer concept of ovarian physiology, which indicates that there are multiple waves of follicular recruitment during each menstrual cycle.[21] Additional clinical studies are needed to assess the efficacy of this strategy, especially regarding the rates of clinical pregnancy and of live-born infants originating from the use of cryopreserved embryos and of oocytes obtained by random start ovarian stimulation.

2) Consider additional safety issues

During COS, there is a potential risk that the supraphysiological estradiol levels as a result of the ovarian stimulation with gonadotropins may promote the growth of estrogen-sensitive tumors. Whereas no study has been able to address whether short-term elevation of estrogen propagates growth of estrogen-receptor positive tumors, there is evidence that acute exposure to estrogen results in increased cell proliferation in vitro in cancer cells.[22] Therefore, alternative and potentially safer protocols have been introduced for fertility preservation in patients with estrogen-sensitive cancers including natural cycle IVF (without ovarian stimulation), stimulation protocols with tamoxifen alone or combined with gonadotropins, and stimulation protocols with aromatase inhibitors, all with the goal of reducing estrogen production.[23]

The most effective treatment to lower the potential risk and maintain a maximum yield from the COS is to administer an aromatase inhibitor, such as letrozole.[24, 25] In a study comparing the efficacy of the letrozole plus gonadotropin protocol in breast cancer patients and the standard IVF protocol in age-matched non-cancer patients with tubal factor infertility, the breast cancer patients started to receive letrozole (5 mg/day) on menstrual cycle day 2 or 3. FSH (150–300 IU/day) was added 2 days later, all medications were discontinued on the day of hCG trigger, and letrozole was reinitiated after oocyte retrieval and continued until estradiol levels fell below 50 pg/mL.[25] This letrozole plus gonadotropin protocol resulted in similar number of total oocytes retrieved and length of ovarian stimulation compared to standard IVF protocol.[25] As expected, peak estradiol levels were significantly lower in the breast cancer patients receiving letrozole plus gonadotropin compared with the standard IVF group (483 ± 278.9 pg/mL vs. 1,464.6 ± 644.9 pg/mL).[25] The studies assessing the effect of letrozole on oocyte maturity and competence demonstrated that the addition of letrozole did not change the number of mature oocytes retrieved and fertilization rates.[25,26] Similarly, in our practice we observed comparable oocyte maturity (MII oocytes/total oocytes retrieved) (0.68 ± 0.19 vs. 0.71 ± 0.23) and fertilization rates (0.77 ± 0.22 vs. 0.78 ± 0.24) in intracytoplasmic sperm injection (ICSI) cycles with and without letrozole (unpublished data). In addition, we and others have found that aromatase inhibitors can be administered with random start COS with no compromise in oocyte yield or fertilization outcomes (data not shown).

The short-term follow-up of breast cancer patients who have undergone ovarian stimulation with letrozole plus gonadotropins has not shown an increase in breast cancer recurrence.[27] In addition, COS with aromatase inhibitors in combination with gonadotropins was also used safely for the embryo cryopreservation in endometrial cancer patients.[28] Therefore, we highly recommend the routine use of letrozole during COS for fertility preservation in patients with estrogen-sensitive cancers.

Letrozole suppresses plasma estradiol levels significantly at doses of 0.1 to 10 mg/day.[29] In our clinic, we start letrozole 2.5 or 5 mg/day, depending on the ovarian reserve of the patient, with the ovarian stimulation (Figure 1).[16] Given the importance of keeping estradiol levels close to that observed in natural cycles in patients with estrogen-sensitive cancers, we check estradiol levels at every clinic visit and titrate letrozole dose up to 10 mg/day to keep estradiol levels lower than 500 pg/mL.[24] These letrozole doses are well-tolerated and the mature oocyte/embryo yield after COS is not affected by letrozole at any dose used in our clinical practice. We also consider continuing letrozole after the oocyte retrieval if serum estradiol levels are still elevated (i.e., estradiol higher than 500 pg/mL). In our experience, even if estradiol levels are above 500 pg/mL prior to retrieval, only a minority of patients requires letrozole post-retrieval. Discontinuation of letrozole can either be at menses or with initiation of chemotherapy.

Ovarian hyperstimulation syndrome (OHSS) is the most serious complication of ovarian stimulation and can be associated with intravascular depletion, ascites, liver dysfunction, pulmonary edema, electrolyte imbalance, and thromboembolic events. While this syndrome is often self-limited with spontaneous resolution within a few days, severe disease may require hospitalization and intensive care. With fertility preservation treatment, balancing the risk of OHSS with the desired maximum chance for successful future pregnancy can make management of the stimulation challenging. The impact of OHSS can be profound in cancer patients, because it may result in delaying or complicating planned lifesaving cancer therapy.[30]

Triggering the final oocyte maturation with hCG carries the well-known risk of inducing OHSS.[31] As an alternative, a GnRH agonist can be used to induce oocyte maturation, in non-down-regulated cycles. GnRH agonist trigger in GnRH antagonist-based protocols dramatically reduces the risk of OHSS due to the short half-life of GnRH agonist-induced endogenous LH surge.[32] In a study comparing GnRH agonist and hCG as the trigger for oocyte maturation in fertility preservation cycles, GnRH agonist trigger resulted in at least a similar number of mature oocytes and cryopreserved embryos compared with the hCG group.[33]

However, in our experience we have observed trigger failures with GnRH agonist trigger at both 1 mg and 4 mg dosing. The likely etiology is that GnRH agonist is able to bind to only a portion of the receptors due to competition with GnRH antagonist yielding a limited LH surge.[34] It is possible that with the increase in dose of GnRH agonist or with hCG supplementation (1,500 IU or less) at the time of trigger, there will be fewer failures. Due to the possibility of failure, we do not routinely recommend GnRH agonist trigger for all patients. In our current practice, 4 mg of leuprolide acetate is being used only in patients with high risk of OHSS.

The number of follicles, more specifically the follicular pattern, in combination with serum estradiol levels, predicts OHSS with high sensitivity and specificity.[35,36] One caveat is that co-treatment with aromatase inhibitors limits the utilization of estradiol level to help predict OHSS. In this scenario, it is important to rely on the follicular pattern and the rate of estradiol rise rather than the absolute serum estradiol levels. If the estradiol levels are rising rapidly while administering letrozole especially in the presence of a high number of small follicles, the patient should be considered as being at risk of OHSS, and GnRH agonist trigger should be used to lower this risk.

In conclusion, we recommend GnRH agonist trigger in GnRH antagonist-based fertility preservation cycles only for women who are at risk for OHSS. The trigger must be confirmed the next morning by measuring serum LH level. In the case of a GnRH agonist trigger failure determined by low post-trigger LH -- in our clinic, we use the cut-off LH level less than 12 mIU/mL, hCG (2,500 to 5,000 IU) -- trigger can be given on the same day.[37] If the patient has relatively low post-trigger LH level, but higher than 12 mIU/mL, the closer attention should be given to the oocyte yield during the oocyte retrieval. If no or an inappropriately low number of oocytes are retrieved after aspirating a couple of mature-size follicles, the oocyte retrieval should be stopped. Maturation should be triggered again by administering hCG (2,500 to 5,000 IU) due to the possibility of failing to trigger oocyte maturation with GnRH agonist and then oocyte retrieval should be attempted again after 34 to 36 hours.[37]

The number of follicles, more specifically the follicular pattern, in combination with serum estradiol levels, predicts OHSS with high sensitivity and specificity.[35,36] One caveat is that co-treatment with aromatase inhibitors limits the utilization of estradiol level to help predict OHSS. In this scenario, it is important to rely on the follicular pattern and the rate of estradiol rise rather than the absolute serum estradiol levels. If the estradiol levels are rising rapidly while administering letrozole especially in the presence of a high number of small follicles, the patient should be considered as being at risk of OHSS, and GnRH agonist trigger should be used to lower this risk.

In conclusion, we recommend GnRH agonist trigger in GnRH antagonist-based fertility preservation cycles only for women who are at risk for OHSS. The trigger must be confirmed the next morning by measuring serum LH level. In the case of a GnRH agonist trigger failure determined by low post-trigger LH -- in our clinic, we use the cut-off LH level less than 12 mIU/mL, hCG (2,500 to 5,000 IU) -- trigger can be given on the same day.[37] If the patient has relatively low post-trigger LH level, but higher than 12 mIU/mL, the closer attention should be given to the oocyte yield during the oocyte retrieval. If no or an inappropriately low number of oocytes are retrieved after aspirating a couple of mature-size follicles, the oocyte retrieval should be stopped. Maturation should be triggered again by administering hCG (2,500 to 5,000 IU) due to the possibility of failing to trigger oocyte maturation with GnRH agonist and then oocyte retrieval should be attempted again after 34 to 36 hours.[37]

Conclusions

Given the importance of reproduction for many young patients faced with cancer, counseling regarding fertility preservation is an essential part of comprehensive cancer care. The unique goals of COS for cancer patients include: 1) maximizing the number of embryos and oocytes for cryopreservation; 2) minimizing any delay to cancer treatment; and 3) safety, with careful consideration for estrogen receptor status and potential for increased risk for OHSS. In emergent settings, random start ovarian stimulation is emerging as a new technique for the purpose of fertility preservation without compromising oocyte yield and maturity. This protocol will minimize delays and as a result enable more patients the opportunity to undergo fertility preservation.

References

1. Loprinzi CL, Wolf SL, Barton DL, Laack NN. Symptom management in premenopausal patients with breast cancer. The lancet oncology. 2008;9(10):993-1001. Epub 2008/12/17. doi: 10.1016/S1470-2045(08)70256-0. PubMed PMID: 19071256.
2. Tschudin S, Bitzer J. Psychological aspects of fertility preservation in men and women affected by cancer and other life-threatening diseases. Human reproduction update. 2009;15(5):587-97. Epub 2009/05/13. doi: 10.1093/humupd/dmp015. PubMed PMID: 19433413.
3. Schover LR. Patient attitudes toward fertility preservation. Pediatric blood & cancer. 2009;53(2):281-4. Epub 2009/03/21. doi: 10.1002/pbc.22001. PubMed PMID: 19301387.
4. Partridge AH, Gelber S, Peppercorn J, Sampson E, Knudsen K, Laufer M, et al. Web-based survey of fertility issues in young women with breast cancer. Journal of clinical oncology : official journal of the American Society of Clinical Oncology. 2004;22(20):4174-83. Epub 2004/10/16. doi: 10.1200/JCO.2004.01.159. PubMed PMID: 15483028.
5. NCIFastStats. Statistics Stratified By Age. Surveillance Epidemiology and End Results (SEER) Program. 2006;Bethesda, MD.
6. Letourneau JM, Smith JF, Ebbel EE, Craig A, Katz PP, Cedars MI, et al. Racial, socioeconomic, and demographic disparities in access to fertility preservation in young women diagnosed with cancer. Cancer. 2012;118(18):4579-88. Epub 2012/03/28. doi: 10.1002/cncr.26649. PubMed PMID: 22451228; PubMed Central PMCID: PMC3387319.
7. Quinn GP, Vadaparampil ST, Lee JH, Jacobsen PB, Bepler G, Lancaster J, et al. Physician referral for fertility preservation in oncology patients: a national study of practice behaviors. Journal of clinical oncology : official journal of the American Society of Clinical Oncology. 2009;27(35):5952-7. Epub 2009/10/15. doi: 10.1200/JCO.2009.23.0250. PubMed PMID: 19826115.
8. Anderson RA, Wallace WH. Fertility preservation in girls and young women. Clinical endocrinology. 2011;75(4):409-19. Epub 2011/05/18. doi: 10.1111/j.1365-2265.2011.04100.x. PubMed PMID: 21575025.
9. The Practice Committee of the American Society for Reproductive Medicine. Fertility preservation and reproduction in cancer patients. Fertility and sterility. 2005;83(6):1622-8. PubMed PMID: 15950628.
10. The Practice Committee of the American Society for Reproductive Medicine. Mature oocyte cryopreservation: a guideline. Fertility and sterility. 2013;99(1):37-43. PubMed PMID: 23083924.
11. McLaren JF, Bates GW. Fertility preservation in women of reproductive age with cancer. American journal of obstetrics and gynecology. 2012;207(6):455-62. Epub 2012/09/11. doi: 10.1016/j.ajog.2012.08.013. PubMed PMID: 22959764.
12. Anderson RA, Kinniburgh D, Baird DT. Preliminary experience of the use of a gonadotrophin-releasing hormone antagonist in ovulation induction/in-vitro fertilization prior to cancer treatment. Hum Reprod. 1999;14(10):2665-8. Epub 1999/10/21. PubMed PMID: 10528005.
13. Humaidan P, Bungum L, Bungum M, Hald F, Agerholm I, Blaabjerg J, et al. Reproductive outcome using a GnRH antagonist (cetrorelix) for luteolysis and follicular synchronization in poor responder IVF/ICSI patients treated with a flexible GnRH antagonist protocol. Reproductive biomedicine online. 2005;11(6):679-84. Epub 2006/01/19. PubMed PMID: 16417730.

14. Nilsson L, Andersen AN, Lindenberg S, Hausken J, Andersen CY, Kahn JA. Ganirelix for luteolysis in poor responder patients undergoing IVF treatment: a Scandinavian multicenter 'extended pilot study'. Acta obstetricia et gynecologica Scandinavica. 2010;89(6):828-31. Epub 2010/05/28. doi: 10.3109/00016341003721029. PubMed PMID: 20504085.
15. Friden BE, Nilsson L. Gonadotrophin-releasing hormone-antagonist luteolysis during the preceding mid-luteal phase is a feasible protocol in ovarian hyperstimulation before in vitro fertilization. Acta obstetricia et gynecologica Scandinavica. 2005;84(8):812-6. Epub 2005/07/20. doi: 10.1111/j.0001-6349.2005.00730.x. PubMed PMID: 16026411.
16. Cakmak H, Rosen MP. Ovarian stimulation in cancer patients. Fertility and sterility. In press.
17. von Wolff M, Thaler CJ, Frambach T, Zeeb C, Lawrenz B, Popovici RM, et al. Ovarian stimulation to cryopreserve fertilized oocytes in cancer patients can be started in the luteal phase. Fertility and sterility. 2009;92(4):1360-5. Epub 2008/10/22. doi: 10.1016/j.fertnstert.2008.08.011. PubMed PMID: 18930226.
18. Sonmezer M, Turkcuoglu I, Coskun U, Oktay K. Random-start controlled ovarian hyperstimulation for emergency fertility preservation in letrozole cycles. Fertility and sterility. 2011;95(6):2125 e9-11. Epub 2011/02/05. doi: 10.1016/j.fertnstert.2011.01.030. PubMed PMID: 21292255.
19. Nayak SR, Wakim AN. Random-start gonadotropin-releasing hormone (GnRH) antagonist-treated cycles with GnRH agonist trigger for fertility preservation. Fertility and sterility. 2011;96(1):e51-4. Epub 2011/05/24. doi: 10.1016/j.fertnstert.2011.04.079. PubMed PMID: 21601193.
20. Cakmak H, Zamah AM, Katz A, Cedars MI, Rosen MP. Effective method for emergency fertility preservation: random-start controlled ovarian hyperstimulation. Fertility and sterility. 2012;98:S170.
21. Baerwald AR, Adams GP, Pierson RA. Characterization of ovarian follicular wave dynamics in women. Biology of reproduction. 2003;69(3):1023-31. Epub 2003/05/16. doi: 10.1095/biolreprod.103.017772. PubMed PMID: 12748128.
22. Platet N, Cathiard AM, Gleizes M, Garcia M. Estrogens and their receptors in breast cancer progression: a dual role in cancer proliferation and invasion. Critical reviews in oncology/hematology. 2004;51(1):55-67. Epub 2004/06/23. doi: 10.1016/j.critrevonc.2004.02.001. PubMed PMID: 15207254.
23. Rodriguez-Wallberg KA, Oktay K. Fertility preservation in women with breast cancer. Clinical obstetrics and gynecology. 2010;53(4):753-62. Epub 2010/11/05. doi: 10.1097/GRF.0b013e3181f96e00. PubMed PMID: 21048442; PubMed Central PMCID: PMC3404603.
24. Testart J, Frydman R, Nahoul K, Grenier J, Feinstein MC, Roger M, et al. Steroids and gonadotropins during the last pre-ovulatory phase of the menstrual cycle. Time relationships between plasma hormones levels and luteinizing hormone surge onset. Journal of steroid biochemistry. 1982;17(6):675-82. Epub 1982/12/01. PubMed PMID: 6217383.
25. Oktay K, Hourvitz A, Sahin G, Oktem O, Safro B, Cil A, et al. Letrozole reduces estrogen and gonadotropin exposure in women with breast cancer undergoing ovarian stimulation before chemotherapy. The Journal of clinical endocrinology and metabolism. 2006;91(10):3885-90. Epub 2006/08/03. doi: 10.1210/jc.2006-0962. PubMed PMID: 16882752.
26. Johnson LN, Dillon KE, Sammel MD, Efymow BL, Mainigi MA, Dokras A, et al. Response to ovarian stimulation in patients facing gonadotoxic therapy. Reproductive biomedicine online. 2013. Epub 2013/02/19. doi: 10.1016/j.rbmo.2013.01.003. PubMed PMID: 23415997.

27. Azim AA, Costantini-Ferrando M, Oktay K. Safety of fertility preservation by ovarian stimulation with letrozole and gonadotropins in patients with breast cancer: a prospective controlled study. Journal of clinical oncology : official journal of the American Society of Clinical Oncology. 2008;26(16):2630-5. Epub 2008/05/30. doi: 10.1200/JCO.2007.14.8700. PubMed PMID: 18509175.
28. Azim A, Oktay K. Letrozole for ovulation induction and fertility preservation by embryo cryopreservation in young women with endometrial carcinoma. Fertility and sterility. 2007;88(3):657-64. PubMed PMID: 17428480.
29. Klein KO, Demers LM, Santner SJ, Baron J, Cutler GB, Jr., Santen RJ. Use of ultrasensitive recombinant cell bioassay to measure estrogen levels in women with breast cancer receiving the aromatase inhibitor, letrozole. The Journal of clinical endocrinology and metabolism. 1995;80(9):2658-60. PubMed PMID: 7673408.
30. Delvigne A, Rozenberg S. Epidemiology and prevention of ovarian hyperstimulation syndrome (OHSS): a review. Human reproduction update. 2002;8(6):559-77. PubMed PMID: 12498425.
31. Humaidan P, Kol S, Papanikolaou EG. GnRH agonist for triggering of final oocyte maturation: time for a change of practice? Human reproduction update. 2011;17(4):510-24. PubMed PMID: 21450755.
32. Engmann L, DiLuigi A, Schmidt D, Nulsen J, Maier D, Benadiva C. The use of gonadotropin-releasing hormone (GnRH) agonist to induce oocyte maturation after cotreatment with GnRH antagonist in high-risk patients undergoing in vitro fertilization prevents the risk of ovarian hyperstimulation syndrome: a prospective randomized controlled study. Fertility and sterility. 2008;89(1):84-91. PubMed PMID: 17462639.
33. Oktay K, Turkcuoglu I, Rodriguez-Wallberg KA. GnRH agonist trigger for women with breast cancer undergoing fertility preservation by aromatase inhibitor/FSH stimulation. Reproductive biomedicine online. 2010;20(6):783-8. PubMed PMID: 20382080.
34. McArdle CA, Franklin J, Green L, Hislop JN. Signalling, cycling and desensitisation of gonadotrophin-releasing hormone receptors. J Endocrinol. 2002;173(1):1-11. PubMed PMID: 11927379.
35. Blankstein J, Shalev J, Saadon T, Kukia EE, Rabinovici J, Pariente C, et al. Ovarian hyperstimulation syndrome: prediction by number and size of preovulatory ovarian follicles. Fertility and sterility. 1987;47(4):597-602. PubMed PMID: 3106098.
36. Papanikolaou EG, Pozzobon C, Kolibianakis EM, Camus M, Tournaye H, Fatemi HM, et al. Incidence and prediction of ovarian hyperstimulation syndrome in women undergoing gonadotropin-releasing hormone antagonist in vitro fertilization cycles. Fertility and sterility. 2006;85(1):112-20. PubMed PMID: 16412740.
37. Cakmak H, Fujimoto VY, Zamah AM, Rosen MP, Tran ND, Cedars MI, et al. Metaphase II (MII) oocytes obtained at different time points in the same in vitro fertilization cycle. J Assist Reprod Genet. 2012;29(11):1203-5. PubMed PMID: 22941385.

Trilogy 3. IFFS/WHO Trilogy: Contraception

Research on male contraception

Regine L. Sitruk-Ware, John Amory** and Eberhard Nieschlag****

*Population Council, New York City, United States
**University of Washington, Seattle, United States
***University Hospitals of Münster, Münster, Germany

Introduction

Men are increasingly expected and willing to share the responsibility for family planning by using contraceptive methods.[1] An ideal male contraceptive must be highly effective, safe, reversible, acceptable, and affordable to men worldwide.

Male contraceptives may be classified as either nonhormonal or hormonal methods. Up to the present, the only available contraceptives for men have been less-than-ideal barrier methods, such as condoms and vasectomy. In the United States, 20.4% of men use condoms (with a failure rate of about 10%) and 10.9% undergo vasectomy. Other contraceptive methods still in the early stages of research attempt to either decrease sperm production or motility or block the ability of sperm to fertilize the ovum.

Research on hormonal methods

Research includes treatment with androgen alone or in combination with progestin or an analog of the gonadotropin-releasing hormone (GnRH) to suppress the pituitary gonadotropins (follicle-stimulating hormone [FSH] and luteinizing hormone [LH]) and result in reduction of sperm output.[2,3] No combinations of testosterone with a progestin has achieved 95% azoospermia so far.[4]

Potential adverse effects on prostate gland growth, when high doses of androgen are used, may be circumvented by combination with a gestagen, such as norethisterone enanthate as recently shown in a non-human primate model[4], or with the development of tissue selective or androgen receptor modulators (SARMs) that could theoretically suppress gonadotropin secretion more profoundly but possess reduced side effects on the prostate due to lack of interaction with the 5α-reductase enzyme.

The Population Council initiated the search for an androgen that would not be a substrate for the 5α-reductase enzyme in order to spare the prostate from the androgenic effect. After screening of several molecules, 7α-methyl-19-nortestosterone (MENT™) was identified, shown to be resistant to 5α reduction in the prostate, and also found to be 10-fold more potent than testosterone (T) in terms of its anabolic effects.[5] MENT™ was identified as an ideal androgen for exogenous administration for contraceptive and/or replacement purposes with health benefits. Therefore, it seems that a new type of molecules should be designed and combinations with newer progestins with SARMs look promising for future development.

In the immature castrated rat, MENT™ had shown a 5 times higher potency than testosterone on levator ani and seminal vesicle weights[5] and appeared to be an appropriate candidate for male contraception as well as for androgen replacement in hypogonadal men.[6,7] Toxicology studies indicated its safety for use in humans and a radioimmunoassay for MENT™ has been developed.[8] Clinical trials showed that MENT™ delivered from one-year implants could induce reversible azoospermia in a high percentage of subjects.[9]

Other approaches include transdermal application of a progestin (Nestorone® [NES]) and an androgen (testosterone gel [T]). Ilani N et al.,[10] evaluated the efficacy of transdermal delivery of both steroid hormones in suppressing spermatogenesis in a 6-month study and showed a high rate of efficacy on sperm suppression.[11] The addition of NES to T resulted in significantly lower sperm concentrations and serum gonadotropin levels compared with T gel alone, with minimal side-effects in all groups. Total and free T serum concentrations remained within normal range during the treatment period in all groups.

Most studies using androgen and progestins were conducted in small groups of volunteers and two large studies testing either a combination of etonogestrel implants and testosterone undecanoate injections[12] or the WHO large efficacy study testing norethisterone enanthate combined with testosterone undecanoate injections (based on a smaller proof-of-principle study[13]) have both shown high efficacy on sperm suppression.[14] However, the former was the result of a collaboration between two pharmaceutical industries that have withdrawn from this field of research, and the WHO study was interrupted due to a high number of side effects, most likely the result of inadequate dose combinations of both hormones.[9,14]

Nonhormonal methods

Research on specific targets of the reproductive system is designed to avoid systemic effects or modifications of the hormonal environment and also to block specific functions such as motility or maturation of sperm. New areas of basic research based on recent progress on genomics and proteomics include studies on genes, proteins, and enzymes involved in the reproductive system.

One approach includes **disruption of the tight junction** between Sertoli cells by analogs of Lonidamine, such as Adjudin™ [Adherens Junction Disruption], which inhibits movement of the germ cells, resulting in release of immature sperm.[15]

Adjudin™ is a lonidamine derivative that disrupts the adhesion of spermatids to the Sertoli cells, causing premature spermiation and infertility.[16,17] The serum testosterone, FSH, and LH levels did not change. Due to findings of some liver inflammation observed in a 29-day chronic toxicology study assessing safety of Adjudin™ administration, Cheng et al. conjugated Adjudin™ to a FSHβ mutant specifically targeting it to Sertoli cells, by-passing the systemic effect, and significantly reducing the dose necessary for contraception.[18] H2-Gamendazole, another lonidamine derivative, works according to the same mechanism as Adjudin™.[19] While it was shown by Tash et al.[19] that a low dose produced 100% infertility after a single oral administration, the reversibility was only 57%. Also, serum levels of LH and testosterone did not change, but FSH levels increased, probably due to a reduction in inhibin B release from Sertoli cells.[20]

Another approach is to target **retinoic acid inhibition** to alter sperm function.[20] Vitamin A (retinol) is required at puberty for the initiation of spermatogenesis and in adults for maintenance of spermatogenesis.[21,22] Retinoic acid binds one of several retinoic acid receptors (RARs), which regulate gene expression. Male RAR knockout animals are sterile due to various defects in spermatogenesis.[20,23] BMS-189453 was identified as an orally active retinoic acid receptor antagonist and a recent study in mice showed that low doses of the molecule might function as a contraceptive without the toxicity seen at higher doses.[24]

Over 50 years ago, it was noted that WIN 18,446, a potential treatment of amoebiasis, displayed anti-spermatogenic activity and was shown to safely, completely, and reversibly inhibit spermatogenesis in many species, including man.[20,25] However, when used orally this molecule induced a "disulfiram reaction" consisting of nausea, vomiting, palpitations, and sweating with concomitant alcohol intake. Therefore the development of WIN 18,446 was abandoned without exploring the mechanism by which it inhibited spermatogenesis.[20]

Amory et al. identified the mechanism as an inhibition of testicular retinoic acid biosynthesis.[26] Studies in the rabbit model indicate that inhibition of the testicular retinoic acid biosynthesis is a promising target for male contraceptive development.[20,26] The development of novel, specific compound that inhibits testicular retinoic acid biosynthesis without interfering with alcohol metabolism is underway and will hopefully identify compounds that reversibly inhibit spermatogenesis without such side effects.

Some other targets have been identified in the last decade:

Recently, Martin Matzuk et al.[27] explored the spermatogenic effects of a selective small-molecule inhibitor (JQ1) of the bromodomain activity during spermatogenesis, providing a lead compound that can cross the blood:testis barrier, targeting the male germ cell for contraception. Treatment of mice with JQ1 reduced seminiferous tubule area, testis size, and spermatozoa number and motility without affecting hormone levels and mating. The inhibitory effects of JQ1 were shown at the spermatocyte and round spermatid stages and cause a complete and reversible contraceptive effect in that animal model.

Previously, other targets have been identified as most promising and advanced in research. M. O'Rand described the epididymal protease inhibitor (EPPIN) localized on the sperm surface and involved in sperm liquefaction as well as gain of sperm function.[28] He showed that blocking EPPIN in monkeys induced infertility in animals, and monkeys' anti-EPPIN antibodies inhibit human spermatozoid motility. These authors confirmed that the EPPIN-semenogelin binding site on the surface of human spermatozoa is an ideal target for a nonsteroidal male contraceptive.[28]

D. Clapham's laboratories identified the "cation channel sperm-associated" (CatSper), which is found only in mature sperm tail.[29] CatSper, a pH-regulated, calcium-selective ion channel, and KSper (Slo3) are core regulators of sperm tail calcium entry and sperm hyperactivated motility. The knock-out (KO) male mice are infertile and sperm lacking the ion channel cannot achieve the hyperactivation required to penetrate the egg. The uniqueness of these sperm ion channels makes them ideal pharmaceutical targets for contraception and using high throughput screening will help to identify inhibitors of CatSper subunits.[29]

Glyceraldehyde 3-phosphate dehydrogenase-S (GAPDS) is the product of a mouse gene expressed only during spermatogenesis and, like its human ortholog (GAPD2), is the sole GAPDH isozyme in sperm.[30] It is tightly bound to the fibrous sheath, a cytoskeletal structure that extends most of the length of the sperm flagellum. Based on Deborah O'Brien's laboratory work, the critical role of glycolysis for sperm motility and its dependence on this sperm-specific enzyme suggest that GAPDS is a potential contraceptive target.[30]

These nonhormonal methods aim at inducing reversible infertility without interfering with hormones secreted by the hypothalamus, pituitary gland, and the testis, targeting specific interactions within the reproductive system at the level of the testes, as well as between spermatozoa and ova.

Conclusion

Despite the unmet need and the interest in developing male contraception, controversy continues about the potential acceptability of a male method by men and whether women would trust their partners to use the method reliably. Glasier et al.[31] showed in a survey of 1,894 women attending family planning clinics in Scotland, China, and South Africa that more than 90% in South Africa and Scotland thought that a 'male pill' was a good idea, with Chinese women only slightly less positive. In addition, the survey from Heineman et al.,[1] indicates that more than 50% of men interviewed in 4 continents would be ready to use a male method.

Nonhormonal methods are less advanced than hormonal male contraception, but new promising targets specific to the male reproductive system have been identified and are still in preclinical research. Innovative strategies to identify selective and druggable targets that will lead to new contraceptive modalities with fewer side effects and possibly with noncontraceptive health benefits still need to be developed.

This futuristic approach still keeps in mind the need for better access to existing contraceptive methods, as well as the discovery of new delivery systems that can deliver the new molecules directly to their specific targets and methods that are simple to use, safe, reversible, and inexpensive, a major challenge for the next decade. In parallel, behavioral assessments/indicators that predict acceptability/successful use of new contraceptives should also be developed.

References

1. Heinemann K, Saad F, Wiesemes M, White S, Heinemann L. Attitudes toward male fertility control: results of a multinational survey on four continents. Hum Reprod 2005;20:549–56.
2. Nieschlag E. Clinical trials in male hormonal contraception. Contraception 2010, 82:457-470.
3. Wang C, Swerdloff RS. Hormonal approaches to male contraception. Curr Opin Urol 2010;20:520-4
4. Wistuba J, Nieschlag E, Semjonow A, Sandhowe-Klaverkamp R, Friedrichs-Gromoll S, Zitzmann M, Simoni M, Luetjens CM. Testosterone-induced prostate growth is blocked by co- and preadministration of norethisterone enanthate in castrated cynomolgus monkeys. Urol Int 2012, 88: 358-364.
5. Kumar N, Didolkar AK, Monder C, Bardin CW, and Sundaram K. The biological activity of 7α-methyl-19-nortestosterone is not amplified in male reproductive tract as is that of testosterone. Endocrinology 1992, 130:3677-83.
6. Kumar, N, Crozat, A, Li F, Catterall JF, Bardin CW, Sundaram K. 7alpha-methyl-19-nortestosterone, a synthetic androgen with high potency. Structure-activity comparisons with other androgens. J Steroid Biochem Molec Biol 1999; 71: 213-22.
7. Sundaram, K, Kumar N. Bardin CW. 7-alpha-methyl-nortestosterone (MENT): the optimal androgen for male contraception. Ann Med 1993; 25:199-205.
8. Kumar N, Didolkar, AK, Ladd, A. Thau, R, Monder, C, Bardin, CW, Sundaram, K. Radioimmunoassay of 7alpha-methyl-19-nortesosterone and investigation of its pharmacokinetics in animals. J Steroid Biochem Molec Biol 1990; 37 587-91.
9. Nieschlag E, Kumar N, Sitruk-Ware R. 7α-methyl-19-nortestosterone (MENT™): the population council's contribution to research on male contraception and treatment of hypogonadism. Contraception. 2013;87(3):288-95.
10. Ilani N, Roth MY, Amory JK, et al. A new combination of testosterone and nestorone transdermal gels for male hormonal contraception. J Clin Endocrinol Metab 2012; 97(10): 3476-86.
11. Mahabadi V, Amory JK, Swerdloff RS, et al. Combined transdermal testosterone gel and the progestin Nestorone suppresses serum gonadotropins in men. J Clin Endocrinol Metab 2009;94:2313-20.
12. Mommers E, Kersemaekers WM, Elliesen J, et al. Male hormonal contraception: a double-blind, placebo-controlled study. J Clin Endocrinol Metab 2008;93:2572-80.
13. Kamischke A, Heuermann T, Krueger K, von Eckardstein S, Schellschmidt I, Ruebig A, Nieschlag E. An effective hormonal male contraceptive using testosterone undecanoate with oral or injectable norethisterone preparations. J Clin Endocrinol Metab 2002, 87: 530-539.
14. WHO. Controlled trials register NET-EN plus TU as a male contraceptive (WHO-HRP ID A25165); 2005, http://www.who.int/reproductive-health/rhl/a25165.html; http://conrad.org/contraception-trials.html

15. Cheng CY, Lie PP, Wong EW, Mruk DD, Silvestrini B. Adjudin disrupts spermatogenesis via the action of some unlikely partners: Eps8, Arp2/3 complex, drebrin E, PAR6 and 14-3-3. Spermatogenesis 2011;1:291-7.
16. Cheng CY, Mruk D. Testin and actin are key molecular targets of adjudin, an anti-spermatogenic agent, in the testes. Spermatogenesis 2011; 1:137-146.
17. Mok K-W, Mruk DD, Lie PPY, Lui W-Y, Cheng CY. Adjudin, a potential male contraceptive, exerts its effects locally in the seminiferous epithelium of mammalian testes. Reproduction 2011;141:571-580.
18. Mruk DD, Wong CH, Silvestrini B, Cheng CY. A male contraceptive targeting germ cell adhesion. Nature Medicine 2006;12:1323-1328.
19. Tash JS, Attardi B, Hild SA, Chakrasali R, Jakkaraj SR, Georg GI. A novel potent indazole carboxylic acid derivative blocks spermatogenesis and is contraceptive in rats after a single oral dose. Biol Reprod. 2008;78:1127-38.
20. Nya-Ngatchou JJ, Amory JK. New approaches to male non-hormonal contraception. Contraception. 2013;87(3):296-9.
21. Vernet N, Dennefeld C, Rochett-Egly C, Oulad-Abdelghani M, Chambon P, Ghyselinck NB, Mark M. Retinoic acid metabolism and signaling pathways in the adult and developing mouse testis. Endocrinology 2006;147:96-110.
22. Koubova J, Menke D, Zhou Q, Capel B, Griswold MD, Page DC. Retinoic acid regulates sex-specific timing of meiotic initiation in mice. Proc Natl Acad Sci USA 2006;103:2472-2479.
23. Kastner P, Mark M, Leid M, Gansmuller A, Chin W, Grondona JM, Décimo D, Krezel W, Dierich A, Chambon P. Abnormal spermatogenesis in RXR beta mutant mice. Genes Dev 1996;10: 80-92.
24. Chung SS, Wang X, Roberts SS, Griffey SM, Reczek PR, Wolgemuth DJ. Oral administration of a retinoic Acid receptor antagonist reversibly inhibits spermatogenesis in mice. Endocrinology. 2011;152: 2492-502.
25. Heller CG, Moore DJ, Paulsen CA. Suppression of spermatogenesis and chronic toxicity in men by a new series of Bis (dichloroacetyl) Diamines. Toxicol Appl Pharmacol 1961;3:1-11.
26. Amory JK, Muller CH, Shimshoni AJ, Isoherranen N, Paik J, Moreb JS, Amory DW, Evanoff R, Goldstein AS, Griswold MD. Suppression of spermatogenesis by bisdichloroacetyldiamines is mediated by inhibition of testicular retinoic acid biosynthesis. J Androl 2011; 32:111-119.
27. Matzuk MM, McKeown MR, Filippakopoulos P, Li Q, Ma L, Agno JE, Lemieux ME, Picaud S, Yu RN, Qi J, Knapp S, and Bradner JE. Small-Molecule Inhibition of BRDT for Male Contraception Cell 2012; 150: 673–84.
28. O'Rand MG, Widgren EE, Beyler S, Richardson RT. Inhibition of human sperm motility by contraceptive anti-eppin antibodies from infertile male monkeys: effect on cyclic adenosine monophosphate. Biol Reprod. 2009; 80(2):279-85.
29. Lishko PV, Kirichok Y, Ren D, Navarro B, Chung JJ, Clapham DE. The control of male fertility by spermatozoan ion channels. Ann Rev Physiol. 2012;74: 453-75.
30. Miki K, Qu W, Goulding EH, Willis WD, Bunch DO, Strader LF, Perreault SD, Eddy EM, O'Brien DA. Glyceraldehyde 3-phosphate dehydrogenase-S, a sperm-specific glycolytic enzyme, is required for sperm motility and male fertility. Proc Natl Acad Sci USA. 2004; 101(47):16501-6.
31. Glasier AF, Anakwe R, Everington D, et al. Would women trust their partners to use a male pill? Human Reprod 2000; 15:646-9.

Evaluation of new approaches to female contraception

Narendra Malhotra, Jaideep Malhotra, Neharika Malhotra Bora, Keshav Malhotra

Rainbow Hospitals, Agra, India

Introduction

Despite the widespread availability of a cafeteria of contraceptive choices, the world still sees a 49% rate of unintended pregnancies, a 22.5% rate of unintended births, and a 26.5% rate of elective abortions in the United States.[1] In the developing world this figure may be much higher.

Unintended pregnancies, elective abortions, and unintended births are a major cause of maternal mortality and morbidity. If the developing world is to achieve United Nations Millennium Development Goal 5 for reduction in maternal mortality, then we need to understand that contraception and contraceptive use is the key.[3]

World Bank and United Nations have projected 80%-90% population growth until 2025 in developing countries. Of this projection, 17% population growth is due to want of another child and 33% from unwanted pregnancies. The remaining 50% is due to better medical care and increased life expectancy[2] (UNFPA: www.unfpa.org, WHO: www.who.int/reproductivehealth/en, UN: The world at six billion www.u.n.org).

Today there is a basket of contraceptive choices available to women, and various studies have shown that today even in the educated and developed world the first-year failure rates are much higher in typical users than perfect users.[4] Therefore, the effectiveness of a contraceptive is not just the effective new methods but is a multiplication of compliance x efficacy; to make a contraceptive effective, a very good and proper counseling is required.[5] Structured counseling includes discussion of side effects and mode of action, educational videos, and patient handouts.

Contraceptions on the horizon

"Technology made large populations possible and large populations make technology indispensable." Joseph Wood Krutch

The 21st century has brought a new era of contraceptive choices. The "pill," when invented, was thought to be the ultimate contraception, giving the woman a power of controlling her own reproduction. The "pill" in its short history has been dominated by many innovations, and newer modalities of hormonal and other contraceptives have been invented and tried.

The newer methods make a formidable list of additions to the current choices.

1. Newer pills
2. Newer barrier methods
3. Implants
4. Patches
5. Rings
6. Injectables
7. Microbicides
8. IUCDs (intrauterine contraceptive devices)
9. Transcervical sterilization
10. Male hormonal contraception
11. Gene-based approaches
12. Immune contraception
13. Antiprogesterone

14. Surgeryless contraception
15. New fertility awareness-based methods

Control of fertility today, and in the future, is and will focus on improving the existing methods. The focus will be (and is already) on[6]:

1. Efficacy
2. Side effects
3. Ease of use
4. Duration of action
5. Manufacturing process
6. Costs
7. Newer mode of actions
8. Additional noncontraceptive benefits
9. Newer nonhormonal methods

The newer research is being done in the world by only two major pharmaceuticals who can afford research (Bayer-Schering-Pharma and MSD). Research for the future is focused on:

1. Female contraception
    a. Ovulation inhibition (new inhibitors) (gene-targeted)
    b. New oral contraceptive (OC) oral regimen
    c. OC with new progestins
    d. OC with estradiol or estradiol esters
    e. Long cycle and continuous delivery
    f. New patches
    g. Vaginal rings
    h. Spray-on contraceptives
2. Fertilization inhibition
    a. Newer intrauterine systems (IUS) (e.g., small Mirena®)
    b. New frameless progestin-releasing systems
    c. Newer barriers
    d. Spermicide and microbicide (dual protection)
    e. New implants
    f. Improved injectables
    g. New approaches to female sterilization and noninvasive tubal occlusion
    h. Immunocontraception for females is not expected to come in near future.
3. Implantation inhibition
    a. SPRMs (selective progesterone receptor modulators)
4. Male contraception
    a. Condoms
    b. Vasectomy

(The development of parenteral hormonal contraceptive for men has been stopped by the pharmaceutical industry). (The search for implant, gels, etc., for men still continues).
(Enovid®/Syntex/US and Anovlar Schering/Germany)

Newer oral pills

Oral pills have been available since 1959 in the United States and 1961 in Europe. The newer oral contraceptive pills offer continuous use, new progestin formulations that reduce the menstrual cycles to four per year, and the newer progestins reduce the side effects.

Oral contraceptive pills are used for (indications):
1. Fertility control
2. Noncontraceptive medical problems
a. Acne vulgaris
b. Dysmenorrhea
c. Premenstrual syndrome (PMS) and premenstrual dysphoric disorder (PMDD)
d. Menstrual irregularities

The newer formulations have shown many benefits and low dose OCP with newer progestogens (drospirenone and cyproterone acetate and the newer regimen of 24/7) have received more acceptance. These formulations have been widely studied for various cancers.

Cancer risks with OCPs

1. Breast cancer: Royal College of General Practitioners study (1968-2007) showed a small decrease in overall risk of developing cancer and a small decrease in mortality.[7,8]
2. Ovarian cancer: According to Holden Comprehensive Cancer Center cancer information (2003), the protective factors for various cancers are OCPs, childbearing, breastfeeding, tubal ligation, and hysterectomy.[9]
3. Endometrial cancer: A meta-analysis by International Association of Cancer Registries (IACR, 1899) showed risk of endometrial cancer in women on OCPs is approximately halved.[10,7]
4. Liver cancer: OCPs do not increase the risk of liver cancers in low-risk populations.[10,7]
5. Cervical cancer: Evidence shows that a long-term use may increase the risk of cervical cancer due to human papillomavirus (HPV) infections.[11]

Various cancer risks of OCPs have been evaluated, researched, and studied, and a recent publication[7] in British Medical Journal shows that "taking contraceptive pills does not increase a woman's chances of developing cancer and may even reduce the risk."

Reduction of dose of ethinyl estradiol (EE)

Lowering the dose of EE adds to many beneficial effects of the pill and removes many side effects.

1. Dose reduction from 50 to 30-35 μg led to reduction of myocardial infarctions, stroke, and deep vein thrombosis (DVT).
2. Lowering the EE dose from 30-35 μg to 20 μg led to further reduction of DVT.
3. Lowering the dose further led to breakthrough bleedings and irregular menstrual patterns without any further benefits.
4. Estrogen-free pills (progesterone only pill, POP) have an advantage of use in breastfeeding women.

Regimen of OCPs

Cochrane analysis[12] of biphasic vs. monophasic and biphasic vs. triphasic shows that probably monophase pills are better, and available trials show no advantage of triphasic for birth control and bleeding pattern. Regimen: Continuous daily OCP for 3 months (ethinyl estradiol and levonorgestrel [LNG, Seasonale® and Seasonique®] 84 pill days with 7 day-hormone free). Continuous daily regimen Lybrel® (90 μg of levonorgestrel/20 μg EE) is not approved in Europe due to intermenstrual spotting. A Cochrane analysis (Edelman et al.)[13] on off-label continuous use of OCP compared with continuous daily use shows equal efficacy.

What is new

Ethinyl estradiol-free contraceptives using estradiol or estradiol esters. In the near future, a new regimen with natural estradiol in combination with nomegestrol acetate (Organon, Schering-Plough now MSD) will be available.[14] Clinical trials for a spray-on contraceptive are ongoing. New progestins are also being tested for contraception (nomegestrol acetate, Nestrone®, trimegestone). These progestins can be used in OCPs, in vaginal rings, and as transdermal contraception (patches or gels).

Once-a-month injectables

Approved by the United States Food and Drug Administration (FDA) in 2000, these injectables are still available in South America even though the production has stopped due to manufacturing problems. Mesigyna® (Bayer-Schering Pharma) and Lunelle™ are given once every 28-33 days (25 mg medroxyprogesterone with 5 mg estradiol cypionate).[15] Combination injectable contraception is a highly effective, reversible method for preventing pregnancy. A new self-injectable (Uniject™/Path) with the same content as Lunelle™ is currently being developed.

Contraceptive patch

Ortho Evra® (Ortho-MacNeil), approved by FDA in 2001, is a patch that releases 150 mg norelgestromin and 20 mg ethinyl estradiol daily, used as a weekly application for 3 weeks with one patch-free week. Cochrane Database[15] has compared skin patches with OCPs, and similar contraceptive benefit was observed with slightly more headaches and breast tenderness with patches. A smaller patch (Fidencia™: Bayer-Schering Pharma) with EE and gestodene will be available soon.

Vaginal ring

Vaginal administration of EE and progestins allows good cycle control at a lower dose. Several rings were developed by WHO and Population Council. Today, NuvaRing® (MSD) is available worldwide with good acceptance (ethylene-vinyl acetate copolymer releasing 15 μg EE and 120 μg etonogestrel). Newer rings with only progestins (nomegestrol acetate) are being developed for lactating mothers.

Emergency contraception (EC)

Postcoital levonorgestrel pills (1,500 μg in 1 tab or 750 μg each in 2 pills) are available as an over-the-counter pill. IUCD introduction after intercourse is also being used as EC. A new emergency contraception pill (ulipristal acetate) has been introduced in Europe and can be used up to 5 days after unprotected coitus. Many other ways of EC are now being tried and studied, including SPRMS, ParaGard® T380A, and gestrinone.

Intrauterine devices

Intrauterine devices have seen a big evolution from inert plastic to copper coils and from horse shoe-shaped frames to T-frames to now LNG-IUS.

Now frameless IUDs (GyneFix®)[16] are also available and can be used in nulliparous women. New IUDs are "Small Mirena®," "Swing" (Copper) releasing with coil stem, IUD releasing a progesterone modulator (CDB 2914), and Copper IUD releasing indomethacin or PG synthetase blocker or inhibitor. Also, in the future we may have a frameless progesterone-releasing IUS.

Barrier methods

Different types of latex diaphragms are available. A Cochrane review found that without spermicide, diaphragms may increase unwanted pregnancies. SILCS are silicone devices placed in the vagina to cover the cervix. Various cervical caps of latex and silicon (Dumas Vault® cap, Vimule®, Lea's Shield®, Prentif Cavity Rim® cap, and FemCap®) have been analyzed by a Cochrane Database review.[17]

Hormonal implants

FDA-approved Norplant® and Jadelle® (6 and 2 rods) (1990) are being used. Implanon™, a non-biodegradable single rod implant, is now available. Implanon NXT® is a radio-opaque implant. Newer implants under trial are elcometrine, nomegestrol acetate (Uniplant® and Surplant®), and new biodegradable capsules or rods.

Depot injections

Depot medroxyprogesterone acetate (DMPA) was approved by FDA in 1992, as was norethisterone oenanthate (NET-EN), and reviewed by a Cochrane analysis.[18] Depo-subQ provera 104™ is a new 3 monthly injectable (Sayana). Several other progesterone-only injectables and combined once-a-month injectables using microspheres or microcapsules are being investigated.

Natural family planning (NFP)

A Cochrane analysis by Grimes et al. compared the NFP methods.[19] Fertility awareness-based methods are a good choice for couples seeking a safe and healthy low-cost method. Cycle monitors detect fertile and infertile days using many markers (Cyclo Test™, Baby Comp®, Bioself). Hormonal-based fertility monitors include Persona and the Home Ovarian Hormone Monitor. Fancy monitoring devices fail to show any extra benefit for contraception and are mainly offered to infertile women for cycle monitoring.

Spermicides

Nonoxynol-9 and octoxinol are available as creams or gels that are used before sexual intercourse. Newer spermicides are being developed with microbicides to provide additional protection against sexually transmitted diseases (STDs) and human immunodeficiency virus (HIV) (algae gel, cellulose gel, molecular condom [smart vaginal drug delivery system]).

Vaginal sponges

Natural sea sponges soaked in spermicide inserted in vagina before intercourse. Sponges are now being re-introduced and three are currently available including Protectaid® and Today Sponge®.

Female condom

Female condoms, according to WHO and Program for Appropriate Technology in Health (PATH), are made of polyurethane and also latex and plastic (Reddy Female Condom™, others). FEMIDOM® (polyurethane), FC2 Female Condom® (nitrile), and V-Amour® (latex) are now also in the market.

Female sterilization

Female and male sterilization is still the most widely used method in the world. A Cochrane analysis (Nardin et al.) analyzed various techniques for tubal occlusions (cutting, tying, clips, rings, and current), but the effectiveness is not clear.[20] Another Cochrane review has analyzed minilaparotomy and endoscopy methods and found laparoscopy had fewer complications while culdoscopy had higher complications.[21] Other methods are quinacrine, Essure®, Adiana®, and Ovabloc®.

Immunocontraception

Immunocontraception is nonhormonal, nonsteroidal contraception targeted at oocyte antigens and sperm antigens and immunization against GnRH, etc. The possible hazards of immunocontraception are cross-reactions of antibody of other nonreproductive tissue leading to prolonged sterilization and safety issues.

Antiprogestins

WHO has suggested use of antiprogestogens in various regimens:

Sequential

1. Mifepristone + Norethisterone
2. Mifepristone + Medroxyprogesterone acetate
3. Mifepristone (day 1-15) + Nomegestrol acetate (16-28 day)
4. Continuous regimen (0.1-10 mg/day)
5. Weekly use – Mifepristone (2.5 – 50 mg)
6. Monthly use – Mifepristone 200 mg 2 days after luteinizing hormone (LH) peak
7. Emergency contraception – Mifepristone – 10 mg

Implantation Inhibition

Immunocontraception

1. WHO-based method against hCG
2. Zygote arrest 1 (ZARI) gene

Anti-implantation agents: If developed this could be a once-a-month or "as-needed" basis contraception.

Summary

Today there are so many choices of contraception available with so many new innovations. It is paramount that today's physicians and maternal health care providers be educated and aware of the benefits of all the newer innovations. Only a well-informed physician can help patients make the best choice while keeping their medical, social, psychological, and philosophical requirements in mind.

WHO concludes: For women to benefit from these new technologies, they need better access to education and income so that they have a greater decision-making power.

Women education, employment, empowerment, and environmental (WEEEEP) problems need to be addressed for saving the world from overpopulation.

References

1. Finer LB, et al. PerspSex Reprod Health 2006.
2. Internet Links (www.unfpa.org; www.worldbank.org; www.who.int, www.un.org, www.wikipedia.org)
3. Frost JJ, Darroch JE, Remez L. In brief 2008.
4. Adapted from Hatches RA, Contraceptive Technology 1998.
5. Structured councelling : Lei Z-W et al., Contraception 1996, 53:357.
6. J Reproduktionsmed Endokrinol 2010; 7 (Special issue 1):18-39.
7. Hannaferd PC, et al. Mortality among contraceptive pill uses: cohort evidence from RC-GPs. Oral contraception study BMJ 2010; 340:927.
8. Silvera SA, Miller Ab, Rohan TE. Oral contraceptive use and risk of breast cancer among women with a family history of breast cancer: a prospective cohort study. Cancer causes control 2005; 16:1059-63.
9. The reduction in risk of ovarian cancer associated with oral contraceptive use. The cancer and sterand Hormone Study N Engl J Med 1987; 316:650-5.
10. Meink O, Farley TV. Risk of Cancer and the Oral Contraceptive pill. BMJ 2007; 335: 651.
11. Franceschi S. The IARC commitment to cancer prevention: the example of papilloma virus and cervical cancer. Resat Results Cancer Res 2005;166:277-97.
12. Vanvliet HA, Grimes DA, et al. Triphasic versus monophasic oral contraceptive for contraception. Cochrome Data Base Syst Rev 2006:(3).
13. Edelman AB, et al. Continuous or extended cycle vs. cyclic use of COC for contraception. Cochrane Database Syt Rev 2005:(3).
14. Astedt B, et al. Clinical trial of a new oral contraceptive pill containing natural oestrogen. Br J Obstet Gynecol 1979:80:732-6.
15. Gallo MF, Grimes DA, Schuls KF. Skin Patch and vaginal rings Vs COC for contraception. Cochrane Data Syst Rev 2003(1).
16. O Brien PA, et al. Frameless Vs Classical IUD for contraception. Cochrane Data base Syste Rev 2005:(1).
17. Gallo M F, et al. Cervical Cap Vs diaphragm for contraception. Cochrane Database Syst Rev 202:(4).
18. Draper BH, et al. DMPA Vs NETEN for long acting progestogenic contraception. Cochrane Database Syst Rev: 2006:(3).
19. Grimes DA, Gallo MF, et al. Fertility awareness-based methods for contraception. Cochrane Database Syst Rev 2004:(4).
20. Nadrin JM, et al. Techniques for the interruption of tubal patency for female sterilization. Cochrane Database Syst Rev 2002:(4).
21. Kulier R, et al. Minilaprotomy and Endoscopic techniques for tubal sterilization Cochrane Database Syst Rev.

Global perspectives on contraception

Sheryl Ziemin van der Poel

World Health Organization, Geneva, Switzerland

Introduction

The rise in prevalence of modern methods of contraceptive use since 1950, on a global level, is a reproductive health success story. "The unmet need for contraception," or the number of women who are married or in a union who are not using but do not desire a child in the ensuing 2 years, has also decreased significantly between 1990 to 2010 (Alkema et al., 2013). However, progress is uneven across countries and territories, and even countries with high prevalence of contraceptive use can still register high levels of unmet need (UN, DESA Population Division, Fertility and Family Planning Section, http://www.un.org/esa/population/publications/wcu2010/WCP_2010/Data.html). Changes in contraceptive prevalence and reducing unintended pregnancies have been clinically linked to increase in maternal survival, averting maternal deaths, decreasing abortion rates, and improving perinatal outcomes (Cleland et al., 2013), but also, a specific but highly used hormonal injectable has more recently been suggested to be potentially linked to a moderate increased human immunodeficiency virus (HIV) acquisition risk (Heffron et al., 2012) - a finding more recent data could not rule out (Morrison et al., 2012). Current public health emphasis has been placed on implementation studies to determine best mechanisms for expanding contraceptive use and decreasing unmet need at country level that will overcome health systems, economic, sociocultural, and religious barriers to access, as well as provide a mix of contraceptive choices (Cleland and Shah, 2013). However, the generation of evidence-based global guidelines based on the best available published evidence is critical in order to address misconceptions and eligibility criteria regarding safe clinical use of contraceptive options, to address potential medical barriers, to improve access to contraceptives, and increase quality of care in family planning practices. Change in clinical classifications of recommendations that define restrictions for use of a contraceptive method are supported by continuous identification of research evidence and debated through global consultations to reach consensus. The clinical guidelines that result and are continuously being updated drive clinical and community level family planning practices.

Contraceptive prevalence and the unmet need for family planning (contraception)

In 2013, a systematic and comprehensive analysis of contraceptive prevalence rates and unmet need for contraception was published with support from the United Nations Population Division and the National University of Singapore (Alkema et al., 2013). Due to the lack of consistency in data collection, variability in sample size, and mix of contraceptive methods, robust modeling and algorithms were needed to harmonize data from reproductive health surveys gathered globally across regions and nations. Prevalence was measured as "the percentage of women who report themselves or their partners as using at least one contraceptive method of any type, modern or traditional. Unmet need for family planning (contraception) was defined as "the percentage of women who want to stop or delay childbearing but who are not using any method of contraception to prevent pregnancy." Country-specific time trends were combined to generate comparisons and also predict projected estimates to the year 2020. Notably, from 1990 to 2010, global contraceptive prevalence rates increased from 54.8% to 63.3%, with the majority occurring in the 1990s, and had a corresponding decrease of "unmet need for contraception" from 15.4% to 12.3% (Alkema et al., 2013). As recently pointed out (Cleland & Shah, 2013), fertility is reduced by one birth per woman for every increase of between 15%-17% of the contraceptive prevalence rate. Small percentage adjustments have profound effects on demographic indicators, and as graphically explained, (Cleland, 2009) "if fertility is half a birth higher or lower than expected between 2005 and 2050, the mid-century population of the planet will be 10.75 or 7.8 billion, respectively." These differences point out the need for continued robust studies and increase in consistency in data collection in order to continuously evaluate contraceptive prevalence rate estimates and project the burden of human populations on development for nations and regions as well as worldwide.

Access to a greater method mix of contraceptives to assure better-related clinical outcomes

Yet, these global differences when unpacked at national level, show where unique and targeted action is required to assist uptake of contraceptive use and to ensure a continual decrease in unmet need. Equally, time trends for both indicators show distinctive differences across and between regions and sub-regions. Current global public emphasis has been suggested to be placed on implementation studies to determine best mechanisms for expanding contraceptive use and decreasing unmet need at country level, which will overcome health systems, economic, socio-cultural, and religious barriers to access, as well as to provide a mix of contraceptive choices (Cleland and Shah, 2013). Most notably, they present that the type of methods, traditional and modern, which were reported to be used by women, differed significantly across regions and uniquely within countries – often with reliance on a "narrow range of methods." Although there is discussion that it is not new contraceptive methods that are required, but rather that expansion to access to more modern methods is critical, there are others who dispute this claim. For example, in this trilogy, new avenues for both hormonal and nonhormonal methods of male contraception are presented as fulfilling a clear, unmet need. Another topic, covering the evaluation of new approaches to female contraception, also clearly addresses bench-to-bedside movement of more advanced innovative discoveries. One of the areas attracting considerable interest is the development of multipurpose technologies to address reproductive health needs of contraception coupled with acquisition of HIV and other sexually transmitted infections, especially with the increasing threats of treatment-resistant strains of disease (Harrison et al., 2013).

Changes in contraceptive prevalence and reducing unintended pregnancies have been clinically linked to increase in maternal survival, averting maternal deaths (Ahmed et al., 2013), decreasing abortion rates, and improving perinatal outcomes. Indeed, if pregnancy levels are decreased, associated maternal mortality rates based on pregnancy outcomes will decrease, as elegantly presented based on DHS data and World Health Organization (WHO) maternal mortality estimates (Cleland et al., 2013). They show that for "each percentage point increase in contraceptive use {there} is an associated … reduction of 8.5 maternal deaths per 100,000 births." Providing a systematic review of literature addressing this clinical health advantage of contraceptive use, they further noted another study in a WHO report (Collumbien et al., 2004) that an estimated "90% of abortion deaths are preventable if all women wanting to stop childbearing use effective contraception." More controversial has been the issue of use of contraceptives to space the time between pregnancies and a subsequent link to maternal mortality; however, a review and meta-analysis, respectively, did find a relationship of spacing with contraceptives to a decrease in subsequent maternal morbidity (Conde-Auidelo & Belizan, 2000) and a decrease in perinatal outcomes (Condo-Auidelo et al., 2006).

The CIRE system and generation of global clinical guidelines

The generation of evidence-based global guidelines based on the best available published evidence is critical in order to address misconceptions and eligibility criteria regarding safe use of contraceptive options, to address potential medical barriers, and to improve access to contraceptives and quality of care in family planning practices. Changes in clinical classifications of recommendations that define restrictions for use of a contraceptive method are supported by a continuous identification of research evidence (CIRE) system. As with most recommendation development systems, published research clinical studies are reviewed and systematic reviews prepared for specific clinical questions, which result in grading on the quality of the evidence, and a global participatory process that informs on existing or generation of new recommendations. Some recommendations that will be reviewed are progestin-only contraception and breastfeeding, contraception during the postpartum period, combined hormonal contraception (COCs) and venous thromboembolism, COCs and cardiac events, and others, including adding new contraceptive methods to the Medical Eligibility Criteria. Some of the existing recommendations that likely have new clinical evidence to evaluate are those associated with the use of levonorgestrel intrauterine system (LNG IUS) for women with breast cancer, COCs with cervical intraepithelial neoplasia, COCs and older age, intrauterine device (IUD) post abortion, COCs for women with known thrombogenic mutations, specific methods of hormonal contraception and forms of cancer. In addition, new recommendations to be considered for adding to the next version of the Selected Practice Recommendations would be addressing how many years a copper or levonorgestrel-containing IUD can be left in place, how many years a woman can use depot medroxyprogesterone acetate (DMPA) continuously, and other contraceptive methods that can be initiated after use of emergency contraceptive pills (WHO Survey Poll for revision of evidence-based contraceptive guidelines, accessed April 2013).

A technical consultation was convened at WHO to specifically address one set of recommendations: hormonal contraception and HIV acquisition, progression and transmission. A specific but highly used hormonal injectable, DMPA has recently been suggested to be potentially linked to a moderate increased HIV acquisition risk (Heffron et al., 2012), which more recent data could not rule out (Morrison et al., 2012). This issue is of particular concern in countries with high burden of HIV, high maternal mortality rates, and where hormonal contraceptives, specifically progestogen-only injectable methods, represent a considerable percentage of the types of modern methods available. Following the global consultation, a technical statement was released on February 16, 2012. An excerpt from the executive summary is presented: "After detailed, prolonged deliberation, informed by systematic reviews of the available evidence and presentations on biological and animal data, GRADE profile summaries on the strength of the epidemiological evidence, and analysis of risks and benefits to country programmes, the group concluded that the World Health Organization should continue to recommend that there are no restrictions (MEC Category 1) on the use of any hormonal contraceptive method for women living with HIV or at high risk of HIV. However, the group recommended that a new clarification (under Category 1) be added to the MEC for women using progestogen-only injectable contraception at high risk of HIV as follows: Some studies suggest that women using progestogen-only injectable contraception may be at increased risk of HIV acquisition, other studies do not show this association. A WHO expert group reviewed all the available evidence and agreed that the data were not sufficiently conclusive to change current guidance. However, because of the inconclusive nature of the body of evidence on possible increased risk of HIV acquisition, women using progestogen-only injectable contraception should be strongly advised to also always use condoms, male or female, and other HIV preventive measures. Expansion of contraceptive method mix and further research on the relationship between hormonal contraception and HIV infection is essential. These recommendations will be continually reviewed in light of new evidence. The group further wished to draw the attention of policy-makers and programme managers to the potential seriousness of the issue and the complex balance of risks and benefits. The group noted the importance of hormonal contraceptives and of HIV prevention for public health and emphasized the need for individuals living with or at risk of HIV to also always use condoms, male or female, as hormonal contraceptives are not protective against HIV transmission or acquisition." Included in the next round of review of WHO recommendations will be the use of hormonal contraception among women with high risk or living with HIV.

Conclusion

Evaluation of contraceptive prevalence rate estimates and projection of the burden of human populations have impact on development and the well-being of low- and middle-income countries, as much as on developed countries. Changes in contraceptive prevalence and reducing unintended pregnancies have been clinically linked to increase in maternal survival, averting maternal deaths, decreasing abortion rates, and improving perinatal outcomes. The generation of evidence-based global guidelines based on the best-available published evidence is critical in order to address misconceptions and eligibility criteria regarding safe use of contraceptives, to address potential medical barriers, to improve access to a greater method mix of contraceptives options, and to increase the quality of clinical care in family planning practices.

References

Ahmed S, Li Q, Liu L, Tsui A. (2012) Maternal deaths averted by contraceptive use; an analysis of 172 countries. Lancet, 380, 111-125

Alkema L, Kantorova V, Menozzi C, Biddlecom A (2013) National, regional and global rates and trends in contraceptive prevalence and unmet need for family planning between 1990 and 2015: a systematic and comprehensive analysis. Lancet (2013) Epub ahead of print.

Cleland J (2008) Contraception in historical and global perspective. Best practice & Research clinical obstetrics and gynaecology, 23, 165-176

Cleland J, Conde-Agudelo A, Peterson H, Ross J, Tsui A (2012) Contraception and health. Lancet, 380, 149-156

Cleland J and Shah I (2013) The contraceptive revolution: focused efforts are still needed. Lancet (2013) Epub ahead of print.

Collumbien M, Gerressu M, Cleland J Non-use and use of ineffective methods of contraception. IN. comparative quantification of health risks, global and regional burden of disease attributable to selected major risk factors. Geneva. World Health Organization. 2004, 1255-1320.

Conde-Agudelo A, Belizan JM (2000) Maternal morbidity and mortality associated with interpregnancy interval: cross sectional study. BMJ 321, 1255-59.

Conde-Agudelo A, Rosas-Bermunez A, Kafury-Goeta AC. (2006) Birth spacing and risk of adverse perinatal outcomes: a meta-analysis. JAMA 295, 1809-23

Harrison PF, Hemmerling A, Romano J, Whaley KJ and Holt B.Young (2013) Developing multipurpose reproductive health technologies: An integrated strategy. AIDS Research and Treatment. Article ID 790154. http:/dx.doi.org/10.1155/2013/790154

Heffron R, Donnell D, Rees H, Celum C, Mugo N, Were E, de Bruyn G, Nakku-Joloba E, Ngure K, Kiarie J, Coombs RW, Baeten JM, Partners in Prevention HSV/HIV Transmission Study Team. (2012) Use of hormonal contraceptives and risk of HIV-I transmission: a prospective cohort study. Lancet Infect Dis 12(1) 19-26

Morrison CS, Skoler-Karpoff S, Kwok C, Chen PL, van der Wijgert J, Gehret-Plagianos M, Patel S, Ahmed K, Ramjee G, Friedland B, Lahteenmaki P. (2012) Hormonal contraception and the risk of HIV acquisition among women in South Africa. AIDS 26(4), 497-504.

Trilogy 4. Obesity and reproduction

Pathophysiological effects of obesity on reproduction

Renato Pasquali

University Alma Mater Studiorum, Bologna, Italy

Introduction

Men and women are characterized by several and specific biologic differences and by different predispositions to develop disease, particularly metabolic and cardiovascular disease, with distinct pathophysiological mechanisms. Obesity, particularly the abdominal phenotype, has negative effects, more in women than in men, on the susceptibility to develop not only metabolic and cardiovascular diseases but also reproductive disorders, with specific differences according to sex.

Obesity and infertility in men

The role of sex hormones

Obesity decreases total testosterone plasma levels in obese men as well as decreasing the levels of sex hormone-binding globulin (SHBG) and altering estrogen production rates and metabolism. The decrease of total testosterone levels parallels with increasing body mass index (BMI), and it is particularly evident in the presence of abdominal obesity (1). Notably, the decrease in SHBG occurs independently of the increase in estrogen production rates that occurs in obese males, and this phenomenon, among others, makes the difference with the age-dependent decrease in testosterone levels that conversely occurs in the presence of progressively increased SHBG concentrations. Other androgen blood levels, chiefly androstenedione and dihydrotestosterone, are conversely unchanged in overweight-obese men, even if in some cases they tend to decrease. It has been clearly demonstrated that androgen and estrogen concentrations in the visceral and subcutaneous adipose tissue significantly correlate with their blood levels, with important regional differences, which supports a specific impact of the sex steroids on adipose function and metabolism of the different fat deposits (2). Moreover, the metabolic syndrome, in which abdominal obesity plays an important role, is always associated with low testosterone blood levels that in turn represent a highly significant independent predictive factor for the presence of the syndrome (3).

The decrease of SHBG levels has an important role in decreasing blood levels of free testosterone; however, it is not exclusive. This is partly due to the fact that, in men, only 53% of testosterone is bound to SHBG, whereas in women the SHBG-bound testosterone is more than 75% (4). This implies that other factors need to be considered in determining low testosterone in obese men.

A typical neuroendocrine derangement may in fact occur in male obesity, characterized by alteration of the gonadotropin-releasing hormone (GnRH) and luteinizing hormone (LH) pulsatility, with reduced pulse number and amplitude, particularly in men with severe obesity. This may be responsible for a hypogonadotropic severe hypotestosteronemia in these individuals (5).

Another factor is the increase in estrogen production rate that, by a negative feedback loop, may inhibit the hypothalamic-pituitary activity in obese males. This is indirectly supported by the increase in testosterone levels and the improvement of spermatogenesis in obese men treated with clomiphene citrate, an anti-estrogenic compound (6). In line with this, other studies have shown that the administration of aromatase inhibitors is capable of increasing testosterone levels in obese individuals (7).

An increase in cortisol production also is able to reduce testosterone levels, as can be frequently shown in patients with Cushing syndrome who usually develop a condition of hypogonadotropic hypogonadism. In fact, obesity, particularly the abdominal-visceral phenotype, may be characterized by a hyperactivity or hyperresponsiveness of the hypothalamic-pituitary-adrenal axis to psychological chronic stress and altered allostatic work (8). In addition, an increased activity of the tissue (mainly visceral fat) 11β-hydroxysteroid dehydrogenase type 1, which is responsible for the conversion of cortisone (inactive steroid) to cortisol, has been confirmed in many studies (8). In addition, some studies have found some decrease in the activity of the 5α- and 5β-reductases, the most important cortisol catabolic system. Finally, there are studies showing an inverse correlation between LH and testosterone levels and the 24h free urinary cortisol excretion in men with abdominal obesity (9).

The excess in circulating blood leptin levels has an additional and important role in determining hypotestosteronemia in obese men. Leptin does, in fact, have specific receptors in the male gonads (10). Moreover, in vitro and in vivo studies have shown that an inverse relationship between leptin and testosterone exists in humans (11, 12). Notably, in patients with hypogonadism, leptin levels are usually low but they return to normal levels after testosterone therapy (13). Interestingly, recent data have also shown that an alteration of the leptin-kisspeptin system may explain the association between the abnormal energy balance and the reproductive function in obesity (14).

Finally, recent studies support the concept that the insulin like factor-3 (INSL3), a member of the relaxin-insulin family that is expressed in testicular Leydig cells and seems to reflect their functional status, may have a role. INSL3 levels are in fact reduced in obese men and are inversely related to BMI but positively with testosterone levels (15).

Male obesity and spermatogenesis

Several studies have shown that an increase in BMI is associated with low testicular volume and particularly a significant alteration in spermatogenic parameters, such as total sperm count and number, as well as modifications of spermatozoa morphology and vitality. This is particularly evident in massive obesity that is associated with a high rate of infertility. Studies in genetically obese mice or in mice fed with a high-fat diet have shown that they had oligospermia and hypomobility of spermatozoa, besides possible abnormalities of morphology and vitality, such as precocious apoptosis, alteration of membrane potential, DNA nemaspermic fragmentation, chromatin integrity, and oxidative stress (16). Notably, not always and not all these abnormalities have been described in obese men. A meta-analysis published in 2008 that considered 5 population studies with a total 2,139 subjects showed that the deterioration of the semen parameters in overweight or obese men was fairly marginal (17). On the contrary, a more recent meta-analysis of 21 studies that included a population of 13,077 subjects showed that the risk of oligospermia and azoospermia increased progressively with gain in body weight with a doubled prevalence in those with massive obesity compared to subjects with normal BMI (18). Therefore, these data seem to confirm a significant prevalence of oligospermia and azoospermia in obese men.

The role of erectile dysfunction (ED) and other factors

ED can be considered a possible contributory cause of infertility. Epidemiological studies have shown that the prevalence of ED is significantly associated with obesity, and the hazard ratios are proportional to BMI values (19), as recently confirmed by the report of the more recent European Male Aging Study (20). Among many potentially involved factors, it has been hypothesized that an important role may be represented by abdominal obesity, which is associated with the production of pro-inflammatory factors responsible for endothelium alteration, one of the first events of atherosclerosis vasculopathy. All factors that interfere with the endothelium function do, in fact, alter the release of nitric oxide and the integrity of the vessels, and may therefore be important in the development of ED. Low testosterone levels are in turn a key factor involved in the development of ED in obese men.

Obesity and infertility in women

Sex steroid hormones, adipose tissue, and reproductive function in women

Sex steroid hormones have an important role in the control of adipose tissue metabolism, differentiation, and morphology, influencing in turn the reproductive system in females. It is known that adipose tissue in the gluteal-femoral region has a specific function promoting fertility in women. This differentiation process starts with the onset of puberty, then tends to stabilize during reproductive age and to regress during menopause. During the reproductive age, there is a higher lipoprotein lipase activity (LPL) in the femoral compared to the abdominal adipose area, whereas the opposite takes place in the lipolytic response to catecholamines (21). These metabolic activities of the adipose tissue tend to markedly change in conditions such as pregnancy and lactation where the lipolysis induced by the catecholamine is reduced in the femoral area and the LPL activity is increased in femoral compared to abdominal adipocytes (22). These data demonstrate that there are specific metabolic processes regulated by different deposits of the adipose tissues.

In women with normal insulin sensitivity, the adipocytes release small amounts of free fatty acid (FFA) and LPL, and testosterone levels at physiological concentrations may support this inhibitory effect mediated by insulin (23). Instead, obese women with insulin resistance have an increased production of FFA that, in turn, further worsens insulin sensitivity. It is possible that the effects of testosterone on abdominal adipose tissue in normal-weight women are adjusted by a protective estrogen effect that causes a down-regulation of the androgen receptor density in the adipose tissue (4). Abdominal obesity is also characterized by a condition of relative functional hyperandrogenism, due to the increased testosterone production rate that in turn may favor an enlargement of the visceral adipose tissue (1). In fact, the administration of testosterone for several months has been shown to increase the visceral fat deposits in women and the same effect has been shown in female-to-males transsexuals receiving testosterone for a long period of time (1). Therefore, a relative or absolute androgen excess may be involved in determining an expansion of visceral fat in women that may in turn lead to alterations in the ovarian function and ovulation.

Obesity, menstrual cycle, and ovulatory disorders

The negative effect of obesity on fertility has been known for a long time (24-27). The excess of adipose tissue developed during adolescence has been found to be associated with menstrual and ovulatory dysfunction in reproductive age. In this scenario, leptin has been shown to play a dominant role (10). Nulliparous women are frequently obese. Obesity represents an important risk factor of anovulatory infertility that increases with gain in body weight, and obese women have an increased risk of infertility 3 times higher than their normal-weight counterpart, besides the lower chance of becoming pregnant (28). This is more evident in the presence of abdominal adipose tissue (29). Moreover, it has been shown that, besides BMI, lifestyle habitudes (smoking, alcohol, and coffee) have a cumulative dose-dependent impact on fecundity (30). In some cases, infertility in obese women may not be related to ovulation disorders, but could be due to other factors such as abnormal oocyte and embryo development or abnormalities of endometrial receptivity.

The relative or absolute androgen excess plays an important role in the development of anovulation in obesity. This may be due to the insulin excess that controls, in physiological condition and in synergy with LH, theca steroidogenesis and several functions of granulosa cells, such as foliculogenesis. In obese women, some adipokines and pro-inflammatory cytokines, such as leptin, tumor necrosis factor alpha (TNFα), and interleukin 6 (IL6), that are increased in the fat tissues, particularly the visceral deposits, as well as reduced adiponectin levels, may have important synergistic negative effects on insulin action, thereby favoring the development of an insulin resistance state and, possibly, favoring androgen excess production (31).

Obesity and assisted reproductive technology (ART)

Obesity reduces the efficiency and effectiveness of ART. For every BMI unit increase in obese women, the probability of pregnancy decreases, whereas loss of BMI units increases the chance of becoming pregnant (32). The abnormal hormonal milieu (sex steroids, insulin) and the actions of several cytokines may affect follicular development, embryo development, and implantation, also after ART. Obese women frequently need higher doses of gonadotropin for IVF. Longer periods of ovarian stimulation, higher cancellation rates, and higher incidence of follicular asynchrony have been found in obese patients undergoing ART (33). In addition, fewer oocytes collected and a higher proportion of poor oocyte and embryo quality have also been reported in obese women. The increased pregnancy failure rate in obese women returns to the normal rate if donor oocytes are used instead of autologous oocytes (33). Unfortunately, the data reported in the literature are discordant because of several methodological limitations of the studies.

The paradigm of polycystic ovary syndrome (PCOS): effect of obesity on fertility and reproduction

The diagnosis of PCOS is made in the presence of at least two of the following criteria: (i) clinical and biochemical hyperandrogenism, (ii) oligo-amenorrhea and anovulation, and (iii) polycystic ovarian morphology, defined by specific parameters (ovarian volume and follicle count), after the exclusion of other conditions and therapies responsible for androgen excess (34). PCOS women are usually characterized by several metabolic abnormalities, chiefly insulin resistance and glucose intolerance, and are affected by very high rates of overweight and obesity. Both compensatory hyperinsulinemia and obesity contribute to the development of physiopathological processes responsible for the PCOS phenotype (35). Hyperinsulinemia does, in fact, play a dominant role in the excessive production of testosterone and both these factors are potentially responsible for the enlargement of visceral fat tissue (36). There are several other factors related to obesity that contribute to the PCOS phenotype. These include alteration of the insulin growth factor system (IGF-1), hyperactivity of the opioid system, a deficiency of vitamin D, an excess or a defect of some cytokines and adipokines, an abnormal control of the antimüllerian (AMH)-gonadotropin releasing hormone (GnRH) system, an increase in INSL3 secretion, and others (35).

The excess of androgen is more pronounced in obese women with PCOS, mainly in those with the abdominal obesity phenotype. Hirsutism itself can be more severe. Finally, menstrual disorders and oligo-anovulation tend to be more common, and infertility is more severe in obese PCOS women. Several cross-sectional and longitudinal clinical studies have shown the negative impact of metabolic abnormalities and obesity on ovulation and fertility in women with PCOS (35, 37). Moreover, PCOS women are characterized by a poor and delayed response to pro-ovulatory therapies such as clomiphene citrate or aromatase inhibitors. They also may have higher miscarriage rates and lower live-birth rates. The ART outcome rate in PCOS women is largely influenced by the higher risk of failure related to body weight gain (38).

PCOS is therefore an excellent model for understanding the negative impact of obesity on fertility in women. This is of specific importance, since approximately 30%-40% of women attending infertility clinics are affected by PCOS.

References

1. Pasquali R. Androgens and obesity: fact and perspectives. Fertil Steril 2006; 85: 1319-40.
2. Bélanger C, Houldc F-S, Lebelc S, Bironc S, Brochuc G, Tchernof A. Omental and subcutaneous adipose tissue steroid levels in obese men. Steroids 2006; 71:674–682.
3. Vermeulen, Giagulli
4. Wajchenberg BL. Subcutaneous and visceral adipose tissue: their relation to the metabolic syndrome. Endocr Rev 2000; 21:697-738.
5. Vermeulen A, Kaufman JM, Deslypere JP, Thomas G. Attenuated luteinizing hormone (LH) pulse amplitude but normal LH pulse frequency, and its relation to plasma androgens in hypogonadism of obese men. J Clin Endocrinol Metab 1993; 76: 1140-1146.
6. Duschek EJ, Gooren LJ, Netelenbos C. Comparison of effects of the rise in serum testosterone by raloxifene and oral testosterone on serum insulin-like growth factor-1 and insulin-like growth factor binding protein-3. Maturitas. 2005; 51:286-93.
7. Leder BZ, Rohrer JL, Rubin SD, Gallo J, Longcope C. Effects of aromatase inhibition in elderly men with low or borderline-low serum testosterone levels. J Clin Endocrinol Metab. 2004; 89:1174-80
8. Pasquali R. The hypothalamic-pituitary-adrenal axis and sex hormones in chronic stress and obesity: pathophysiological and clinical aspects. Ann N Y Acad Sci. 2012; 1264:20-35
9. Vicennati V, Ceroni L, Genghini S, et al. Sex difference in the relationship between the hypothalamic-pituitary-adrenal (HPA) axis and sex hormones in obesity. Obes Res 2006; 14: 235-43.
10. Moschos S, Chan JL, and Mantzoros CS. Leptin and reproduction: a review. Fertil Steril 2002; 77: 433-44.
11. Caprio M, Isidori AM, Carta AR, et al. Expression of functional leptin receptors in rodent Leydig cells. Endocrinology 1999; 140: 4939-47.
12. Isidori AM, Caprio M, Strollo F, et al. Leptin and androgens in male obesity: evidence for leptin contribution to reduced androgen levels. J Clin Endocrinol Metab 1999; 84:.3673-80.
13. Jockenhovel F, Blum WF, Vogel E, et al. Testosterone substitution normalizes elevated serum leptin levels in hypogonadal men. J Clin Endocrinol Metab. 1997; 82: 2510-3.
14. Roa J, Navarro VM, Tena-Sempere M. Kisspeptins in reproductive biology: consensus knowledge and recent developments. Biol Reprod. 2011; 85:650-60.

15. Foresta C, Di Mambro A, Pagano C, Garolla A, Vettor R, Ferlin R. 2009 Insulin-like factor 3 as a marker of testicular function in obese men. Clin Endocrinol (Oxf). 71:722-6
16. Vigueras-Villaseñor RM, Rojas-Castañeda JC, Chávez-Saldaña M, et al. Alterations in the spermatic function generated by obesity in rats. Acta Histochem. 2011; 113:214-20.
17. Aggerholm AS, Thulstrup AM, Toft G, Ramlau-Hansen CH, Bonde JP. 2008 Is overweight a risk factor for reduced semen quality and altered serum sex hormone profile? Fertil Steril. 90:619-26
18. Sermondade N, Faure C, Fezeu L, et al. 2012 BMI in relation to sperm count: an updated systematic review and collaborative meta-analysis.. Hum Reprod Update. Dec 12. Epub ahead of print
19. Corona G, Lee DM, Forti G,et al. 2010 Age-related changes in general and sexual health in middle-aged and older men: results from the European Male Ageing Study (EMAS). J Sex Med. 7:1362-80
20. Palmer NO, Bakos HW, Fullston T, Lane M. Impact of obesity on male fertility, sperm function and molecular composition. Spermatogenesis. 2012; 2:253-263.
21. Norman RJ and Clark AM. Obesity and reproductive disorders: a review. Reprod Fertil Dev, 199810: 55-63.
22. Rebuffé-Scrive M, Enk L, Crona N, Lönnroth P, Abrahamsson L, Smith U, Björntorp P. Fat cell metabolism in different regions in women. Effect of menstrual cycle, pregnancy, and lactation. J Clin Invest. 1985; 75:1973-6.
23. Wu FC, von Eckardstein A. Androgens and coronary artery disease. Endocr Rev. 2003; 24:183-217.
24. Rogers J, and Mitchell GW. The relation of obesity to menstrual disturbances. N Engl J Med 1952; 247: 53-56.
25. Hartz AJ, Barboriak PN, Wong A, et al. The association of obesity with infertility and related menstrual abnormalities in women. Int J Obes Rel Metab Dis1979; 3: 57-77
26. Lake JK, Power C, and Cole TJ. Women's reproductive health: the role of body mass index in early and adult life. Int J Obes Rel Metab Dis 1997; 21:432-438.
27. Rich-Edwards JA, Goldman MB, Willet WC, et al. Adolescent body mass index and infertility caused by ovulatory dysfunction. Am J Obstet Gynecol 1994; 71: 171-177.
28. Moran LJ, Dodd L, Nisenblat V, Norman RJ. 2011 Obesity and reproductive dysfunction in women. Endocrinol Metab Clin North Am 40:895-906
29. Zaadstra BM, Seidell JC, Van Noord PA, et al. Fat and female fecundity: prospective study of effect of body fat distribution on conception rates. Br Med J, 1993; 306: 484-487.
30. Hassan MA, Killick SR Negative lifestyle is associated with a significant reduction in fecundity. Fertil Steril 2004; 81:384-92.ì
31. Chen X, Jia X, Qiao J, Guan Y, Kang J. Adipokines in reproductive function: a link between obesity and polycystic ovary syndrome. J Mol Endocrinol. 2013; 50:R21-37.
32. Fedocksák P, Dale P, Storeng R et al. 2004 Impact of overweight on assisted reproduction treatment. Hum Reprod 11:2523-252
33. Bellver J, Busso C, Pellicer A, et al. 2006 Obesity and assisted reproductive technology outcomes. Reprod Biomed Online. 12:562-8.
34. The Rotterdam ESHRE/ASRM-Sponsored PCOS consensus workshop group. Revised 2003 consensus on diagnostic criteria and long-term health risks related to polycystic ovary syndrome (PCOS). Hum Reprod. 2004: 19:41-7.
35. Usadi RS, Legro RS. Reproductive impact of polycystic ovary syndrome. Curr Opin Endocrinol Diabetes Obes. 2012; 19:505-11.

36. Dunaif, A. Insulin resistance and the polycystic ovary syndrome: mechanisms and implications for pathogenesis. Endocr Rev 1997; 18.774-800.
37. Diamanti-Kandarakis E, Dunaif A. Diamanti-Kandarakis E, Dunaif A. 2012 Insulin resistance and the polycystic ovary syndrome revisited: an update on mechanisms and implications. Endocr Rev. 33:981-1030.
38. Nahuis MJ, Oosterhuis GJ, Hompes PG, van Wely M, Mol BW, van der Veen F. The basic fertility workup in women with polycystic ovary syndrome: a systematic review. Fertil Steril. 2013 Apr 12. doi:pii: S0015-0282(13)00416-0. 10.1016/j.fertnstert.2013.03.015. [Epub ahead of print]

Reproductive outcomes after bariatric surgery

Roland Devlieger, Goele Jans, Matthias Lannoo, Bart Van der Schueren, Christophe Matthys

University Hospitals Leuven, Leuven, Belgium

Introduction

Bariatric, or obesity, surgery offers, in combination with the necessary lifestyle modifications, an effective treatment for morbid obesity. It results in a significant long-term weight loss and in improvement of obesity-associated comorbidities. A surgical intervention is considered when conventional interventions have failed in patients with a body mass index (BMI) $\geq$ 40 kg/m² or with a BMI $\geq$ 35 kg/m² with co-morbidities such as sleep apnea, diabetes, joint disease, and cardiopulmonary problems.

Worldwide, approximately 340,768 bariatric procedures were performed in 2011.[1] Eighty-five percent of the patients are women of reproductive age.[2] Bariatric surgery is increasingly considered as a treatment option for adolescents with morbid obesity. Consequently, an increasing number of women with a history of bariatric surgery are getting pregnant or attending fertility treatment services.

Bariatric surgery

The most commonly performed procedures nowadays are the sleeve gastrectomy (SG), adjustable gastric banding (AGB), and Roux-en-Y Gastric Bypass (RYGB). Both the SG and AGB lead to a restricted food intake by reducing gastric storage capacity. A gastric pouch is created by the use of staples or a band. The silicon gastric band of the AGB is inflated or deflated with fluid, creating a smaller or larger opening to the gastric pouch. The RYGB is a mixed procedure that limits both energy intake and absorption. A gastric pouch is created, but is separated from the remaining stomach by stapling or transection. The pouch empties directly into the distal jejunum, bypassing the remaining stomach, duodenum, and most of the proximal jejunum.

Worldwide, the most commonly performed procedures in 2011 were RYGB (46.6%), SG (27.8%), and AGB (17.8%). In Europe, the total number of procedures increased from 2003 to 2011, with a decrease of AGB and a rise in SG and RYGB. In the United States/Canada, the total number of procedures increased from 2003 to 2008, but decreased from 2008 to 2011. Less RYGBs and more SGs were performed, and AGB rose from 2003 to 2008 and then decreased.[1]

Fertility after bariatric surgery

In general, the weight loss as a result of the surgery reverses the adverse effects of obesity on fertility.

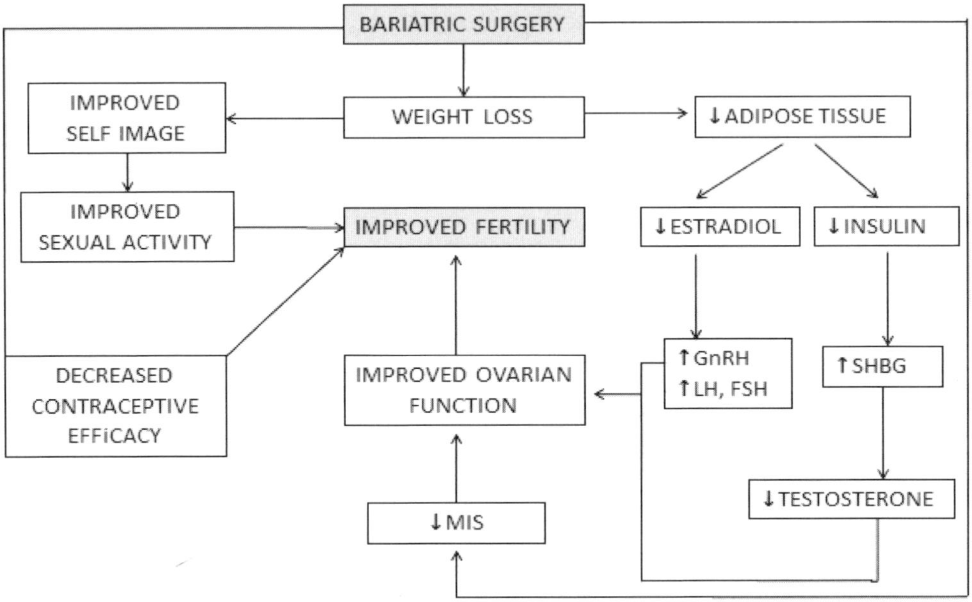

Figure 1. Effects of bariatric surgery on fertility. Abbreviations: FSH Follicular Stimulating Hormone, GnRH Gonadotropin Releasing Hormone, LH Lutenising Hormone, MIS Müllerian Inhibiting Substance, SHBG Sex Hormone Binding Globuline. Source: *Maternal Obesity, chapter 17, Pre-pregnancy bariatric surgery: improved fertility and pregnancy outcome?*[3]

Hormonal alterations in non-pregnant woman after bariatric surgery are the result of decreased adipose tissue mass, resulting in lower estradiol levels, stimulating the hypothalamic release of gonadotropin-releasing hormone (GnRH) and luteinizing hormone (LH) and the follicle-stimulating hormone (FSH) secretion by the pituitary gland. Weight loss also lowers insulin levels, resulting in increased sex hormone binding globulin (SHBG) and decreased peripheral testosterone concentrations. Finally, müllerian inhibiting substance (MIS) levels are decreased after bariatric surgery (Figure 1).[3] Comparing the pre- and postoperative fertility status, an improvement in spontaneous pregnancy rates is found. In anovulatory obese women, up to 71% regained cyclicity of menstrual blood loss in proportion to the amount of weight loss.[4] Sexual interest, activity, and function also appear to improve after weight loss.[5]

As most fertility units use BMI cut-offs to restrict access to fertility treatment for morbidly obese women, surgery is increasingly being considered as a fertility treatment option. After surgery, most guidelines advise to wait for at least one year before starting fertility treatment, although this remains an area of debate.[6-8]

Pregnancy after bariatric surgery

Conclusions about the consequences of bariatric surgery on pregnancy outcomes need to be drawn with caution since literature is limited by the number and quality of the available studies.[3,9,10]

Pregnancy outcomes

The weight loss after surgery results in a significantly lower rate of obesity-related maternal morbidities, approaching those of non-obese women.[11] Bariatric surgery does not seems to be an indication for cesarean delivery.[12] It seems to protect against excessive gestational weight gain (GWG) and the rate of postpartum weight loss is similar to the rate of postoperative weight loss in non-pregnant women.[13,14]

An internal hernia, created by the increased intra-abdominal pressure, is the most described surgical complication during pregnancy. The reported incidence of intestinal obstruction after RYGB is up to 5%.[15] A bowel obstruction is more likely to develop at mid pregnancy when the uterus becomes an abdominal organ and puts pressure on the intestine, at term when the fetal head descends, and in postpartum period with rapid uterus involution.[16] Prevention, early recognition, and intervention are crucial since a hernia or obstruction could progress to bowel strangulation, anastomotic disruption, dilation of the bypassed stomach, necrosis, and perforation. Other reported surgical complications are band migration, gastric ulceration, and strictures.

Fetal and neonatal outcome

Reports suggest that the higher risk for miscarriage in obese women declines after bariatric surgery.[5,6] Theoretically, the surgery itself leads to an increased risk of developing congenital malformations compared with normal weight, overweight, and obese women, since vitamin and mineral deficiencies are common postoperatively. However, eating habits and a changed absorption in both the obese and the bariatric population need to be taken into account. A study by Sheiner et al. (2004) observed no difference between the post-surgery group and the obese control group.[17] A study of Weintraub et al. reported a higher rate of fetal malformations than in pregnancies before surgery.[18] Two case series observed high rates of neural tube defect (NTD), but the mothers were non-adherent with recommended vitamin supplementation.[19,20] Regarding perinatal mortality, no increase was seen after laparoscopic adjustable gastric banding (LAGB), RYGB, or biliopancreatic diversion.

A systematic review found no difference in the incidence of low birth weight after both the restrictive and malabsorptive type of surgery, but only four articles in the review reported on low birth weight.[12] Since there are case series and cohort studies mentioning high incidences of intrauterine growth restriction (IUGR), this aspect certainly requires more attention.[21,22] More preterm deliveries are reported in pregnancies conceived within the first year after bariatric surgery compared to later pregnancies.[22] Babies show lower mean birth weights, and the prevalence of macrosomia and large for gestational age (LGA) babies is reduced compared to obese and non-obese controls. The incidence of IUGR and small for gestational age (SGA) babies appears to be increased.[9]

Nutritional deficiencies

The risk for preterm births and NTDs due to, respectively, maternal iron-deficient anemia and folic acid deficiency may be increased. More specific complications due to nutritional deficiencies have also been reported, independent of the time between surgery and conception: IUGR, oligohydramnios, electrolyte imbalances, cerebral hemorrhage, bilateral microphthalmia, permanent retinal damage, and even fetal deaths.[23-26] Vitamin B12 deficiency can be expected after all procedures since vitamin B12 uptake requires intrinsic factor, the production of which is reduced after surgery. Vitamin B12 deficiency can also cause maternal anemia. This maternal deficit is also reflected in the concentration in the breast milk and can result in vitamin B12 insufficiency in the baby.[27-29]

Clinical recommendations

The specific needs of these high-risk pregnancies are best addressed by a multidisciplinary team including obstetricians, surgeons, endocrinologists, pediatricians, psychiatrists, and nutritionists. Recommendations regarding preconceptional, prenatal, and postpartum follow-up are summarized in Table 1.[3]

Management recommendations
Preconception • Post-operative detection and correction of nutritional deficiencies • Supplementation tailored to type of bariatric procedure performed with specific attention for folic acid, vitamin B12, iron and fat-soluble vitamins • Visits to a nutritionist/lifestyle coach to ensure a healthy and varied diet and healthy level of physical activity • Fertility counselling, advice on reliable contraception to delay pregnancy for 12 months.
Prenatal care • Early prenatal consultation to determine baseline nutritional status, followed by regular check-ups • Nutritional supplementation tailored to the individual patient and the type of bariatric procedure. A standard prenatal vitamin daily is the minimum requirement. • Serial ultrasound examination with specific attention for correct dating and detection of fetal growth restriction and malformations • Advise gestational weight gain within OIM guidelines for preconceptional BMI. • For an adjustable gastric banding procedure, active band management is advisable according to GWG and individual health status *Removal of all band fluid as early as possible in the pregnancy to minimize the effect on emesis. After 14 weeks gestation or later, fluid can be inserted again in cases of excessive GWG. To minimize the impact of delivery on the gastric band and vice versa, the fluid is removed again at 36 weeks of gestation.* • Awareness for possible intestinal obstruction during pregnancy • Fasting and 2h postprandial glucose level monitoring instead of glucose challenge test or oral glucose tolerance test to detect gestational diabetes mellitus
Postpartum care • Recommend and support breastfeeding • Inform paediatrician of maternal bariatric surgery history and possible effects on the newborn. • Postpartum follow-up and correction of nutritional deficiencies. • Visits to a nutritionist to ensure a healthy and varied diet

Permitted adaptation from *Maternal Obesity, chapter 17, Pre-pregnancy bariatric surgery: improved fertility and pregnancy outcome?*[3]

Time between surgery and conception

The American College of Obstetricians and Gynecologists (ACOG) advises to wait at least 12 months before becoming pregnant, as this is the period of rapid weight loss.[30] After a LAGB, pregnancy shortly post-surgery may predispose to band revisions. Also, a trend towards more miscarriages and preterm delivery was reported in a group conceiving within the first year after surgery compared to a group conceiving later.[14] However, delaying pregnancy too long also may incur risks. The need for intravenous iron therapy or packed red cell transfusion was more frequent among women pregnant after four years compared to less than four years after

RYGB.[31] In contrast, studies found similar pregnancy outcomes in women conceiving during vs. after the period of maximal weight loss.[32]

No conclusive evidence exists to suggest that pregnancy during the first postoperative year is safe. Until more research is performed, clinicians should advise postoperative patients to delay pregnancy until a stable weight is reached.

Contraception

Postponing conception at least 12 months implies providing advice on safe and effective contraceptive use. However, unintended pregnancies are frequently reported and are at the highest risk for nutritional deficiencies during the period of embryogenesis. Previously obese women with anovulatory cycles not requiring contraception should be informed that fertility will likely be improved after surgery.

As many postoperative patients are still obese, safety concerns arise regarding the possibility of increased post-surgery risk of venous thromboembolism when using combined oral contraceptives. Concerns also exist around the effectiveness of oral contraception.[33] Effectiveness could be decreased by the surgically induced gastrointestinal malabsorption, but also by postoperative complications such as sustained diarrhea and/or vomiting. Second, there could be a fracture risk due to bone loss with the use of depot medroxyprogesterone acetate in a population already losing bone mass as a consequence of weight loss and nutritional deficiencies.[34]

Until more evidence is available, physicians should recommend oral contraception with prudence after bariatric surgery and should consider non-oral administration of hormonal contraception.

Nutritional advice

Ideally a woman with bariatric surgery starts off with a good nutritional status in the preconception period. During pregnancy, prevention of nutritional deficiencies remains a priority. Although some general recommendations exist, no controlled trials are available to determine the type and dosage of supplements. A pregnancy-specific multivitamin supplement is usually prescribed. However, one does not know the proportion absorbed, especially in patients with a malabsorptive type of surgery. Therefore it is reasonable to assess nutritional status every trimester and adapt a prescription to the patient's plasma micronutrient profile. In case of a deficiency, a monthly check-up is required. Also, the pharmaceutical formulation needs to be taken into consideration. A patient with a LAGB could prefer a tablet, syrup, drinkable solution, or an intramuscular injection, rather than a capsule that can cause dysphagia at the level of the band. A dose of 400 μg folate daily is recommended as for all women of reproductive age. A higher dose could be considered if the woman after surgery is still obese, since maternal obesity is a risk factor for malformations such as NTD.[35]

Concluding remarks

In women of reproductive age, fertility is often enhanced after bariatric surgery. Many pregnancy outcomes are improved, but risks related to nutritional deficiencies and surgical complications are increased.

References

1. Buchwald H, Oien DM. Metabolic/Bariatric surgery worldwide 2011. Obes Surg 2013;23:427-36.
2. Samuel I, Mason EE, Renquist KE, Huang YH, Zimmerman MB, Jamal M. Bariatric surgery trends: an 18-year report from the International Bariatric Surgery Registry. Am J Surg 2006;192:657-62.
3. Devlieger R, Guelinckx I. Pre-pregnancy bariatric surgery: improved fertility and pregnancy outcome? In: Gillman MW, Poston L, eds. Maternal obesity. 2012:209-21.
4. Teitelman M, Grotegut CA, Williams NN, Lewis JD. The impact of bariatric surgery on menstrual patterns. Obes Surg 2006;16:1457-63.
5. Merhi ZO. Impact of bariatric surgery on female reproduction. Fertil Steril 2009;92: 1501-8.
6. Shah DK, Ginsburg ES. Bariatric surgery and fertility. Curr Opin Obstet Gynecol 2010;22:248-54.
7. Sheiner E, dri A, Balaban E, Levi I, Aricha-Tamir B. Pregnancy outcome of patients who conceive during or after the first year following bariatric surgery. Am J Obstet Gynecol 2011;204:50e1-6.
8. Devlieger R, Vansant G, Guelinckx I. Bariatric surgery. Am J Obstet Gynecol 2011;205:e7-e8.
9. Guelinckx I, Devlieger R, Vansant G. Reproductive outcome after bariatric surgery: a critical review. Hum Reprod Update 2009;15:189-201.
10. Guelinckx I, Devlieger R, Vansant G. Pregnancy following bariatric surgery. In: Ovesen PG, Jensen DM, eds. Maternal Obesity and Pregnancy. 2012.
11. Bennett WL, Gilson MM, Jamshidi R, et al. Impact of bariatric surgery on hypertensive disorders in pregnancy: retrospective analysis of insurance claims data. BMJ 2010;340:c1662.
12. Maggard MA, Yermilov I, Li Z, et al. Pregnancy and fertility following bariatric surgery: a systematic review. JAMA 2008;300:2286-96.
13. Dixon JB, Dixon ME, O'Brien PE. Birth outcomes in obese women after laparoscopic adjustable gastric banding. Obstet Gynecol 2005;106:965-72.
14. Dao T, Kuhn J, Ehmer D, Fisher T, McCarty T. Pregnancy outcomes after gastric-bypass surgery. Am J Surg 2006;192:762-6.
15. Wax JR, Wolff R, Cobean R, Pinette MG, Blackstone J, Cartin A. Intussusception complicating pregnancy following laparoscopic Roux-en-Y gastric bypass. Obes Surg 2007;17:977-9.
16. Kakarla N, Dailey C, Marino T, Shikora SA, Chelmow D. Pregnancy after gastric bypass surgery and internal hernia formation. Obstet Gynecol 2005;105:1195-8.
17. Sheiner E, Levy A, Silverberg D, et al. Pregnancy after bariatric surgery is not associated with adverse perinatal outcome. Am J Obstet Gynecol 2004;190:1335-40.
18. Weintraub AY, Levy A, Levi I, Mazor M, Wiznitzer A, Sheiner E. Effect of bariatric surgery on pregnancy outcome. Int J Gynaecol Obstet 2008;103:246-51.
19. Haddow JE, Hill LE, Kloza EM, Thanhauser D. Neural tube defects after gastric bypass. Lancet 1986;1:1330.
20. Martin L, Chavez GF, Adams MJ, Jr, et al. Gastric bypass surgery as maternal risk factor for neural tube defects. Lancet 1988;1:640-1.
21. Friedman D, Cuneo S, Valenzano M, et al. Pregnancies in an 18-Year Follow-up after Biliopancreatic Diversion. Obes Surg 1995;5:308-13.
22. Patel JA, Patel NA, Thomas RL, Nelms JK, Colella JJ. Pregnancy outcomes after laparoscopic Roux-en-Y gastric bypass. Surg Obes Relat Dis 2008;4:39-45.

23. Cools M, Duval EL, Jespers A. Adverse neonatal outcome after maternal biliopancreatic diversion operation: report of nine cases. Eur J Pediatr 2006;165:199-202.
24. Gurewitsch ED, Smith-Levitin M, Mack J. Pregnancy following gastric bypass surgery for morbid obesity. Obstet Gynecol 1996;88:658-61.
25. Eerdekens A, Debeer A, Van Hoey G, et al. Maternal bariatric surgery: adverse outcomes in neonates. Eur J Pediatr 2010;169:191-6.
26. Van Mieghem T, Van Schoubroeck D, Depiere M, Debeer A, Hanssens M. Fetal cerebral hemorrhage caused by vitamin K deficiency after complicated bariatric surgery. Obstet Gynecol 2008;112:434-6.
27. Celiker MY, Chawla A. Congenital B12 deficiency following maternal gastric bypass. J Perinatol 2009;29:640-2.
28. Grange DK, Finlay JL. Nutritional vitamin B12 deficiency in a breastfed infant following maternal gastric bypass. Pediatr Hematol Oncol 1994;11:311-8.
29. Wardinsky TD, Montes RG, Friederich RL, Broadhurst RB, Sinnhuber V, Bartholomew D. Vitamin B12 deficiency associated with low breast-milk vitamin B12 concentration in an infant following maternal gastric bypass surgery. Arch Pediatr Adolesc Med 1995;149:1281-4.
30. ACOG. practice bulletin no. 105: bariatric surgery and pregnancy. Obstetrics & Gynecology 2009;113:1405-13.
31. Nomura RM, Dias MC, Igai AM, Paiva LV, Zugaib M. Anemia during pregnancy after silastic ring Roux-en-Y gastric bypass: influence of time to conception. Obes Surg 2011;21:479-84.
32. Wax JR, Cartin A, Wolff R, Lepich S, Pinette MG, Blackstone J. Pregnancy following gastric bypass for morbid obesity: effect of surgery-to-conception interval on maternal and neonatal outcomes. Obes Surg 2008;18:1517-21.
33. Paulen ME, Zapata LB, Cansino C, Curtis KM, Jamieson DJ. Contraceptive use among women with a history of bariatric surgery: a systematic review. Contraception 2010;82:86-94.
34. Coates PS, Fernstrom JD, Fernstrom MH, Schauer PR, Greenspan SL. Gastric bypass surgery for morbid obesity leads to an increase in bone turnover and a decrease in bone mass. J Clin Endocrinol Metab 2004;89:1061-5.
35. Centers for Disease Control and Prevention. CDC Grand Rounds: additional opportunities to prevent neural tube defects with folic acid fortification. MMWR Morb Mortal Wkly Rep 2010;59:980-4.

Weight management to improve outcomes in infertility

Lisa Moran

The Robinson Institute, Adelaide, Australia

Introduction

Overweight (body mass index [BMI] 25-29.9 kg/m^2) and obesity (BMI $\geq$ 30 kg/m^2) are issues of increasing prevalence in Western society and are estimated to affect 66% of adults in the United States (1). Overweight and obesity are associated with a variety of clinical complications including an elevated risk of metabolic conditions such as impaired glucose tolerance, type 2 diabetes, the metabolic syndrome, and cardiovascular disease. They are also associated with an increased prevalence of other disorders including sleep apnea, cancers, and worsened psychological health (2). In women, being overweight or obese is also associated with worsened reproductive health and infertility (3,4). With specific regards to women, the prevalence of overweight and obesity in women is estimated at 30% and 22%, respectively, in Australia (5) with a 2.5% increase from 1980 to 2000 in women of reproductive age (6). Recent US 2009-2010 data similarly report that 31.9% of women of reproductive age (20-39 years) are obese (7). Given the adverse effects of overweight and obesity on reproductive dysfunction, this indicates a significant proportion of women of reproductive age who may suffer adverse effects of infertility related to excess adiposity.

Overweight and obesity and infertility

The association between female weight and infertility in the general population is well recognized, and reproductive dysfunction occurs in women who are underweight or overweight or obese (3,4). With regards to excess adiposity, overweight or obese women have an increased risk of menstrual problems, are less likely to conceive after 12 months of unprotected intercourse (8), and have an increased risk of menstrual irregularity, ovulatory dysfunction, or ovulatory infertility (3, 4, 9, 10). It is estimated that 25% of ovulatory infertility in the United States can be attributed to being overweight (4), and the relative risk of anovulation increases from 1.3 times in women with a BMI of 24-31 kg/m^2 to 2.7 times in women with a BMI > 32 kg/m^2 compared with women of normal weight (11). Overweight and obesity also are associated with reduced pregnancy and live birth rate in assisted reproductive technology (ART) and increased duration of ovulation induction, higher clomiphene citrate and gonadotropin doses to achieve ovarian response, impaired response to ovarian stimulation, decreased follicle number and oocytes retrieved, and increased cycle cancellation rate (12-16). There is also a recognized contribution specifically of abdominal adiposity to reproductive dysfunction and infertility in women. Women with elevated upper body fat (as assessed by methods including the waist to hip ratio or waist circumference) have an elevated risk of menstrual irregularity, a history of infertility, and a decrease in the probability of conception with ART (17-20).

Overweight and obesity and infertility and PCOS

Overweight and obesity can be associated with infertility in women first through the common condition of polycystic ovary syndrome (PCOS), which affects up to 18% of women of reproductive age (21). PCOS is associated reproductively with the diagnostic features of clinical or biochemical hyperandrogenism, anovulation or menstrual disturbances, or the presence of polycystic ovaries on ultrasound (22). PCOS is the most common cause of anovulatory infertility in women. It also is associated with the metabolic features of elevated risk factors and prevalence of impaired glucose tolerance (IGT), type 2 diabetes mellitus (DM2), and cardiovascular disease (CVD) and the psychological features of worsened anxiety, depression, and quality of life (23, 24). Insulin resistance is a key pathophysiological feature of PCOS and augments ovarian androgen production and reduces hepatic sex hormone-binding globulin production, overall contributing to hyperandrogenism (25). Insulin resistance also is associated with an elevated prevalence of cardiometabolic disease risk factors in both women with and without PCOS (26, 27). Insulin resistance is proposed to be present in PCOS in a form that is mechanistically distinct from obesity-associated insulin resistance and occurs even in lean women with PCOS (28). Where a woman with PCOS is overweight or obese, she may therefore have both PCOS-specific insulin resistance and obesity-associated insulin resistance. This then contributes to a worsening of the clinical features of PCOS (29). This is particularly relevant for central or visceral adiposity, which is strongly associated with insulin resistance in PCOS (30) or the general population (31). Overweight and obesity therefore contribute to reproductive abnormalities and infertility in women.

Overweight and obesity and infertility independent of PCOS

While overweight and obesity can contribute to anovulatory infertility or PCOS through disturbances to the hypothalamic pituitary ovarian axis, the association of overweight and obesity and infertility is not entirely explained by ovulatory disorders or PCOS. While PCOS is associated with reproductive dysfunction, menstrual irregularity, anovulation, and infertility, an elevated risk of primary ovulatory infertility has been observed for women with an elevated body mass index (BMI) at 18 years of age either with or without PCOS (11). Obesity also is associated with reduced conception rates and fecundability in women with regular cycles or normal ovulation (32-34). This indicates that while overweight and obesity may worsen the reproductive consequences of PCOS including ovulatory or menstrual disorders and ART outcomes such as ovulation induction, pregnancy rate, and pregnancy outcomes including stillbirth (35-37) and the diagnosis or prevalence of PCOS (38) an association between overweight and obesity and infertility in women is also present independent of PCOS. Overweight or obese women also have an increased risk of miscarriage (13, 15, 16, 39, 40). Additional effects of obesity may include impaired oocyte development, embryo development, and endometrial receptivity, and psychological features including sexual dysfunction and reduced sexual frequency (41, 42). These reproductive abnormalities may be associated with a variety of metabolic alterations that occur with obesity including insulin resistance, hyperandrogenism, altered hypothalamic pituitary ovarian axis function, gonadotropin regulation, altered oocyte lipid profile and inflammatory markers, and alterations in emerging novel circulating markers including leptin, adiponectin, interleukin-6, plasminogen-activator inhibitor-1, tumor necrosis factor-α, and ghrelin (41, 43).

Weight management and infertility

Given the association between overweight and obesity and infertility in women, either in PCOS, anovulatory women, or ovulatory women, weight management is a logical treatment strategy. This can be defined as prevention of excess weight gain, achieving a modest weight loss, and sustaining a reduced weight long-term. This is best achieved through lifestyle management, which traditionally refers to a complex multidisciplinary approach that combines dietary modification, physical activity, and behavioral interventions including attention to psychological adjustment, behavior modification, and stress management strategies (44, 45). Furthermore, maternal overweight and obesity are also associated with worsened maternal and infant pregnancy outcomes (46) and childhood obesity and obesity-associated metabolic outcomes (47, 48). This highlights the importance of optimal weight management on not only improving fertility but optimizing maternal obstetric and infant and child health.

The importance of weight management for infertility in women was highlighted by a number of programs conducted for obese anovulatory infertile women, either with or without PCOS, who undertook a 6-month multidisciplinary lifestyle management program after unsuccessful ovulation induction (49, 50). Weight loss of 6.3-10.2 kg was associated with resumption of ovulation and spontaneous or medical treatment-associated pregnancies in the majority of women and over two thirds of the women achieving a live birth. Similar results were reported for obese infertile women with or without menstrual irregularities or PCOS who were treated with a dietary and exercise weight reduction program. In obese infertile women, a 10.2 kg weight loss was associated with improvements in menstrual function for 80% of women and a 29% pregnancy rate in association with improvements in insulin resistance and hyperandrogenism (51). A lifestyle program during ART resulted in a significant reduction in weight (3.8±3.0 kg) and no adverse effects for pregnancy or live birth outcome compared to no treatment. An overall pregnancy rate of 53% (20/38 participants) was reported compared to 10%/month for spontaneous pregnancies in this population. While there were no differences in fertility outcomes between the intervention and control groups, for all women a waist circumference reduction was associated with increased odds of pregnancy (odds ratio [OR] 1.286, P=0.042), and an intention to treat analysis of women who achieved pregnancy had greater reductions in waist circumference compared to women who did not become pregnant (-5.5±3.7 compared to -2.6±4.1 cm).

Weight management and infertility in PCOS

A recent Cochrane review in PCOS identified n=6 studies in n=164 women assessing the effect of lifestyle interventions on the reproductive, metabolic, and psychological features with studies aimed at either specifically inducing or not inducing weight loss or examining lean or overweight participants. On meta-analysis, lifestyle intervention or modest weight loss was associated with decreased insulin resistance and hyperandrogenism. However, there were limited data reported on menstrual patterns and ovulation and no data reported on pregnancy outcomes, live birth, or miscarriage (52). Additional studies in PCOS lacking a defined control group have reported that modest weight loss (5%-10% of initial body weight) is associated with improvements in menstrual cycle regularity and ovulation (53,54) associated with reductions in central fat, intra-abdominal fat, or insulin resistance (55,56). With regards to the effects of weight loss or lifestyle management on clinical reproductive outcomes, a 6 month dietary intervention in overweight and obese anovulatory women with PCOS resulted in a ≥ 5% weight loss over 6 months in 25/33 women and resumption of regular menstrual cycles for n=18, spontaneous ovulation for n=15 women, spontaneous pregnancies for n=10, and live births for n=8 women (57). Similarly, a dietary intervention over 6-7 months in obese women with PCOS resulted in ≥ 5% weight loss in 78/144 women and improvement in menstrual function in 18/48 women with menstrual dysfunction, resumption of regular menstrual cycles in 6/48 previously amenorrheic women and spontaneous conception in 30/54 previously infertile women (58). Lifestyle management and weight loss in PCOS therefore improves reproductive and metabolic parameters and clinical reproductive outcomes although there is a lack of higher quality data for menstrual function, ovulation, pregnancy, and birth outcome data.

Bariatric surgery and infertility

While lifestyle interventions for weight management are recognized as logical initial treatment strategies for infertility in women with or without PCOS, it is recognized that maintaining a reduced weight long term is very difficult and weight regain is common (59). Alternative obesity treatments are therefore increasingly assessed, particularly in combination with lifestyle (diet, exercise, and behavioral) strategies or after lifestyle strategies have proved unsuccessful. Surgical treatments include bariatric surgery procedures such as gastrointestinal surgical procedures (gastric banding, gastric bypass including Roux-en-Y, biliopancreatic diversion, and sleeve gastrectomy). These have been associated with the resolution of clinical conditions including infertility and PCOS (60, 61). Improvements in menstrual regularity, ovulation, and fertility are also reported following bariatric surgery (62, 63), which may be related to postsurgery improvements in the hormonal profile, specifically decreased insulin resistance, hyperandrogenism, and estradiol or increased luteinizing hormone (LH) and follicle-stimulating hormone (FSH) in women with or without PCOS (61, 64-66), luteal function (67), and sexual function (66). A number of guidelines for bariatric surgery recommend eligibility with a BMI ≥ 40 kg/m2 or ≥35 kg/m2 if present with other comorbid conditions in conjunction with prior weight management programs (68, 69). However, the 2009 American Congress of Obstetricians and Gynecologists clinical practice guidelines do not specifically recommend bariatric surgery for fertility (70). It also is crucial to follow clinical practice points. Women are recommended to not conceive for a period of 12-24 months following bariatric surgery (70) due to concerns of fetal undernutrition and poor fetal growth (63), and contraceptive counseling post-bariatric surgery should be widely disseminated.

International guidelines for weight management through lifestyle interventions and infertility in women

International guidelines for weight management prior to pregnancy advise women to achieve a healthy weight prior to conception with obese women advised to lose at least 5%-10% of weight before becoming pregnant (71). Our group was recently instrumental in developing the first Evidence-Based Guidelines for the Assessment and Management of PCOS (72), which were conducted in accordance with national (Australia) and international (National Institute of Clinical Excellence) criteria for best practice in clinical guideline development. These stated that lifestyle management (single or combined approaches of diet, exercise, and/or behavioral interventions) for weight loss, prevention of weight gain, or for general health benefits should be recommended in PCOS (Level B evidence) and should target weight loss in overweight or obese women and prevention of weight gain in lean women, should include both reduced dietary energy intake and exercise, and should be first line therapy for all women (Level C evidence). Psychological factors should be considered and managed to optimize engagement and adherence with lifestyle interventions (Clinical Practice Point); face to face, tailored dietary advice, including education, behavioral change techniques, and ongoing support should be utilized for weight loss (Level C evidence) or prevention of weight gain (Clinical Consensus Recommendation). Healthy food choices should be used irrespective of diet composition for weight loss (Level C evidence) or prevention of weight gain (Level D evidence) and exercise participation of at least 150 minutes per week should be recommended with 90 minutes per week aerobic activity at moderate to high intensity (60%-90% of maximum heart rate) (Level D evidence). All health professionals should partner jointly with women with PCOS and referral to appropriate allied health professionals (e.g., dieticians, exercise physiologists) should be utilized where appropriate (Clinical Practice Point). Lifestyle management should be used to alleviate the clinical severity of infertility (Level C evidence) and should be the first line therapy in obese women with PCOS for 3-6 months to determine if ovulation is induced prior to pharmacological ovulation induction therapy. Bariatric surgery also could be considered second line therapy to improve fertility outcomes in adult women who are anovulatory with a BMI > 35 kg/m2 and who remain infertile despite undertaking an intensive lifestyle management program for a minimum of 6 months (72).

Conclusion

Overweight and obesity are associated with infertility in women, either in conjunction with or independent of the common condition PCOS. Weight management is crucial for not only improving the fertility of women but also in reducing obesity-associated maternal and infant outcomes during pregnancy and optimizing childhood obesity-associated disease risk. Modest weight loss improves reproductive hormone profiles, menstrual regularity and ovulation, and conception and birth outcomes in overweight or obese women with or without PCOS. International evidence-based guidelines recommend achieving a healthy weight prior to conception and aiming for modest weight loss if obese.

References

1. CDCP. Prevalence of Overweight and Obesity Among Adults: United States, 2003-2004.: US Department of Health and Human Services, 2003.
2. World Health Organisation. Obesity: Preventing and managing the global epidemic. Geneva: World Health Organisation, 1997.
3. Grodstein F, Goldman MB, Cramer DW. Body mass index and ovulatory infertility. Epidemiology 1994;5:247-50.
4. Rich-Edwards JW, Spiegelman D, Garland M, et al. Physical activity, body mass index, and ovulatory disorder infertility. Epidemiology 2002;13:184-90.
5. Cameron AJ, Welborn TA, Zimmet PZ, et al. Overweight and obesity in Australia: the 1999-2000 Australian Diabetes, Obesity and Lifestyle Study (AusDiab). Med J Aust 2003;178:427-32.
6. AIHW. Health, well-being and bodyweight:characteristics of overweight and obesity in Australia, 2001. Australian Institute of Health and Welfare Bulletin No. 13 2001.
7. Ogden CL, Carroll MD, Kit BK, Flegal KM. Prevalence of obesity in the United States, 2009-2010. NCHS Data Brief 2012:1-8.
8. Lake JK, Power C, Cole TJ. Women's reproductive health: the role of body mass index in early and adult life. Int J Obes Relat Metab Disord 1997;21:432-8.
9. Green BB, Weiss NS, Daling JR. Risk of ovulatory infertility in relation to body weight. Fertil Steril 1988;50:721-6.
10. Hartz AJ, Barboriak PN, Wong A, Katayama KP, Rimm AA. The association of obesity with infertility and related menstural abnormalities in women. Int J Obes 1979;3:57-73.
11. Rich-Edwards JW, Goldman MB, Willett WC, et al. Adolescent body mass index and infertility caused by ovulatory disorder. Am J Obstet Gynecol 1994;171:171-7.
12. Tamer Erel C, Senturk LM. The impact of body mass index on assisted reproduction. Curr Opin Obstet Gynecol 2009;21:228-35.
13. Wang JX, Davies M, Norman RJ. Body mass and probability of pregnancy during assisted reproduction treatment: retrospective study. Bmj 2000;321:1320-1.
14. Dodson WC, Kunselman AR, Legro RS. Association of obesity with treatment outcomes in ovulatory infertile women undergoing superovulation and intrauterine insemination. Fertil Steril 2006;86:642-6.
15. Fedorcsak P, Dale PO, Storeng R, et al. Impact of overweight and underweight on assisted reproduction treatment. Hum Reprod 2004;19:2523-8.
16. Rittenberg V, Seshadri S, Sunkara SK, Sobaleva S, Oteng-Ntim E, El-Toukhy T. Effect of body mass index on IVF treatment outcome: an updated systematic review and meta-analysis. Reprod Biomed Online 2011;23:421-39.
17. Hartz AJ, Rupley DC, Rimm AA. The association of girth measurements with disease in 32,856 women. Am J Epidemiol 1984;119:71-80.

18. Kaye SA, Folsom AR, Prineas RJ, Potter JD, Gapstur SM. The association of body fat distribution with lifestyle and reproductive factors in a population study of postmenopausal women. Int J Obes 1990;14:583-91.
19. Zaadstra BM, Seidell JC, Van Noord PA, et al. Fat and female fecundity: prospective study of effect of body fat distribution on conception rates. Bmj 1993;306:484-7.
20. Wass P, Waldenstrom U, Rossner S, Hellberg D. An android body fat distribution in females impairs the pregnancy rate of in-vitro fertilization-embryo transfer. Hum Reprod 1997;12:2057-60.
21. March WA, Moore VM, Willson KJ, Phillips DI, Norman RJ, Davies MJ. The prevalence of polycystic ovary syndrome in a community sample assessed under contrasting diagnostic criteria. Hum Reprod 2010;25:544-51.
22. Norman RJ, Dewailly D, Legro RS, Hickey TE. Polycystic ovary syndrome. Lancet 2007;370:685-97.
23. Moran LJ, Misso ML, Wild RA, Norman RJ. Impaired glucose tolerance, type 2 diabetes and metabolic syndrome in polycystic ovary syndrome: a systematic review and meta-analysis. Hum Reprod Update 2010;16:347-363.
24. Barry JA, Kuczmierczyk AR, Hardiman PJ. Anxiety and depression in polycystic ovary syndrome: a systematic review and meta-analysis. Hum Reprod 2011;26:2442-51.
25. Teede H, Hutchison SK, Zoungas S. The management of insulin resistance in polycystic ovary syndrome. Trends Endocrinol Metab 2007;18:273-9.
26. Haffner SM, Stern MP, Mitchell BD, Hazuda HP, Patterson JK. Incidence of type II diabetes in Mexican Americans predicted by fasting insulin and glucose levels, obesity, and body-fat distribution. Diabetes 1990;39:283-8.
27. Ehrmann DA, Liljenquist DR, Kasza K, et al. Prevalence and predictors of the metabolic syndrome in women with polycystic ovary syndrome. Journal of Clinical Endocrinology & Metabolism 2006;91:48-53.
28. Dunaif A, Finegood DT. Beta-cell dysfunction independent of obesity and glucose intolerance in the polycystic ovary syndrome. J Clin Endocrinol Metab 1996;81:942-7.
29. Lim SS, Norman RJ, Davies MJ, Moran LJ. The effect of obesity on polycystic ovary syndrome: a systematic review and meta-analysis. Obes Rev 2012.
30. Goverde AJ, van Koert AJ, Eijkemans MJ, et al. Indicators for metabolic disturbances in anovulatory women with polycystic ovary syndrome diagnosed according to the Rotterdam consensus criteria. Hum Reprod 2009;24:710-7.
31. Yamashita S, Nakamura T, Shimomura I, et al. Insulin resistance and body fat distribution. Diabetes Care 1996;19:287-91.
32. Jensen TK, Scheike T, Keiding N, Schaumburg I, Grandjean P. Fecundability in relation to body mass and menstrual cycle patterns. Epidemiology 1999;10:422-8.
33. van der Steeg JW, Steures P, Eijkemans MJ, et al. Obesity affects spontaneous pregnancy chances in subfertile, ovulatory women. Hum Reprod 2008;23:324-8.
34. Gesink Law DC, Maclehose RF, Longnecker MP. Obesity and time to pregnancy. Hum Reprod 2007;22:414-20.
35. Balen AH, Conway GS, Kaltsas G, et al. Polycystic ovary syndrome: the spectrum of the disorder in 1741 patients. Hum Reprod 1995;10:2107-11.
36. Kiddy DS, Sharp PS, White DM, et al. Differences in clinical and endocrine features between obese and non-obese subjects with polycystic ovary syndrome: an analysis of 263 consecutive cases. Clin Endocrinol (Oxf) 1990;32:213-20.
37. Al-Azemi M, Omu FE, Omu AE. The effect of obesity on the outcome of infertility management in women with polycystic ovary syndrome. Arch Gynecol Obstet 2004;270:205-10.

38. Teede HJ, Joham AE, Paul E, et al. Longitudinal weight gain in women identified with Polycystic Ovary Syndrome: Results of an observational study in young women. Obesity 2012;In press.
39. Bohrer M, Kemmann E. Risk factors for spontaneous abortion in menotropin-treated women. Fertil Steril 1987;48:571-5.
40. Boots C, Stephenson MD. Does obesity increase the risk of miscarriage in spontaneous conception: a systematic review. Semin Reprod Med 2011;29:507-13.
41. Brewer CJ, Balen AH. The adverse effects of obesity on conception and implantation. Reproduction 2010;140:347-64.
42. Robker RL. Evidence that obesity alters the quality of oocytes and embryos. Pathophysiology 2008;15:115-21.
43. Robker RL, Wu LL, Yang X. Inflammatory pathways linking obesity and ovarian dysfunction. J Reprod Immunol 2011;88:142-8.
44. NHMRC. Clinical guidelines for weight control and obesity management in adults. 2002.
45. Clinical guidelines on the identification, evaluation, and treatment of overweight and obesity in adults: executive summary. Expert Panel on the Identification, Evaluation, and Treatment of Overweight in Adults. Am J Clin Nutr 1998;68:899-917.
46. Dodd JM, Grivell RM, Ngyuen MA, Chan A, Robinson JS. Maternal and perinatal health outcomes by maternal body mass index category. . ANZJOG 2011;51:136-40.
47. Schack-Nielsen L, Michaelsen KF, Gamborg M, Mortensen EL, Sorensen TI. Gestational weight gain in relation to offspring body mass index and obesity from infancy through adulthood. Int J Obes (Lond) 2010;34:67-74.
48. Oken E, Taveras EM, Kleinman KP, Rich-Edwards JW, Gillman MW. Gestational weight gain and child adiposity at age 3 years. American Journal of Obstetrics & Gynecology 2007;196:322.e1-322.e8.
49. Clark AM, Ledger W, Galletly C, et al. Weight loss results in significant improvement in pregnancy and ovulation rates in anovulatory obese women. Hum Reprod 1995;10:2705-12.
50. Clark AM, Thornley B, Tomlinson L, Galletley C, Norman RJ. Weight loss in obese infertile women results in improvement in reproductive outcome for all forms of fertility treatment. Hum Reprod 1998;13:1502-5.
51. Hollmann M, Runnebaum B, Gerhard I. Effects of weight loss on the hormonal profile in obese, infertile women. Hum Reprod 1996;11:1884-91.
52. Moran LJ, Hutchison SK, Norman RJ, Teede HJ. Lifestyle changes in women with polycystic ovary syndrome. Cochrane Database of Systematic Reviews 2011;2.
53. Moran LJ, Noakes M, Clifton PM, Tomlinson L, Galletly C, Norman RJ. Dietary composition in restoring reproductive and metabolic physiology in overweight women with polycystic ovary syndrome. J Clin Endocrinol Metab 2003;88:812-9.
54. Moran LJ, Noakes M, Clifton PM, Wittert GA, Williams G, Norman RJ. Short-term meal replacements followed by dietary macronutrient restriction enhance weight loss in polycystic ovary syndrome. Am J Clin Nutr 2006;84:77-87.
55. Huber-Buchholz MM, Carey DG, Norman RJ. Restoration of reproductive potential by lifestyle modification in obese polycystic ovary syndrome: role of insulin sensitivity and luteinizing hormone. J Clin Endocrinol Metab 1999;84:1470-4.
56. Kuchenbecker WK, Groen H, van Asselt SJ, et al. In women with polycystic ovary syndrome and obesity, loss of intra-abdominal fat is associated with resumption of ovulation. Hum Reprod 2011;26:2505-12.
57. Crosignani PG, Colombo M, Vegetti W, Somigliana E, Gessati A, Ragni G. Overweight and obese anovulatory patients with polycystic ovaries: parallel improvements in anthropometric indices, ovarian physiology and fertility rate induced by diet. Hum Reprod 2003;18:1928-32.

58. Tolino A, Gambardella V, Caccavale C, et al. Evaluation of ovarian functionality after a dietary treatment in obese women with polycystic ovary syndrome. Eur J Obstet Gynecol Reprod Biol 2005;119:87-93.
59. Ayyad C, Andersen T. Long-term efficacy of dietary treatment of obesity: a systematic review of studies published between 1931 and 1999. Obes Rev 2000;1:113-9.
60. Neto RM, Herbella FA, Tauil RM, Silva FS, de Lima SE, Jr. Comorbidities Remission After Roux-en-Y Gastric Bypass for Morbid Obesity is Sustained in a Long-Term Follow-up and Correlates with Weight Regain. Obes Surg 2012;22:1580-5.
61. Escobar-Morreale HF, Botella-Carretero JI, Alvarez-Blasco F, Sancho J, San Millan JL. The polycystic ovary syndrome associated with morbid obesity may resolve after weight loss induced by bariatric surgery. J Clin Endocrinol Metab 2005;90:6364-9.
62. Maggard MA, Yermilov I, Li Z, et al. Pregnancy and fertility following bariatric surgery: a systematic review. JAMA 2008;300:2286-96.
63. Guelinckx I, Devlieger R, Vansant G. Reproductive outcome after bariatric surgery: a critical review. Hum Reprod Update 2009;15:189-201.
64. Bastounis EA, Karayiannakis AJ, Syrigos K, Zbar A, Makri GG, Alexiou D. Sex hormone changes in morbidly obese patients after vertical banded gastroplasty. Eur Surg Res 1998;30:43-7.
65. Gerrits EG, Ceulemans R, van Hee R, Hendrickx L, Totte E. Contraceptive treatment after biliopancreatic diversion needs consensus. Obes Surg 2003;13:378-82.
66. Legro RS, Dodson WC, Gnatuk CL, et al. Effects of gastric bypass surgery on female reproductive function. J Clin Endocrinol Metab 2012;97:4540-8.
67. Rochester D, Jain A, Polotsky AJ, et al. Partial recovery of luteal function after bariatric surgery in obese women. Fertil Steril 2009;92:1410-5.
68. Dixon JB, le Roux CW, Rubino F, Zimmet P. Bariatric surgery for type 2 diabetes. Lancet 2012;379:2300-11.
69. SIGN. Management of Obesity: A national clinical guideline. Edinburgh, Scotland, 2010.
70. ACOG. Bariatric Surgery and Pregnancy. ACOG Practice Bulletin No. 105. . Obstet Gynecol 2009;113:1405-13.
71. NICE. Dietary interventions and physical activity interventions for weight management before, during and after pregnancy. London, UK.: National Institute for Health and Clinical Excellence 2010.
72. Teede HJ, Misso ML, Deeks AA, et al. Assessment and management of polycystic ovary syndrome: summary of an evidence-based guideline. Med J Aust 2011;195:S65-112.

Trilogy 5. Adhesions and reproductive surgery

Molecular biologic regulation of peritoneal repair and adhesion development

Michael P. Diamond and Ghassan M. Saed***

*Georgia Regents University, Augusta, United States
**Wayne State University, Detroit, United States

Postoperative adhesions represent tissue adherence at locations where there should be no such attachments. Adhesions can be bands that are plastic wrap-like transparent bands, or they can be more opaque and dense, with or without vascularity. Additionally, adhesions can be "cohesive," meaning that there are direct connections from one tissue to another without an intervening adhesive band.

Teleologically, adhesions represent a means by which the body tries to re-establish a supply of oxygen and nutrients as well as remove metabolic wastes from tissue that has been injured by pathologic processes and/or surgery per se. Surgery, with its associated disruption of blood supply to tissue, coagulating, and ligating of vessels, results in deprivation of tissue perfusion. The pathways leading to adhesion development include histamine release, generation of cytokines and growth factors, enhanced expression of extracellular matrix material, inhibition of plasminogen activator activity, and stimulation of angiogenesis.

Following tissue injury, histamine release enhances cellular migration to the wounded sites, with vascular leakage leading to accumulation of tissue exudate that accumulates at the tissue surface, mixing with any blood that has collected from local or distant vascular disruption. Whether or not this fibrinosis persists is a key factor in determining whether an adhesion develops at that location. A major determinant of persistence is the degree of plasminogen activator activity. Plasminogen activator activity (PAA), which can be determined by the ratio of tissue plasminogen activator (tPA) to its inhibitor plasminogen activator inhibitor-1 (PAI-1), resides in both the peritoneal mesothelial cells as well as the underlying fibroblasts. If these cells are functioning normally, PAA persists, with dissolution of the fibrinous mass. Then fibroblasts, which begin to migrate to the site of tissue injury, must stop at the tissue surface. Any extracellular matrix produced may contribute to fibrosis, but without development of an adhesive band. This tissue surface is remesothelialized within 3 to 5 days. In contrast, in the presence of tissue hypoxia, there is a reduction in expression of tPA and an increase in PAI-1 expression, resulting in an impairment of PAA. Under these conditions, the fibrinous mass persists. Fibroblasts, which migrate towards the site of tissue injury, are able to migrate into the persisting fibrinous mass via a mechanism that is in part transforming growth factor-beta (TGF-β) mediated, with subsequent deposition of extracellular matrix material, including collagens I and III and fibronectin. As this developing adhesion continues to be relatively hypoxic, there is continuing production of pro-oxidants, such as superoxide and nitric oxide, which maintain continuing signaling by hypoxia inducible factor-alpha (HIF-1α), which continues to stimulate the cascading pathways. This includes continued increased expression of TGF-β1, tumor necrosis factor alpha (TNFα), and interleukin 6 (IL-6), as well as increased expression of vascular endothelial growth factor (VEGF). Of note, this enhancement of VEGF expression is also associated with neoangiogenesis, which develops within the now-established adhesion. Similar changes for many of these parameters have also been observed in mesothelial cells and macrophages.

Concurrently with fibroblast migration into the fibrinous mass is remesotheliazation of the injured tissue surface, as well as deposition of mesothelial cells surrounding the fibroblast-infiltrated fibrinous mass, resulting in a monolayer mesothelial cell covering the adhesive bands. Importantly, this process of remesotheliazation is thought to be completed in 3 to 5 days after tissue injury (unless there is persisting tissue injury). In situations where one injured tissue surface is in contact with another, initiation of cohesive adhesion development at these sites has been documented to occur as early as 8 hours after injury in an animal model. Such a process is also likely mediated in part by integrins.

An important attribute of the injured tissues and adhesions is the anaerobic metabolism that is in part necessitated by the lack of oxygen supply for oxidative metabolism through the Kreb's cycle. Consequently, adhesions manifest collection of lactic acid with a tendency for lowering of tissue pH, which if severe enough could interfere with protein and enzyme functions. Adhesions, and adhesion fibroblasts, also manifest increased oxidative stress. This is characterized by increased generation of toxic reactive oxygen and reactive nitrogen species, which can bind to DNA, proteins, and lipids with resultant deterioration in cellular function.

Utilizing isolated fibroblasts from normal peritoneum and adhesions of the same patients, we have identified that adhesion fibroblasts manifest the inflammatory-like milieu described above, including the aforementioned changes in extracellular matrix, growth factors, and cytokines. Additionally, there is increased expression of cyclooxygenase (COX-2), P53, and alpha smooth muscle actin. Additionally, the adhesion fibroblasts have decreased rates of apoptosis (programmed cell death), which has been demonstrated by multiple complementary approaches, including mRNA expression and protein levels of BAX, BCL2, and caspase 3, as well as by flow cytometry.

Importantly, the cell culture model has allowed examination not only of the impact of hypoxia on these cells, but also the effect of reoxygenation. Surprisingly, when examining the expression of collagen I and TGF-β, the elevation in expression identified with exposure to hypoxia (2% oxygen) was not restored to that of normal peritoneal fibroblasts by reoxygenation. Thus, the inflammatory-like changes manifested by hypoxia (e.g., after surgical injury and revascularization) persist! Persistence of these changes, in combination with the reduction in apoptosis, thus provides a molecular biology mechanism for the previously identified high rate of adhesion development after surgery, as well as the greater rates of adhesion reformation after adhesiolysis than de novo adhesion formation after primary surgery.

In fact, approximately 70%-90% of women develop adhesions after gynecology surgery performed at laparotomy, with occurrence at specific anatomic locations after surgical procedures such as myomectomy, ovarian cystectomy, and treatment of endometriosis in the same range. While it had been hoped that minimally invasive laparoscopic surgery would be associated with a reduction in adhesion development, examination of the incidence of adhesions after laparoscopic surgery has shown rates that appear to be equivalent to those seen after laparotomy.

When examining the time it takes for peritoneal repair (e.g., remesotheliazation) after surgery, it appears that it is completed within 3 to 5 days of surgical injury. Thus, approaches to reduce postoperative adhesions (including mode of entry into the abdomen, surgical instrumentation, and anti-adhesion adjuvants) need to effect peritoneal repair processes during this early short time interval. This observation is consistent with clinical evaluations of adhesion development at early second-look laparoscopies that have shown no difference in adhesion incidence, severity, or extent over a time interval of 1 to 12 weeks after the initial surgical procedure. The observation that adhesions become denser and more vascular over a time interval of 1 to 2 years is consistent with the concept that the adhesion continues to be relatively hypoxic over this time period, with increasing vascularity as a teleological effort of the body to re-establish the supply of oxygen and nutrients to these tissues.

Improved understanding of the pathogenesis will be important to identify approaches to reduce or eliminate postoperative adhesions. While approaches identified to reduce adhesions may be able to be administered systemically, it is likely that local delivery, such as with an anti-adhesion adjuvant that has its own inherent ability to reduce postoperative adhesions, will allow for prolonged delivery during the healing process, thereby improving efficacy.

Decision-making in reproductive surgery

Luk Rombauts

Monash IVF, Melbourne, Australia

Introduction

"To decide" derives from the Latin decider, which literally means "to cut off," from de- "off," and caedere "to cut." The sense of loss conveyed in the original meaning of the Latin verb is also apparent in many other languages, for example, the beautiful French expression 'Choisir c'est mourir un peu' (to choose is to die a little) or the English version 'You can't have your cake and eat it.'

These idioms illustrate the concept of trade-offs. A trade-off is a situation that involves losing one quality or aspect of something in return for gaining another quality or aspect. It often implies a decision to be made with full comprehension of both the upside and downside of a particular choice (1).

Decision-makers and their environment

Decisions are made by decision-makers who are influenced by the decision environment they operate in. In medicine, health-related trade-off decisions are made by patients - and healthy people, for that matter - who are the real decision-makers as they provide the ultimate consent to proceed with screening, examination, diagnostic testing, and treatment. These medical decisions may be less frequent than other decisions, but they generally are of much greater importance. Doctors should be thought of as facilitators of this process and in that sense they are part of the patient's decision environment. The decision environment sphere includes not only other facilitators such as family and support staff, but also regulators such as governments, professional societies, and colleges, which set competency standards, guidelines, and health budgets, and also more abstract social constructs such as moral principles (e.g., first, do no harm).

Defining good decisions

Ultimately, good decisions should lead to a good outcome, use all relevant information, be derived after a deliberative process, be able to be justified to others, and be consistent with the life goals of the decision-maker.

Defining a good outcome, however, is not always straightforward. Having restored tubal patency following a microsurgical tubal reanastomosis without complications can be defined as a successful surgical outcome in a narrow sense, but in a broader sense the patient will define success as a live birth. Similarly, endometriosis patients may not be interested so much in a complete clearance of all lesions as in a restoration of their overall quality of life. In other words, there are many layers or dimensions that make up a good health outcome and the importance of these may vary significantly among individuals. Another problem for patients is that it may be difficult for them to have a realistic view of what to expect following surgery.

Different methodologies, including deconstructive and holistic approaches, have been developed to facilitate the communication between surgeons and patients so that both can define better what health dimensions are valued most. As an example, the Endometriosis Health Profile-30 contains a core questionnaire with 30 items and 5 scales for pain, control and powerlessness, emotional well-being, social support, and self-image (2). Other methods assume that patients may not always explicitly deconstruct their decisions in many dimensions and use a more intuitive holistic approach, such as the time trade-off or the standard gamble. In the time trade-off the patient is asked whether he/she would rather not have treatment or a treatment that delivers a chance of perfect health but with a reduced life expectancy (e.g., 5 years less). In the standard gamble the patient is asked whether he/she would rather not have treatment or a treatment that delivers a chance of perfect health (e.g., 95%) but also a chance of death (e.g., 5%). The point at which the patient is willing to accept the trade-off or gamble is called the utility. For treatments where death or reduced life expectancy is an extremely unlikely outcome, the gambles may need to be adjusted to different adverse outcomes. These methods make the assumption that patients have no difficulty processing probabilities, but despite these and other disadvantages, these methods force the patient to think more deliberately about what they value in health.

A typical outcome following surgery is that the patient will go through a recovery period during which her health state will temporarily deteriorate. Furthermore, the improved health state that the patient eventually expects to achieve may not be permanent; surgery for endometriosis-related pain has a reported recurrence rate of between 10%-55% in the first 12 months. The way a patient's health quality is expected to vary over time can be plotted on a graph with the resulting area under the curve (AUC) calculated as the quality-adjusted life years (QALY). Although different treatments can thus be compared and communicated more accurately, not everything is captured by the QALY. For example, two treatments may have an equal QALY (same AUC), and yet one may be strongly preferred by patients because its associated health quality is expected to increase compared to the alternative where it decreases over time.

Communicating information

The principle of informed consent requires the patient to make decisions based on the best available evidence. Clinicians already have access to a large body of knowledge summarized in Cochrane reviews, evidence-based guidelines, and consensus statements, but not all relevant questions have been adequately covered with good-quality studies. Furthermore, even when the evidence is very solid, outcomes are often expressed as probabilities with a certain degree of uncertainty. Unfortunately, the human mind does not come with a natural ability to compute probabilities easily. Even very numerate people, including medical specialists, often make significant errors when interpreting such information (3). Not surprisingly, understanding and addressing the pitfalls of communicating expected outcomes and probable risks to patients with varying levels of education is a science in itself.

It is well known that people are generally better at dealing with frequencies rather than probabilities (e.g., 1 in 10,000 versus 0.01%), even though they represent the same probability (4). Information regarding treatment effects can also be presented in ways that are mathematically equivalent, but some formulations may appear more favorable to both patients and doctors (5). This point can be illustrated with the findings of the Endocan study, which demonstrated that laparoscopic ablation of minimal to mild endometriosis increases the chance of a pregnancy lasting longer than 20 weeks. The relative risk (RR) was 1.71, or 71% more pregnancies in the treatment arm. The absolute risk (AR) was 0.12, which means that there were 12 extra pregnancies (> 20 weeks) for every 100 women who underwent laparoscopic ablation. The most relevant statistic for patients perhaps is the number needed to treat (NNT): in this study 9 patients needed to be treated to achieve 1 extra pregnancy (6). Nevertheless, patients and clinicians are more likely to opt for the surgery after being presented with the relative risk, which leads them to overestimate the real treatment effect.

Heuristics and their biases

When we make decisions, we like to believe that our decisions are well-considered and free of bias. Much work has been done in the field of behavioral science showing that this belief is misplaced. The studies of Kahneman and Tversky and many others have identified many biases that lead us to make poor judgments. Kahneman and Tversky developed a conceptual model of the functioning brain, showing through clever experiments that there are two processes at work: System 1 and System 2 (7). System 1 or fast thinking is the sort of automatic thinking we associate with intuition, snap decisions, and rule of thumb. System 2 or slow thinking involves those thought processes that require deep analysis and effort, such as complex algebra. System 2 is not only slow but also lazy and is often more than happy to accept the 'advice' from System 1. These mental shortcuts to ease the cognitive load of decision-making are called heuristics. In many situations they are very helpful, but sometimes they can lead to significant errors of judgment and bias. A further problem is that it does not always help to know that these heuristics are at work. The well-known Müller-Lyer illusion (Figure 1) serves as a good analogy. Although we know that the lines are the same length we cannot avoid seeing them being different lengths.

It is good to highlight here some of the more important biases that influence medical decision-making.

The availability bias occurs when we confuse the ease with which we recall events as a proxy for the likelihood that they will occur. For example, the probability of certain events happening in new patients is generally overestimated because a surgeon may recall similar cases or events more easily if they were unusual (rare condition) or memorable (the 'close shave'). When patients have had a previous bad experience with a procedure they are also likely to show an aversion towards the intervention even when the alternative options are more risky.

The representativeness bias occurs when we are too quick to assume that something that seems similar to other things in a certain category (stereotype) is itself more likely a member of that category: if it looks like a duck, walks like a duck, and quacks like a duck, then it is a duck. It is the heuristic that often leads us to be convinced that a 'textbook' set of symptoms represents a very rare condition, even though it is more probable that the symptoms can be explained by other conditions that are far more prevalent. Immediate recognition of the stereotype leads us to ignore the base rate frequency.

The anchoring bias refers to the tendency to rely too much on the first available information (the anchor) without adjusting appropriately when further facts are presented. In medicine, doctors tend to focus too strongly on features in the patient's initial presentation without reviewing the working diagnosis when more information becomes available. A referral letter can, for example, provide a strong anchor if it contains the referring doctor's provisional diagnosis.

Confirmatory bias can further aggravate this problem with our tendency to look for, recognize, and recall information that fits our tentative diagnosis. This bias also leads us to disregard information that contradicts our hypothesis and stops us from completing our mental check list because we are convinced we have already established a firm diagnosis. Patients increasingly self-diagnose and can also be guilty of confirmation bias. Many are very adept at fitting a square peg in a round hole, especially now that access to information on the internet has become so easy. These patients also tend to seek out advice from doctors who confirm their bias.

The effects of superiority bias have been well documented in many situations. A well-known example is the study of Svenson et al. (8) who showed that 93% of survey respondents in a sample of US drivers rated themselves better than an average driver. In medicine, clinicians also tend to overestimate their ability to make correct diagnoses and good treatment decisions (9).

Another major problem that affects both patients and their doctors is the framing effect. The framing effect, described first by Tversky and Kahneman (10), is an important cognitive bias that leads people to make different decisions depending on how the information is presented. Tversky and Kahneman illustrated this effect with what has now become known as the "Asian disease problem."

Subjects were asked to imagine that the United States is preparing for the outbreak of an unusual Asian disease, which is expected to kill 600 people. Two alternative programs to combat the disease have been proposed. Subjects were told to assume that the exact scientific estimation of the consequences of the programs is as follows (subjects were randomized to receive a 'positive' frame or a 'negative frame'):

Positive frame (lives saved):
- If Program A is adopted, 200 people will be saved.
- If Program B is adopted, there is a one-third probability that 600 people will be saved and a two-thirds probability that no people will be saved.

Negative frame (lives lost):
- If Program C is adopted, 400 people will die.
- If Program D is adopted, there is a one-third probability that no one will die and a two-thirds probability that 600 people will die.

Subjects presented with the positive frame were more likely to choose Program A (the certain option), whereas subjects offered the negative frame preferred Program D (the gamble), even though the consequences of A and C on the one hand and C and D on the other are exactly the same. Loss aversion is a primary tenet of Prospect Theory as formulated by Tversky and Kahneman (11). It states that the pain of loss is often greater in magnitude than the pleasure of gain, and this helps to explain why people faced with a loss are more likely to engage in risky behaviors (e.g., the gamble in the Asian disease problem) designed to offset that loss than if they are faced with a gain.

The relevance for patients is that they may opt for one treatment over another depending on whether the outcomes are stated as a loss or a gain. And to make matters more complex, the impact of the frame depends on the type of treatment being decided on. Invasive treatments are generally more preferred in a positive frame than in a negative frame, whereas the opposite applies for medical treatments.

Framing also occurs when a decision is based on a process of selection rather than elimination. When selecting the best treatment for endometriosis-related pain from a number of possible options, the gynecologist will be inclined to make the selection by comparing the benefits of each alternative, such as efficacy and affordability. On the other hand, when asked to exclude options from the same set, (s)he will be more likely to focus on a comparison of the risks or disadvantages of each.

At any given time the decision process may involve complex interactions between many different heuristics, some of which are helpful and some of which introduce bias. Teaching metacognition, or thinking about the thinking, has been advocated as one way to reduce the effect of heuristic bias in decision-making processes (12).

Decisions under pressure

The decision process that leads to a diagnosis or the selection of the most suitable treatment generally occurs in a controlled environment where time is on the surgeon's side. In emergency situations, however, the decision process is not aimed at making the best decision, but at gaining satisfactory control of the situation in the available time. The response in these emergencies thus centers around three key concerns: 1) the nature of the problem, 2) the level of risk, and 3) the available time. Surgeons and anesthetists tend to use an analytical approach if more time is available, and a rule-based (check-list) or intuitive approach (learned behaviors) if the risk is very high and there is little time to think (13). The level of experience of the surgeon often dictates which approach will dominate and the approach may shift dynamically from an intuitive one to a rule-based or analytical one once the critical emergency (e.g., catastrophic bleeding) has been brought under control.

Conclusion

Medical decisions require informed consent and put the patient at the center of almost all such decisions. Doctors, therefore, need to understand what the patient values and expects from her treatment and need to be adept at tailoring the most appropriate communication strategy to each individual patient. Cognitive heuristics can be powerful assistants in decision-making, but the best protection against the biases they are also associated with is being mindful that they exist.

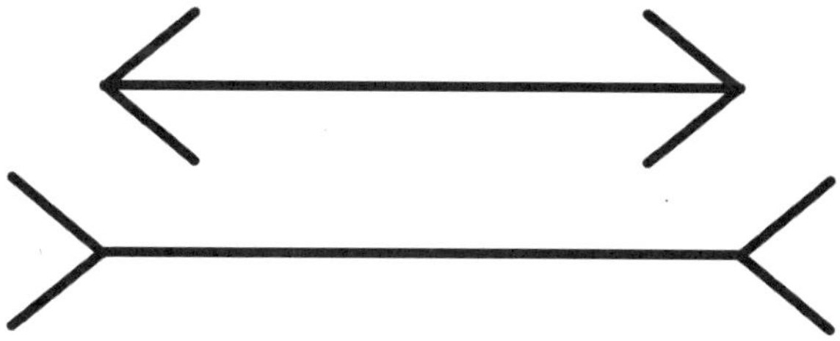

Figure 1. The Müller-Lyer illusion

References

1. "Trade-off." Wikipedia. Wikimedia Foundation, Inc, 2 Mar. 2013. Web. 10 Mar. 2013. <en.wikipedia.org/wiki/Trade-off>.
2. Jones G, Kennedy S, Barnard A, Wong J, Jenkinson C. Development of an endometriosis quality-of-life instrument: The Endometriosis Health Profile-30. Obstet Gynecol. 2001;98(2):258-64.
3. Gigerenzer G, Hoffrage U. How to improve Bayesian reasoning without instruction: Frequency formats. Psychological Review 1995;102:684-704.
4. Tversky A, Kahneman D. Extensional versus intuitive reasoning: The conjunction fallacy in probability judgment. Psychological Review 1983;90:293-323.
5. Carling CL, Kristoffersen DT, Montori VM, Herrin J, Schünemann HJ, Treweek S, Akl EA, Oxman AD. The effect of alternative summary statistics for communicating risk reduction on decisions about taking statins: a randomized trial. PLoS Med 2009;6(8):e1000134.
6. Interpretation of clinical trial results. The Practice Committee of the ASRM, F&S 2008;90:S114-120.
7. Kahneman D. A perspective on judgement and choice. American Psychologist 2003; 58:697-720.

8. Svenson O. Are we all less risky and more skillful than our fellow drivers?. Acta Psychologica 1981;47 (2): 143–148.
9. Berner ES, Graber ML. Overconfidence as a cause of diagnostic error in medicine. Am J Med. 2008 May;121(5 Suppl):S2-23.
10. Tversky A, Kahneman D. The framing of decisions and the psychology of choice. Science 1981;211:453–458.
11. Kahneman D, Tversky A. Prospect theory: an analysis of decision under risk. Econometrica 1979;47:263–291.
12. Croskerry P. Cognitive forcing strategies in clinical decision making. Ann Emerg Med. 2003;41:110-20.
13. Pauley K, Flin R, Yule S, Youngson G. Surgeons' intraoperative decision making and risk management. Am J Surg 2011;202:375-81.

New technologies in reproductive surgery

Geoffrey H. Trew

Hammersmith & Queen Charlotte's Hospital, London, United Kingdom

Introduction

Adhesion formation is almost inevitable after any form of gynecological surgery. Adhesions are now the most frequent complication of abdominopelvic surgery, representing one of the greatest unresolved problems in surgery today (1, 2, 3). They pose serious quality-of-life issues for many patients, with associated social and health care costs. Although adhesiolysis remains the main treatment, adhesions reform in most patients and reformed adhesions tend to be more dense and severe than de novo adhesions (4, 3).

Despite advances in surgical techniques, the health care and patient-related burden of adhesion-related complications has not changed. While laparoscopy has been commonly believed to be less adhesiogenic compared to laparotomy, the comparative risk of adhesion-related complications following open and laparoscopic gynecological surgery is similar for most procedures (5).

An Expert Working Party of the European Society of Gynaecological Endoscopy (ESGE) comprehensively reviewed the evidence on adhesions, their health impact, and adhesion-reduction strategies and published broad practice consensus proposals on adhesions and their prevention in gynecological surgery (2, 3). This work was then further extended by various expert groups at a national level including Spain (6), Italy (7), France (8, 9), Poland (10), Germany (11), and Canada (12).

Despite the high risk and serious consequences of adhesions, few patients receive information even as part of informed consent (13, 14, 15, 16, 17). This is important as medico-legal interest in adhesion-related complications is rising (18).

In the United Kingdom formal guidance has been issued to surgeons that all risks over 1%–2% should be discussed as part of consent or failure of notification could be deemed to be negligent. It advises that patients should be informed in writing even if the likelihood of serious adverse outcomes 'is small' (19, 20). Authorities in various countries including Australia, Canada, and France have also adopted high standards emphasizing the need for patients to be better informed (21, 22). 'Common sense is the key' (23).

As well as improvements in surgical technique, developments in adhesion-reduction strategies and new agents offer a realistic possibility of reducing adhesions and improving outcomes for patients. General consensus from a number of groups is that use of adhesion reduction agents should now be considered, particularly in high-risk surgery and in patients with adhesiogenic conditions (2, 3, 6, 7, 9, 10, 11, 12). Additionally, however, it is clear that further and more robust clinical studies are required, including research on new, innovative strategies to prevent adhesions more effectively through an improved surgical environment, new and combination devices, and pharmacological agents.

Measures to reduce adhesions

Preoperative and intraoperative considerations

Preoperative identification of patients with adhesions allows for surgical planning to both reduce potential intraoperative complications and improve outcomes. Given the significant risks associated with laparoscopic entry (24, 25), the number of prior surgeries and type of incisions used are of importance. Current imaging techniques do not allow adequate pre-assessment of adhesions, but it is hoped technology will be improved in the future.

Central to any intraoperative adhesion reduction strategy is meticulous surgical technique. Key steps following the fundamental principles of 'microsurgical technique' have been published by various Expert Groups and are summarized in Table 1 (3, 26, 27).

General principles
Focus on planned surgery and if secondary pathology is identified, question the risk benefit of surgical treatment before proceeding
Reduce duration of surgery
Reduce bleeding as blood increases adhesion formation • Ensure diligent hemostasis • But also reduce cautery time and frequency causing peritoneal trauma and thus stimulating adhesion formation
Aspirate aerosolized tissue following cautery
Excise tissues to reduce fulguration
Avoid incisions through highly vascularized structures such as muscle layers
Use magnification to allow a better view and thus gentler handling and more precise dissection of tissues
Whenever possible avoid manipulation of structures distant to the operative site
Avoid contamination
Any risk of infection needs to be reduced as the resulting inflammatory cascade escalates adhesion formation
Prevent foreign body contamination
Reduce drying of tissues Limit heat and light Use frequent irrigation solutions but ensure the solution used does not have an irritant effect on the peritoneum Phosphate-buffered saline solution has been shown to result in a 150% increase in adhesions compared to no irrigation (28)
Regularly aspirate irrigants in laparoscopic as well as open surgery
Limit use of sutures Choose fine nonreactive sutures Consider fibrin glue as a useful alternative
In laparotomy:
• Avoid bowel packing
• Minimize the use of dry towels or sponges
• Use starch- and latex-free gloves
In laparoscopy:
• Reduce pressure and duration of the laparoscopic pneumoperitoneum
• Consider insufflation with humidified gas

Table 1. Surgical steps to reduce adhesions.

However, many of the traumas that cause adhesions are a routine and inevitable part of surgery; to achieve meticulous hemostasis, for example, while limiting the use of cautery can be difficult. Even with careful surgical technique, postoperative adhesions occur and some conditions and procedures, including endometriosis and myomectomy, are particularly adhesiogenic (6, 7, 8, 9, 29).

Adhesion-reduction agents

Clinical outcome studies in surgery are complex (30). The multi-factorial nature of pregnancy as a clinical outcome makes it a difficult outcome to measure. The number of patients required to demonstrate a reduction in small bowel obstruction (SBO) is very large (30), requiring many centers and lengthy study periods with associated biases from inter-center and surgeon variables and changes in surgical practice (31). The focus of research has thus been on secondary end-point evidence that in reducing adhesions there will be an associated impact on improved clinical outcomes. This has largely been accepted by the US Regulatory Authority – the Food and Drug Administration (FDA) (32).

Compared to FDA requirements for approval, the European CE medical devices accreditation system is not as demanding. It only requires preclinical evidence of safety, some animal model efficacy, and some evidence of clinical safety from small pilot studies, which sometimes include a modest assessment of efficacy in, or in some instances only extrapolation of data on agents previously available for use in humans – not necessarily for the reduction of adhesions – or from similar agents that had been previously used for the reduction of adhesions but subsequently withdrawn. Because of these differences in approval systems, there are many more products available in Europe, most of which, however, have little if any robust clinical safety let alone efficacy evidence.

Pharmacological agents

The pathophysiology of adhesions presents various theoretical opportunities for pharmacological treatments. A wide range of agents has been investigated - including antibiotics, nonsteroidal anti-inflammatory drugs, corticosteroids, antihistamines, progestogens, gonadotropin-releasing hormone (GnRH) agonists, heparin, and fibrinolytics (33-38). While some have shown promising preclinical results, to date no clinical studies have shown benefits and there have been safety concerns associated with normal healing (33). Research continues on a range of agents but their potential is experimental and theoretical only.

Physical barriers

Actions during surgery and the physical separation of traumatized peritoneal surfaces in the critical 3-5 day period of adhesion development after surgery are currently the only practical ways to reduce adhesion formation.

Abdominopelvic adhesion-reduction agents with published evidence of clinical safety and efficacy in the reduction of abdominopelvic agents, and approved by the FDA or European CE medical devices accreditation system, and which are available at the time of writing, are discussed. Although there are other agents approved in Europe, at the time of writing they do not have published clinical evidence. Many experimental agents having shown promising preclinical evidence were then abandoned due to issues in the clinical setting. Evidence of impact on clinical outcomes as well as reduction of adhesions is considered along with studies in patients with cancer or those undergoing caesarean deliveries. Of the agents currently approved in Europe, only three have been researched to the robust standards required by the US FDA and are approved for use in North America: Interceed®, Seprafilm®, and Adept®.

Site-specific mechanical barriers

Interceed® (Gynecare, Johnson & Johnson, Somerville, NJ, USA)

Interceed® is approved for use by the FDA in open surgery only. In Europe it is approved in open and laparoscopic surgery. It is an oxidized regenerated cellulose material in a knitted weave that when applied to raw peritoneum following surgery and in contact with fluids, forms a viscous gel barrier coating within 8 hours, preventing fibrin band formation and subsequent fibroblast invasion, and is completely resorbed after 4 weeks. Use in laparoscopy requires some skill. Meticulous hemostasis is crucial. Interceed's® efficacy reduces in the presence of blood and may increase adhesion formation (39, 40).

There is a substantial literature on gynecological use and a Cochrane review concluded it reduces adhesion formation while not affecting wound healing (40). It reported there was no research on pregnancy but omitted a 2-year follow-up study of infertile patients which demonstrated an increase in pregnancy rate compared to surgical controls (41).
No published studies have been identified on reduction of pelvic pain or SBO or use following cancer surgery. One Korean study published as proceedings indicated that prior use of Interceed® in women having repeat caesareans had a significantly lower adhesion rate.

Seprafilm® (Genzyme, Cambridge MA, USA)

Seprafilm® is approved for use by the FDA in open surgery. In Europe it is approved for use in open and laparoscopic surgery. It is a transparent absorbable film of hyaluronic acid – carboxymethylcellulose – that is absorbed spontaneously within 7 days and excreted within 28 days. Efficacy is not affected by blood (42). Seprafilm® is not very malleable and therefore usually used as a barrier placed between the bowel or omentum and anterior abdominal wall at wound closure, where it can prevent adherence and potentially reduce the risk of enterotomy at subsequent surgery. Although there is some work in laparoscopy (43, 44), its use is not realistic in routine surgery.

Efficacy was assessed in two pivotal laparotomy studies – myomectomy and colorectal surgery (42, 45). A Cochrane review criticized the validity of the statistical findings in the myomectomy study (40) and, while there is now a broader mounting literature on its use, this is largely in general surgery (46). Seprafilm® showed a significant but limited efficacy in reducing adhesive SBO, requiring reoperation by laparotomy (47). However, a mean of 4.4 sheets per patient was required and the study highlighted use at the site of an anastomosis led to increased anastomotic leaks.

In a retrospective study in a gynecological oncology setting, Seprafilm® was associated with a higher rate of postoperative intra-abdominal collections, greatest in those undergoing a debulking procedure (48). Another retrospective study in gynecological oncology did not show this (49), nor did an earlier small prospective study (50). Seprafilm® has been evaluated in 1 study of 52 primary caesarean deliveries. Published in Japanese (41), the incidence and severity of adhesions at subsequent caesarean delivery was significantly less in Seprafilm® patients (46, 52). Two recent reviews by Genzyme comprehensively present the extensive clinical evidence of use of Seprafilm® (53, 54).

Prevadh® (Covidien, Mansfield, MA, USA/Sofradim, Trevoux, France)

Prevadh® is a hydrophilic film presented on a hemostatic collagen sponge with two surfaces – a fleece surface and a smooth nonporous surface composed of porcine oxidized type-1 atelocollagen. It is designed to be used on plane surfaces where it can be fixed onto the adhesiogenic surface using an association of oxidized starch and phosphate tampon solution. When there is inadequate hemostasis, the fleece lyophilized side is placed onto the bleeding area and the film side then prevents blood from crossing the fleece – thus creating a barrier to help reduce adhesions forming.

Currently there is only one published open clinical study – a pilot safety study of 78 patients (one gynecological) – that suggested it is safe with respect to foreign body reaction, abdominal abscess, and pulmonary embolism. Efficacy assessments were limited and inconclusive (55).

Gel barriers

As site-specific film barriers are generally difficult to use in laparoscopic surgery, a number of gel barriers have also been developed.

Hyalobarrier® (Nordic Pharma, Paris, France/Fidia Advanced Biopolymers, Abano Terme, Padova Italy)

Hyalobarrier® is a highly viscous auto-crosslinked hyaluronan gel that stays at the site to which it is applied, dissolving some days later. Two small-scale randomized, controlled studies in patients undergoing laparoscopic myomectomy showed a reduction in adhesions (56, 57). The first study (56) reported a pregnancy rate significantly greater than in the surgical control group (58).

There are no published data on Hyalobarrier® in cancer or in caesarean deliveries.

Intrauterine use

Hyalobarrier® has been researched for use in reducing intrauterine adhesions following hysteroscopic surgery with success and may be useful in this situation (33, 59, 60). A recent meta-analysis concluded that the incidence of adhesions was significantly reduced with use of the agent compared to surgery alone, but that further studies were required (61).

Intercoat®/Oxiplex®/AP (Ethicon/Gynecare, Johnson & Johnson, Somerville, NJ, USA/ FzioMed, San Luis Obispo, CA, USA)

Intercoat®, is a viscoelastic carboxymethylcellulose (CMC) and polyethylene oxide (PEO) composite gel approved for use in Europe as an adhesion-reduction barrier for abdominopelvic surgery. Two small-scale pilot studies in gynecological laparoscopy assessed safety and demonstrated improvements in American Fertility Society (AFS) scores (62, 63). Intercoat® has been evaluated in a small study in endometriosis and was effective in reducing adhesions in all groups, compared to surgery controls (64).

There are no studies on clinical outcomes, cancer patients, or caesarean deliveries.

Coseal® (Baxter BioSurgery, Baxter Healthcare Corporation, Deerfield IL, USA)

Coseal® is a resorbable hydrogel polyethylene glycol polymer solution that has European approval for use in abdominopelvic surgery. A clinical study in myomectomy patients concluded that when used alongside good surgical technique in both open and laparoscopic myomectomy, Coseal® significantly reduced the incidence, extent, and severity of adhesions at sites of application with no apparent safety issues (65).

No further clinical research in abdominopelvic surgery is yet published.

Broad coverage fluid agents

Adept® (Baxter BioSurgery, Baxter International, Deerfield IL, USA)

Adept® is the only agent approved by the FDA for use in laparoscopic surgery. In Europe it is approved for use in open and laparoscopic abdominopelvic surgery.
Adept® is a nonviscous, iso-osmotic, clear solution of 4% icodextrin that handles like normal saline and persists in the abdominopelvic cavity throughout the critical period of adhesion formation. Clinical studies have used a combined approach as an irrigant/wash throughout surgery, with a 1,000 mL instillate then left postoperatively.

An initial pilot study provided safety data as well as some evidence of efficacy (66). A registry study in routine surgery in Europe (ARIEL) provided data on use, acceptability, and safety in 4,620 patients – 2,882 gynecological (2,069 laparoscopy, 813 laparotomy) (67, 68). It demonstrated that Adept® was easy to use in routine surgical practice and had a good safety profile (67, 68).

A major US pivotal randomized study in patients undergoing laparoscopic gynecological surgery with adhesiolysis (69) concluded that Adept® patients had a significant reduction in adhesions throughout the peritoneal cavity. It reduced clinically important adhesions, including in patients with severe endometriosis and with a high burden of pre-existing adhesions and in patients with infertility and pelvic pain.

Adept® was compared against lactated Ringer's solution (LRS). Although LRS had some clinical benefit, Adept® provided a significant benefit over and above LRS throughout the peritoneal cavity and in more complex cases (69).

An RCT in Europe of de novo adhesions after laparoscopy for removal of fibroids or endometriosis cysts further confirmed the safety of Adept® in laparoscopic surgery (70). The proportion of patients with de novo adhesion formation was considerably higher than previous literature suggested. Overall, the study provided no evidence of a clinical effect, but various surgical covariates including surgery duration, blood loss, number and size of incisions, suturing and number of knots were found to influence de novo adhesion formation.

Adept® has been researched in the management of SBO where it is reported it significantly reduced the reoccurrence of adhesive small bowel obstruction (71, 72).

While there are no specific studies in oncology, icodextrin 4% solution is approved in 13 European countries as an intraperitoneal carrier solution for chemotherapeutic agents in cancer patients. In the ARIEL registry, Adept® was used in 182 gynecological and 518 general surgery patients with cancer with no issues (67, 68).

At present there are no studies of Adept® in caesarean deliveries.

Areas of future research

Laparoscopic pneumoperitoneum

Emerging data suggest that the entire peritoneal cavity may be a cofactor in adhesion formation, especially during laparoscopy, and that the CO2 pneumoperitoneum may be the important adhesiogenic factor (73). Preclinical research indicates that a variety of factors are involved, including laparoscopic gas, temperature, pressure, humidity, and time. CO2 may induce intraperitoneal acidosis or mesothelial desiccation. The intraperitoneal pressure associated with prolonged pneumoperitoneum may cause adverse effects on the microcirculation inducing hypoxemia, which, together with other mesothelial insult from the surgical process, may stimulate expression of factors such as the plasminogen system (PAI-1), vascular endothelial growth factor (VEGF), and placental and transforming growth factors, resulting in an increase in adhesion formation (33, 74). Research for potential adhesion-reduction strategies involving the pneumoperitoneum is progressing.

Combining techniques

The future of anti-adhesion strategies will probably use different methods at different levels. It is apparent that available agents reduce but are limited in their efficacy to prevent adhesions and there is therefore a growing focus on combining agents, including the potential to combine a barrier device (film, gel, or solution) with an active pharmacological agent – the barrier acting as an anti-adhesion agent and a carrier to deliver an active pharmacological agent(s) to the peritoneum to more effectively reduce adhesions through interruption of the primary mechanisms of adhesion formation. Various agents including growth factors, reactive-oxygen species (ROS), scavengers, 5-fluorouracil, statins, and various anti-inflammatory agents have been considered. Currently this is hypothesis and experimental research only.

Better studies

Of key importance is the need for better-designed, more robust clinical studies of anti-adhesion agents. While the costs may be high, it is an imperative that there is more investment in assessing the safety and efficacy of adhesion-reduction strategies if they are to be adopted in routine surgery. Without this, surgeons will remain sceptical, health care systems will remain reluctant to fund, and – most importantly – patients will remain at serious risk of postoperative abdominopelvic adhesions and their associated complications.

Acknowledgments: No funding was received from any commercial, research, or other organization for the development of this work.

References

1. Diamond MP, El-Hammady E, Wang R, Kruger M, Saed G. Regulation of expression of tissue plasminogen activator and plasminogen activator inhibitor-1 by dichloroacetic acid in human fibroblasts from normal peritoneum and adhesions. Am J Obstet Gynecol 2004;190:926-34.
2. DeWilde RL, Trew G, on behalf of the Expert Adhesions Working Party of the European Society of Gynaecological Endoscopy (ESGE). Postoperative abdominal adhesions and their prevention in gynaecological surgery. Expert consensus position. Gynecol Surg 2007;4:161-8.
3. De Wilde, Trew G, on behalf of the Expert Adhesions Working Party of the European Society of Gynaecological Endoscopy (ESGE). Postoperative abdominal adhesions and their prevention in gynaecological surgery. Expert consensus position. Part 2 – steps to reduce adhesions. Gynecol Surg 2007;4:243-53.
4. Diamond MP, Freeman ML. Clinical implications of postsurgical adhesions. Hum Reprod Update 2001;7:567-76.
5. Lower AM, Hawthorn RJS, Clark D, Boyd JH, Finlayson AR, Knight AD, Crowe AM, on behalf of the Surgical and Clinical Adhesions Research (SCAR) Group. Adhesion-related readmissions following gynaecological laparoscopy or laparotomy in Scotland: an epidemiological study of 24,046 patients. Hum Reprod 2004;19:1877-85.
6. Pérez Medina T, Álvarez Bernardi J, Degollada M, de Santiago J, González L, Pascual A, Pérez Milán P, Crowe AM. Documento de consenso del grupo de trabajo sobre las adherencias de la sección de endoscopia de la SEGO. Progresos de Obstetricia y Ginecología 2010;53:454-475.

7. Mais V, Angioli R, Coccia E, Fagotti A, Landi S, Melis GB, Pellicano M, Scambia G et al. Aderenze addominali postoperatorie e loro prevenzione in chirurgia ginecologica Documento di consenso di una "task force" di ginecologi italiani sulle aderenze. Minerva Ginecologica 2011;63:47-70.
8. Audebert A, Darai E, Bénfla JL, Yazbeck C, Dechaud H, Wattiez A, Crowe AM, Pouly JL. Adherences postoperatoires et leur prevention en chirurgie gynecologique: 1. Ce qu'il faut savoir. Gynécologie Obstétrique & Fertilité 2011 DOI: 10.1016/j.gyobfe.2011.10.002.
9. Pouly JL, Darai E, Yazbeck C, Bénifla JL, Dechaud H, Watiez A, Crowe AM, Audebert A. Adherences postoperatoires et leur prevention en chirurgie gynecologique: II. Comment les prevenir? Gynécologie Obstétrique & Fertilité 2011 DOI: 10.1016/j.gyobfe.2011.10.001.
10. Polish Gynecological Society. Polish Gynecological Society Consensus in Adhesion Reduction Management. Ginekol Pol 2010;81:235-6.
11. Hirschelmann A, Tchartchian G, Wallwiener M, Hackethal A, DeWIlde, DL. A review of the problematic adhesion prophylaxis in gynaecological surgery. Arch Gyneol Obstet 2012;285:1089-1097.
12. SOGC Clinical Practice Guidelines. Adhesion prevention in gynaecological surgery. Int J Gynecol Obstet 2010;111:193-197.
13. Wiseman D (2003) Adhesions and informed consent: Patients awareness of adhesions prior to surgery. V1th International Symposium on Peritoneum (PAX), Amsterdam. PAX Abstracts pp 21:VII(4).
14. Trew G, Cooke I, Lower A, McVeigh E. Post-operative abdominal adhesions – awareness of UK gynaecologists – a survey of members of the Royal College of Obstetricians and Gynaecologists. Gynecol Surg 2009;6:25-37.
15. Hackethal A, Sick C, Brueggmann D, Tchartchian G, Wallwiener M, Muenstedt K et al. Awareness and perception of intra-abdominal adhesions and related consequences: survery of gynaecologists in German hospitals. Eur J Obstet Gynecol Reprod Biol 2010;150:180-9.
16. Schreinmacher MHF, ten Broock RP, Bakkum EA, van Goor H, Bouvy ND. Adhesion Awareness: A national survey of surgeons. World J Surg 2010;34:2805-12.
17. Rajab TK, Wallwiener M, Talukdar S, Kraemer B. Adhesion-related complications are common, but rarely discussed in preoperative consent: a multicenter study. World J Surg 2009;33:748-50.
18. Ellis H, Crowe A. Medico-legal consequences of post-operative intra-abdominal adhesions. Int J Surg 2009;7:187-91.
19. NHS Litigation Authority. Informed Consent NHSLA Risk Alert. 2004;4. Available from: http://www.nhsla.com/NR/rdonlyres/AD7A7848-E9A3-4668-839F-43E54BBFA3A1/0/RiskManagementAlert4.pdf .
20. Cole A. GMC asks doctors to take greater care over consent after introduction of mental capacity Act 2005. BMJ 2008;336:1152-3.
21. Skene L, Smallwood R. Informed consent: lessons form Australia. BMJ 2002;324:39-41.
22. Moumjid N, Callu MF. Commentary: informed consent and risk communication in France. BMJ 2003;327:734-5.
23. Sokol DK, How can I avoid being used? Common sense is the key. BMJ 2011;343:7827 doi: 10.1136/bmj.d7827 (published 14 December 2011).
24. Audebert AJ, Gomel V. Role of microlaparoscopy in the diagnosis of peritoneal and visceral adhesions and in the prevention of bowel injury associated with blind trocar insertion. Fertil Steril 2000;73:631-5
25. Dubuisson J, Botchorischvili R, Perrette S, Bourdel N, Jardon K, Rabischong B et al. Incidence of intraabdominal adhesions in a continuous series of 1000 laparoscopic procedures. Am J Obstet Gynecol 2010;203:111.e1-3.

26. Gomel V. Microsurgery in female infertility. Boston USA: Little, Brown and Co; 1983;p.225-44.
27. Robertson D, Lefebvre G, Leyland N, Wolfman W, Allaire C, Awadalla A et al. Adhesion prevention in gynaecological surgery. J Obstet Gynaecol Can 2010;32:598-608.
28. van Westreenen M, van den Tol PM, Pronk A, Marquet RL, Jeekel J, Leguit P. Perioperative lavage promotes intraperitoneal adhesion in the rat. Eur Surg Res 1999;31:196-201.
29. Brochhausen C, Schmitt VH, Planck CNE, Rajab TK, Holleman et al. Current strategies and future perspectives for intraperitoneal adhesion prevention. J Gastrointest Surg 2012;16:1256-74.
30. Wilson MS, Menzies D, Knight AD, Crowe AM. Demonstrating the clinical and cost effectiveness of adhesion reduction strategies. Colorectal Dis 2002;4:355-60.
31. Salum M, Wexner SD, Nogueras JJ, Weiss E, Koruda M, Behrens S et al. Does sodium hyaluronate- and carboxymethylcellulose-based bioresorbable membrane (Seprafilm) decrease operative time for loop ileostomy closure? Tech Coloproctol 2006;10:187-91.
32. FDA (US Food and Drug Administration) Center for Devices and Radiological Health. Guidance for resorbable adhesion barrier devices for use in abdominal and/or pelvic surgery. DHHS/FDA. 2002 http://www.fda.gov/MedicalDevices/DeviceRegulationandGuidance/GuidanceDocuments/ucm072879.htm
33. Nappi C, Di Spiezio Sardo A, Greco E, Guida M, Bettocchi S, Bifulco G. Prevention of adhesions in gynaecological endoscopy. Hum Reprod Update 2007;13:379-94.
34. Metwally ME, Watson A, Lilford R, Vanderkerchove P. Fluid and pharmacological agents for adhesion prevention after gynaecological surgery. Cochrane Database of Systematic Reviews 2006, Issue 2. Art No.: CD001298. DOI: 10.1002/14651858.CD001298.pub3.
35. Pados G, Venetis CA, Almaloglou K, Tarlatzis BC. Prevention of intra-peritoneal adhesions in gynaecological surgery: theory and evidence. Reprod Biomed Online 2010;21:290-303. Epub 2010 Apr 27.
36. Attar R, Yildirim G, Kumbak B et al. Efficacy of melatonin and hyaluronate/carboxymethylcellulose membrane in reventing adhesion formation following adhesiolysis in a rat uterine model. J. Obstet Gynecol Res 2011;37:125-31.
37. Atta HM Prevention of peritoneal adhesions: A promising role for gene therapy. World J Gastroenterol 2011;17:5049-58.
38. Lalountas M, Ballas KD, Michalakis A et al. Postoperative adhesion prevention using a statin-containing cellulose film in an experimental model. Brit j Surg 2012;99:423-29.
39. Liakakos T, Thomakos N, Fine PM, Dervenis C, Young RL. Peritoneal adhesions: aetiology, pathophysiology and clinical significance – recent advances in prevention and management. Dig Surg 2001;18:260-73.
40. Ahmad G, Duffy JMN, Farquhar C, Vail A, Vanderkerchove P, Watson A et al. Barrier agents for adhesion prevention after gynaecological surgery. Cochrane Database of Systematic Reviews 2008, Issue 2. Art No.:CD000475. DOI: 10.1002/14651858.CD000475. pub2.
41. Sawada T, Nishizawa H, Nishio E, Kadowaki M. Postoperative adhesion prevention with an oxidized regenerated cellulose adhesion barrier in infertile women. J Reprod Med 2000;45:387-9.
42. Diamond MP and the Seprafilm Adhesion Study Group. Reduction of adhesions after uterine myomectomy by Seprafilm* membrane (HAL-F): a blinded, prospective, randomized, multicenter clinical study. Fertil Steril 1996;66:904-10.
43. Takeuchi H, Kitade M, Kikuchi I, Shimanuki H, Kinoshita K. A novel instrument and technique for using Seprafilm hyaluronic acid/carboxymethylcellulose membrane during laparoscopic myomectomy. J Laparoendosc Adv Surg Tech 2006;16:497-502.

44. Chuang Y-C, Fan C-N, Cho F-N, Kan Y-Y, Chang Y-H, Kang H-Y. A novel technique to apply a Seprafilm (hyaluronate-carboxymethylcelluslose) barrier following laparoscopic surgeries. Fertil Steril 2008;90:1959-63.
45. Becker JM, Dayton MT, Fazio VW, Beck DE, Stryker SJ, Wexner SD et al Prevention of postoperative abdominal adhesions by a sodium hyaluronate-based bioresorbable membrane: a prospective, randomized, double-blind multicenter study. J Am Coll Surg 1996;183:297-306.
46. González-Quintero VH, Cruz-Pachano FE. Preventing adhesions in obstetric and gynecologic surgical procedures. Rev Obstet Gynecol 2009;2:38-45.
47. Fazio VW, Cohen Z, Fleshman JW, van Goor H, Bauer JJ, Wolff BG et al. c. Dis Colon Rectum 2006;49:1-11.
48. Leitao MM Jr, Natenzon A, Abu-Rustum NR, Chi DS, Sonoda Y, Levine DA et al. Postoperative intra-abdominal collections using a sodium hyaluronate-carboxymethylcellulose (HA-CMC) barrier at the time of laparotomy for ovarian, fallopian tube, or primary peritoneal cancers. Gynecol Oncol 2009;115:204-8.
49. Tan A, Argenta P, Ramirez R, Bliss R, Geller M. The use of sodium hyaluronate-carboxymethylcellulose (HA-CMC) barrier in gynecologic malignancies: a retrospective review of outcomes. Ann Surg Oncol 2009;16:499-505.
50. Bristow RE, Montz FJ.Pevention of adhesion formation after radical oophorectomy using a sodium hyaluronate-carboxymethylcellulose (HA-CMC) barrier. Gynecol Oncol 2005;99:301-8.
51. Fushiki H, Ikoma T, Kobayashi H, Yoshimoto H. Efficacy of Seprafilm as an adhesion prevention barrier in Caesarean sections: availability of anti-adhesion film (Seprafilm) for Caesarean section. Obstetric and Gynaecologic Treatment [Japanese] 2005;91:557-61.
52. Sbarra M, Boyd M, Dardarian TS. Complications due to adhesion formation following cesarean sections: a review of deliveries in three cases. Fertil Steril 2009;92:394.e13-6.
53. Diamond MP, Burns EL, Accomando, Mian S, Holmdahl L. Seprafilm adhesion barrier: a review of preclinical, animal, and human investigational studies. Gynecol Surg 2012;9:237-45.
54. Diamond MP, Burns EL, Accomando, Mian S, Holmdahl L. Seprafilm adhesion barrier: a review of the clinical literature on intraabdominal use. Gynecol Surg 2012;9:247-57.
55. Mabrut JY, Favre JP, Desrousseaux B, Chipponi J, Arnaud JP, Domergue J et al. Safety and long-term outcome of a new concept for surgical adhesion-reduction strategies (Prevadh): a prospective, multicenter study. Hepatogastroenterology 2008;55:517-21.
56. Pellicano M, Bramante S, Cirillo D, Palomba S, Bifulco G, Zullo F et al. Effectiveness of autocrosslinked hyaluronic acid gel after laparoscopic myomectomy in infertile patients: a prospective, randomized, controlled study. Fertil Steril 2003;80:441-4.
57. Mais V, Bracco GL, Litta P, Gargiulo T, Melis GB. Reduction of postoperative adhesions with an auto-crosslinked hyaluronan gel in gynaecological laparoscopic surgery: a blinded, controlled, randomized, multicentre study. Hum Reprod 2006;21:1248-54.
58. Pellicano M, Guida M, Bramante S, Acunzo G, Di Spiezio Sardo AG, Tommaselli GA et al. Reproductive outcome after autocrosslinked hyaluronic acid gel application in infertile patients who underwent laparoscopic myomectomy. Fertil Steril 2005;83;498-500.
59. Acunzo G, Guida M, Pellicano M, Tommaselli GA, Di Spiezio Sardo A, Bifulco G et al. Effectiveness of auto-cross-linked hyaluronic acid gel in the prevention of intrauterine adhesions after hysteroscopic adhesiolysis: a prospective, randomized, controlled study. Hum Reprod 2003;18:1918-21.
60. Guida M, Acunzo G, Di Spiezio Sardo A, Bifulco G, Piccoli R, Pellicano M et al. Effectiveness of auto-crosslinked hyaluronic acid gel in the prevention of intrauterine adhesions after hysteroscopic surgery: a prospective, randomized, controlled study. Hum Reprod 2004;19:1461-4.

61. Mais V, Cirronis MG, Peiretti M et al. Efficacy of auto-crosslinked hyaluronan gel for adhesion prevention in laparoscopy and hysteroscopy: a systematic review and meta-analysis of randomized controlled trials. Eur J Obstet Gynecol Reprod Biol 2012;160:1-5.
62. Lundorff P, Donnez J, Korell M, Audebert AJM, Block K, diZerega GS. Clinical evaluation of a viscoelastic gel for reduction of adhesions following gynaecological surgery by laparoscopy in Europe. Hum Reprod 2005;20:514-20.
63. Young P, Johns A, Templeman C, Witz C, Webster B, Ferland R et al. Reduction of postoperative adhesions after laparoscopic gynecological surgery with Oxiplex/AP Gel*: a pilot study. Fertil Steril 2005;84:1450-6.
64. diZerega GS, Coad J, Donnez J. Clinical evaluation of endometriosis and differential response to surgical therapy with and without application of Oxiplex/AP* adhesion barrier gel. Fertil Steril 2007;87:485-9.
65. Mettler L, Hucke J, Bojahr B, Tinneberg H-R, Leyland N, Avelar A. A safety and efficacy study of a resorbable hydrogel for reduction of post-operative adhesions following myomectomy. Hum Reprod 2008;23:1093-1100.
66. diZerega GS, Verco SJS, Young P, Kettel M, Kobak W, Martin D et al. A randomized, controlled pilot study of the safety and efficacy of 4% icodextrin solution in the reduction of adhesions following laparoscopic gynaecological surgery. Hum Reprod 2002;17:1031-8.
67. Sutton C, Minelli L, Garcia E, Korell M, Pouly JL, Pados G et al. Use of icodextrin 4% solution in the reduction of adhesion formation after gynaecological surgery. Gynecol Surg 2005;2:287-96.
68. Menzies D, Hildago Pascual M, Walz MK, Duron JJ, Tonelli F, Crowe A et al. Use of icodextrin 4% solution in the prevention of adhesion formation following general surgery: from the multicentre ARIEL Registry. Ann R Coll Surg Engl 2006;88:375-82.
69. Brown CB, Luciano AA, Martin D, Peers E, Scrimgeour A, diZerega GS, on behalf of the Adept Adhesion Reduction Study Group. Adept (icodextrin 4% solution) reduces adhesions after laparoscopic surgery for adhesiolysis: a double-blind, randomized, controlled study. Fertil Steril 2007;88:1413-26.
70. Trew G, Trew G, Pistofidis G, Pados G, Lower A, Mettler L, et al. Gynaecological endoscopic evaluation of 4% icodextrin solution: a European, multicentre, double-blind, randomized study of the efficacy and safety in the reduction of de novo adhesions after laparoscopic gynaecological surgery. Hum Reprod 2011. doi: 10.1093/humrep/der135.
71. Catena F, Ansaloni L, Pinna A. Prospective controlled randomized trial on prevention of postoperative abdominal adhesions by Icodextrin 4% solution after laparotomic operation for small bowel obstruction caused by adherences. Eur J Trauma Emerg Surg 2010;36(Suppl. 1):7.
72. Catena F, Di Saverio S, Kelly MD, Biffl WL, Ansaloni L, Mandala V, et al. Bologna Guidelines for diagnosis and management of adhesive small bowel obstruction (ASBO): 2010 evidence-based guidelines of the world society of emergency surgery. World J Emerg Surg 2011;6:5.
73. Schonman R, Corona R, Bastidas A, De Circco C, Koninckx PR. Effect of upper abdomen tissue manipulation on adhesion formation between injured areas in a laparoscopic mouse model. J Minim Invasive Gynecol 2009;16:307-12.
74. Binda MM, Molinas CR, Hansen P, Koninckx PR. Effect of desiccation and temperature during laparoscopy on adhesion formation in mice. Fertil Steril 2006;86:166-75.

Trilogy 6. Endometrial receptivity

Science of implantation

Jan J. Brosens

Warwick Medical School, Coventry, United Kingdom

Introduction

The prevalence of chromosomal instability in human preimplantation embryos is exceptional. Array-based analyses of individual blastomeres have shown that the chromosomal error rate in top-quality embryos is at least 70% (1, 2). These large-scale structural chromosomal imbalances are caused predominantly by mitotic non-disjunction rather than meiotic errors. Thus, human beings generate exceptionally diverse preimplantation embryos, which are occasionally entirely diploid, mostly mosaic, and not uncommonly completely chromosomally chaotic. These observations pose some important questions. For example, if transient instability is the norm during human embryonic development, what could be the possible biological advantages? What are the mechanisms that subsequently restore chromosomal order? And – perhaps most pertinently – how can humans be reproductively successful when faced with such extraordinary prevalence of highly invasive abnormal embryos?

A good starting point to answer the latter is the maternal-fetal conflict hypothesis, as described in detail by Haig (3). This hypothesis is predicated on the idea that the inborn conflict between the needs of parents and offspring drives reproductive evolution and innovation. It predicts that reproductive success depends on a constant homeostatic rebalancing of embryonic and maternal traits. In other words, the maternal-fetal conflict hypothesis predicts that a strategy must have emerged to safeguard the mother against investing in invasive but developmentally abnormal embryos. It also predicts that the diversity ingrained in human embryos must be met by an intrinsic ability to adapt the maternal response to an individual conceptus.

Recent studies have provided evidence that the human endometrium engages in embryo quality control and natural selection at implantation (4, 5). Unraveling the molecular basis of these hitherto unrecognized uterine functions promises to fundamentally overhaul our understanding of the implantation process as well as shed new light on the pathological pathways that underpin reproductive failure.

Spontaneous decidualization

The most striking feature of the human reproductive cycle is 'spontaneous' decidualization. This process is defined by mesenchymal to epithelial transformation of endometrial stromal cells into secretory decidual cells (6). Among other functions, decidualization confers maternal immunotolerance to the semi-allogeneic embryo, rendering it an obligatory process for successful pregnancy in all species with invading placentae. Importantly, in all but a handful of species, decidualization of the endometrium is triggered by embryonic signals. One of those exceptions is the human uterus where the decidual process is 'spontaneous,' meaning it occurs in each cycle in response to elevated circulating progesterone levels and rising tissue cyclic adenosine monophosphate (cAMP) concentrations.

The term 'spontaneous' is somewhat misleading in so far as decidualization of the endometrium is tightly controlled. It is initiated in the mid-luteal phase of the cycle first in stromal cells surrounding the terminal spiral arteries and underlying the luminal epithelium. During the late secretory phase, it will have encompassed most of the superficial endometrial layer. The expression of decidual genes is coordinated and hardwired by the presence of regulatory transposable elements found only in placental mammals. The insertion of these mobile DNA elements in the genome established new boundaries between inactive and active chromatin in stromal cells and introduced novel cis-regulatory elements (enhancer/repressor elements) that co-opted the cAMP and progesterone signaling pathways to drive expression of decidua-specific genes (7).

A key feature of the decidual process is that it bestows a secretory phenotype on human endometrial stromal cells (HESCs). The spatial and temporal pattern of differentiation ensures that decidualizing cells are strategically placed to induce a microenvironment conducive to implantation. The nature of this microenvironment will change dynamically as the decidual process unfolds. Initially, it resembles an acute-phase pro-inflammatory response, characterized by endogenous production of free radicals and by coordinated expression of chemokines and other inflammatory mediators (8). At a functional level, the duration of this pro-inflammatory decidual response determines the length of the window of implantation. This notion is based on the observation that, only during the pro-inflammatory decidual response, the secretome of human endometrial stromal cells induces the expression of key receptivity genes when flushed through the lumen of a mouse uterus. Amongst the implantation genes that are regulated in the mouse uterus in response to signals from decidualizing human endometrial stromal cells are Hbegf, Lif, Bmp2, and Wnt4 (8).

Activation of feedback pathways curtails the inflammatory decidual response and triggers a profound anti-inflammatory response, characterized by simultaneous down-regulation of various chemokines and other inflammatory mediators. Elegant studies in mice have shown that by silencing chemokine expression, decidual cells ensure that T cells cannot migrate into the feto-maternal interface (9). Continued progesterone signaling will profoundly up-regulate 11β-hydroxysteroid dehydrogenase type 1 (11βHSD1), the enzyme that converts inert cortisone to active cortisol (10). Interestingly, inhibition of 11βHSD1 activity abolishes the induction of this enzyme in decidualizing cells, indicating that local cortisol signaling reinforces 11βHSD1 expression through an autocrine mechanism. Indeed, apart from the progesterone receptor (PR) and androgen receptor, human stromal cells also express cortisol-responsive glucocorticoid and mineralocorticoid receptors (GR and MR, respectively). Upon decidualization, GR expression declines whereas MR levels increase (10). Knockdown experiments showed that activation of this 11βHSD1/MR axis induces the expression of several enzymes involved in lipid metabolism and retinoid acid storage pathway. Thus, local cortisol biosynthesis and activation of MR-dependent target genes are likely important for histotrophic support for the developing fetus prior to the onset of placental perfusion around 10-11 weeks' gestation. Combined, these observations illustrate how a single process - 'spontaneous' decidualization - ensures that the window of implantation is coupled to an early pregnancy environment that is both supportive and tolerant of the embryonic semi-allograft.

Embryo encapsulation and biosensoring

Based on mouse models, implantation is viewed as a step-wise process that starts with apposition and adherence of a developmentally competent blastocyst to a receptive endometrium. The embryo then breaches the luminal epithelium and invades maternal tissues. As a direct consequence of this model, there has been a relentless search for markers predictive of a receptive human endometrium (e.g., αvβ3 integrin staining, pinopodes, expression of HOXA10, LIF, etc.). Despite tremendous efforts of numerous investigators, attempts at predicting and reliably manipulating endometrial receptivity, especially in the context of in vitro fertilization (IVF) treatment, have so far been unsuccessful.

In fact, there are a number of reasons to doubt this implantation paradigm. The foremost challenge in mice is to achieve synchronized implantation of multiple embryos. Unlike their human counterparts, murine embryos do not carry gross chromosomal abnormalities and are capable of temporarily suspending development, a process termed diapause, while awaiting a maternal signal for implantation. This maternal signal in the mouse is a surge in ovarian estradiol (11). By contrast, human embryos do not normally exhibit diapause, are highly invasive, and – as aforementioned – are often chromosomally unstable. In view of these species-specific differences, the luminal epithelium of the human endometrium may perhaps not be such a defining barrier for implantation.

Notably, decidualizing human endometrial stromal cells exhibit two important traits that are probably more fundamental to the likelihood of successful implantation. First, several studies have shown that decidual cells have an intrinsic propensity to migrate in response to embryonic and trophoblast signals. Inhibition of the migratory activity of decidualizing stromal cells suppresses embryo trophoblast invasion in co-culture models, indicating that active endometrial tissue remodeling must take place before an embryo can embed in the stroma (5, 12). Rather than being a passive matrix, these observations suggest that decidualizing stromal cells actively encapsulate the early conceptus. Placed in the context of an evolutionary maternal-fetal conflict hypothesis, it seems that decidualizing HESCs are programmed to mount a counter-invasive attack in response to the invasive nature of human embryos.

Second, compelling evidence has emerged to suggest that decidual cells are responsible for quality control of embryos that have breached the luminal epithelium (4, 5). Again this notion is based on co-culture experiments, demonstrating that decidualizing – but not undifferentiated – HESCs are exquisitely sensitive to signals derived from developmentally incompetent embryos. The notion that the endometrium is capable of sensing and adapting its response to individual embryos was in fact first reported in ruminants. Microarray analyses in the bovine have shown that endometrial gene expression will adapt to the developmental origins (e.g., somatic cell nuclear transfer, IVF, artificial insemination) and potential of the embryo (13). Thus, endometrial plasticity, here defined as the ability to mount a maternal response tailored to individual embryos, seems to be critical for reproductive success in mammals. If so, the maternal-fetal conflict hypothesis predicts that endometrial plasticity must be an evolutionarily enhanced reproductive trait of the human uterus.

Rejection and renewal

The concept of biosensoring and natural embryo selection at implantation only make sense if mechanisms exist for prompt rejection of an unwanted conceptus. A cardinal feature of the decidual cells is that they are poised to self-destruct in response to defined cues (14). In the absence of pregnancy, the principle trigger is a fall in circulating progesterone levels, which in turn reactivates the expression of inflammatory mediators, triggering apoptosis, influx of immune cells, extracellular matrix breakdown, and ultimately menstrual shedding. In pregnancy, human chorionic gonadotropin (hCG) produced by the invading trophoblast will drive ovarian progesterone production until this function is taken over by the placenta. It is conceivable that decidual cells employ several pathways to induce a menstruation-like response when censoring signals from developmentally compromised human embryos. For example, by shutting down the expression of key implantation factors, decidual cells may induce a microenvironment that, directly or indirectly, interferes with trophoblast hCG production. However, it also is conceivable that signals emanating from developmentally impaired embryos interfere with PR activity in decidual cells, thus triggering menstruation-like disposal of the conceptus regardless of the level of hCG production or circulating progesterone. Whatever the underlying mechanism, it has been estimated that half of all human embryos are disposed of this way before any clinical signs of pregnancy (15).

An inevitable consequence of spontaneous decidualization in the absence of pregnancy is menstruation. At first glance, this seems rather a hefty price for resolving the maternal-embryonic conundrum in human beings. However, menstruation also imposes a need for cyclic renewal of the endometrium. In fact, the regenerative capacity of the endometrium is nothing but remarkable and this in turn reflects the abundance of adult stem cells (16-19). They reside predominantly around the vessels and are reportedly immune-privileged compared to other types of stem cells, rendering them a promising resource for cell-based therapies. These stem cells are the progenitors of the stromal cells that will mount a decidual response in pregnancy. In fact, molecular phenotyping has shown that endometrial stromal cells, mesenchymal stem cells, and follicular dendritic cells are closely related (20). Thus, plasticity on the endometrium depends on differentiating stromal cells akin to stem cells and capable of exerting specialist immune functions.

Conclusions and perspective

The human uterus is characterized by extraordinary plasticity. The primary driver is spontaneous decidualization and cyclic menstruation, which bestow several innovative functions on the human endometrium, such as the propensity to migrate towards the embryo, to engage in quality control, and to timely reject an unwanted conceptus. Deregulation of these evolutionary innovative uterine functions has been shown to underpin clinical miscarriage (5, 8, 15, 21), the most common complication of pregnancy. It is conceivable that other defects during the peri-implantation period become amplified as pregnancy unfolds, leading to pre-eclampsia, fetal growth restriction, or preterm labor. Targeting the endometrium prior to conception and harnessing the mechanisms responsible for uterine plasticity may hold the key to improving pregnancy outcome in women at risk of reproductive failure.

References

1. Mertzanidou A, Wilton L, Cheng J, Spits C, Vanneste E, Moreau Y et al. Microarray analysis reveals abnormal chromosomal complements in over 70% of 14 normally developing human embryos. Human reproduction. 2013;28:256-64.
2. Vanneste E, Voet T, Le Caignec C, Ampe M, Konings P, Melotte C et al. Chromosome instability is common in human cleavage-stage embryos. Nat Med. 2009;15:577-83.
3. Haig D. Genetic conflicts in human pregnancy. The Quarterly review of biology. 1993;68:495-532.
4. Teklenburg G, Salker M, Molokhia M, Lavery S, Trew G, Aojanepong T et al. Natural selection of human embryos: decidualizing endometrial stromal cells serve as sensors of embryo quality upon implantation. PLoS One. 2010;5:e10258.
5. Weimar CH, Kavelaars A, Brosens JJ, Gellersen B, de Vreeden-Elbertse JM, Heijnen CJ et al. Endometrial stromal cells of women with recurrent miscarriage fail to discriminate between high- and low-quality human embryos. PLoS One. 2012;7:e41424.
6. Gellersen B, Brosens IA, Brosens JJ. Decidualization of the human endometrium: mechanisms, functions, and clinical perspectives. Seminars in reproductive medicine. 2007;25:445-53.
7. Lynch VJ, Leclerc RD, May G, Wagner GP. Transposon-mediated rewiring of gene regulatory networks contributed to the evolution of pregnancy in mammals. Nat Genet. 2011;43:1154-9.
8. Salker MS, Nautiyal J, Steel JH, Webster Z, Sucurovic S, Nicou M et al. Disordered IL-33/

ST2 Activation in Decidualizing Stromal Cells Prolongs Uterine Receptivity in Women with Recurrent Pregnancy Loss. PLoS One. 2012;7:e52252.

9. Nancy P, Tagliani E, Tay CS, Asp P, Levy DE, Erlebacher A. Chemokine gene silencing in decidual stromal cells limits T cell access to the maternal-fetal interface. Science. 2012;336:1317-21.
10. Kuroda K, Venkatakrishnan R, Salker MS, Lucas ES, Shaheen F, Kuroda M et al. Induction of 11beta-HSD 1 and Activation of Distinct Mineralocorticoid Receptor- and Glucocorticoid Receptor-Dependent Gene Networks in Decidualizing Human Endometrial Stromal Cells. Molecular endocrinology. 2013;27:192-202.
11. Hamatani T, Daikoku T, Wang H, Matsumoto H, Carter MG, Ko MS et al. Global gene expression analysis identifies molecular pathways distinguishing blastocyst dormancy and activation. Proceedings of the National Academy of Sciences of the United States of America. 2004;101:10326-31.
12. Grewal S, Carver JG, Ridley AJ, Mardon HJ. Implantation of the human embryo requires Rac1-dependent endometrial stromal cell migration. Proceedings of the National Academy of Sciences of the United States of America. 2008;105:16189-94.
13. Mansouri-Attia N, Sandra O, Aubert J, Degrelle S, Everts RE, Giraud-Delville C et al. Endometrium as an early sensor of in vitro embryo manipulation technologies. Proceedings of the National Academy of Sciences of the United States of America. 2009;106:5687-92.
14. Brosens JJ, Gellersen B. Death or survival--progesterone-dependent cell fate decisions in the human endometrial stroma. Journal of molecular endocrinology. 2006;36:389-98.
15. Salker M, Teklenburg G, Molokhia M, Lavery S, Trew G, Aojanepong T et al. Natural selection of human embryos: impaired decidualization of the endometrium disables embryo-maternal interactieons and causes recurrent pregnant loss. PLoS One. 2010;April 22.
16. Du H, Taylor HS. Stem cells and reproduction. Curr Opin Obstet Gynecol. 2010;22:235-41.
17. Gargett CE, Nguyen HP, Ye L. Endometrial regeneration and endometrial stem/progenitor cells. Rev Endocr Metab Disord. 2012;13:235-51.
18. Gargett CE, Ye L. Endometrial reconstruction from stem cells. Fertil Steril. 2012;98:11-20.
19. Du H, Naqvi H, Taylor HS. Ischemia/reperfusion injury promotes and granulocyte-colony stimulating factor inhibits migration of bone marrow-derived stem cells to endometrium. Stem Cells Dev. 2012;21:3324-31.
20. Munoz-Fernandez R, Prados A, Leno-Duran E, Blazquez A, Garcia-Fernandez JR, Ortiz-Ferron G et al. Human decidual stromal cells secrete C-X-C motif chemokine 13, express B cell-activating factor and rescue B lymphocytes from apoptosis: distinctive characteristics of follicular dendritic cells. Human reproduction. 2012;27:2775-84.
21. Salker MS, Christian M, Steel JH, Nautiyal J, Lavery S, Trew G et al. Deregulation of the serum- and glucocorticoid-inducible kinase SGK1 in the endometrium causes reproductive failure. Nat Med. 2011;17:1509-13.

Hormonal conditioning of the endometrium

Claire Bourgain

Vrije Universiteit Brussel, Brussels, Belgium

Introduction

In the human natural cycle endometrium, estrogen and progesterone are the main drivers towards a luteal transformation and establishment of a receptive implantation window in the menstrual cycle. This window is characterized by definite morphological changes in the endometrial tissue, albeit difficult to report with consistent reproducibility (1, 2). Rather than daily dating (3), gene expression analysis confirms a shift in up- and down-regulated genes from late follicular towards three distinct luteal endometrial development stages (Figure 1) (4). Progesterone effect on the endometrium is a complex phenomenon involving endocrine, paracrine, and intracrine pathways that orchestrate timely differentiation of the endometrial epithelial, stromal, and vascular components as well as the endometrial immune system (5). To date, however, the endometrial receptivity is still not unequivocally characterized at the molecular level (6).

In assisted reproductive technology (ART), the endometrial development is modified by the ovarian stimulation protocol (7). This phenomenon has been well documented in histological, immunological, gene expression, and proteomic studies. The normal process of mid-luteal transformation is thus altered by supra-physiological and untimely increase in steroid concentrations. Moreover, the type of pituitary down-regulation, gonadotropin stimulation, final oocyte maturation, and luteal support regimen also affect the endometrial development. Pregnancy rates in ART cycles are considerably lower compared to cycles transferring embryos into a natural cycle (8). This adds circumstantial evidence that ART-induced microenvironment changes may induce a diminished capacity or even failure of the endometrium to achieve a receptive status.

Ovarian stimulation and premature endometrial secretory transformation

One of the most consistent endometrial features induced by ovarian stimulation is a significant alteration in endometrial development on the day of oocyte retrieval (hCG+2). In former studies, an attempt was made to classify these changes according to the standard 'gold' Noyes criteria (8, 9, 10, 11, 12, 13). The performance of classical dating of the endometrial biopsy has been questioned (2). In ART cycles, these criteria are even more challenged, as they apply to natural cycles and do not reflect the specific alterations that occur in stimulated cycles. In a recent publication, besides conventional dating, Evans et al. (13) made an attempt to describe and quantify the specific endometrial morphological patterns on the day of oocyte retrieval. Ovarian stimulation induced profound endometrial maturation alterations, and these were reported consistently in all studies. Moreover, the phenomenon has been observed both in gonadotropin-releasing hormone (GnRH)-agonist and -antagonist stimulation regimens. The glands showed prominent signs of active secretion, characterized by a premature presence of subnuclear vacuolization. Stromal and vascular changes were also evident. This contrasts with the narrow straight mitotically active glands and compact stroma typically seen in natural cycle peri-ovulatory endometria. Another peculiar finding was the induction of an even more advanced glandular secretory transformation with prominent stromal edema presence in subgroups of patients with identical inclusion criteria receiving identical ART regimens. This maturation pattern was reported either as extremely advanced (10, 11) or mixed fragile (13) endometrial maturation. The biological confirmation of such a subgroup was demonstrated when gene expression analysis was performed in these endometria (14). On the day of oocyte retrieval, morphologically extreme advanced endometria differentially expressed 2,550 genes compared to endometria with early secretory changes. By principal component analysis, endometria with severe advanced glandular maturation clustered in a separate gene expression group.

Several factors may contribute to the phenomenon of precocious endometrial secretion.

In GnRH-antagonist cycles, the severity of precocious endometrial secretory changes seems related to variables in the follicular phase of the ART cycle. Endometrial advanced maturation was positively correlated with the serum luteinizing hormone (LH) concentrations at initiation of the stimulation, the duration of follicle-stimulating hormone (FSH) stimulation before starting the antagonist (11), and prolongation of the follicular phase by a delayed hCG ovulatory trigger (15).

In a study comparing a stimulated cycle for IVF to the natural cycle in the same patient, up-regulation of the progesterone receptor in stimulated cycles was initiated already at the end of the proliferative phase, even before the ovulatory trigger was administered (16). On the day of oocyte retrieval, the glandular and stromal endometrial progesterone receptors were less expressed in stimulated cycles when evaluated by immunohistochemistry (17). This is likely resulting from increased progesterone receptor priming by the elevated estradiol concentrations in the follicular phase followed by a rapid progesterone raise after hCG administration.

Ovarian stimulation also leads to frequent premature serum progesterone elevation, associated with lower pregnancy and implantation rates (18). The severity of endometrial secretory changes at oocyte retrieval could, however, not be predicted by the absolute serum progesterone concentration values (10). Recently, a study evaluating the endometrial gene expression on the day of oocyte retrieval according to the concentration of serum progesterone on the day of hCG administration in GnRH-antagonist cycles demonstrated a distinct difference in endometrial gene expression profile between patients with a progesterone serum concentration above and below the threshold of 1.5 ng/mL on the day of hCG administration (19).

Prolonged exposure of hCG in the follicular phase in stimulated cycles leads to down-regulation of the LH-choriogonadotropin (CG) receptor and may be another factor detrimentally affecting the endometrial receptivity (20). This finding was, however, not supported by a study with low-dose hCG replacing recombinant FSH during the late follicular phase in a GnRH-antagonist protocol. Clinically, similar pregnancies were achieved (21). When endometrial biopsies on the day of oocyte retrieval were compared in the low-dose hCG and a conventional GnRH-antagonist protocol, morphologically identical endometria with only minimal difference in gene expression were observed (12).

The type of ovulatory trigger and luteal phase support in in vitro fertilization (IVF) stimulation protocols also affects the endometrial development. Luteal phase support has proven to be mandatory in most protocols using pituitary down-regulation (22). Final oocyte maturation with GnRH agonist instead of hCG resulted in a significant endometrial gene expression difference on day 5 following oocyte retrieval. By Ingenuity® pathway analysis, these genes where involved in several biological functions related to natural killer cell and integrin signaling, as well as arachidonic acid metabolism. In unsupplemented cycles, premature activation of genes related to endometrial stromal breakdown and menstruation was noticed (23).

Endometrial conditioning in ART and subsequent pregnancy outcome

An endometrial biopsy procedure in the cycle with embryo transfer is difficult to implement due to evident ethical concern related to a possible negative interference with the implantation process.

Studies evaluating biopsies on the day of oocyte retrieval with subsequent embryo transfer have been performed in GnRH-agonist and -antagonist cycles (10, 11, 12, 13). Non-pregnant patients displayed a heterogeneous morphology that varied from subtle secretory changes to severely advanced secretory maturation. Implantation correlated negatively with the latter group, as throughout all reports, no clinical pregnancies ensued in this patient subgroup. Pregnant patients showed a histology that was consistently secretory and could be considered intermediate between the natural cycle morphology and the severe alterations seen in non-pregnant patients. Immunohistochemical markers for steroid receptors, quantification of immune cells, and vascularization of endometria in ART showed variable results according to the type of stimulation but could not be related to subsequent pregnancy outcome.

To decipher the receptive endometrial molecular signature on the day of oocyte retrieval, a study was conducted by gene expression analysis and real time polymerase chain reaction (RT-PCR) in two distinct GnRH-antagonist protocols (24). Pregnant and non-pregnant patients were matched for histological dating, cycle characteristics, age, and embryo quality. The endometrial RNA was extracted and gene expression was analyzed. The differentially expressed genes were further studied for biological network analysis. From this study emerged one biological network involving molecules within the COX-2 pathway. Increased gene expression of cyclooxygenase-2 (COX-2) coincided with a lower probability to conceive. Other consistently differentially expressed genes in pregnant and non-pregnant patients involved a specific type of metalloprotease. This finding is of particular interest, as COX-2 is a known crucial reproductive factor in mice, involved in ovulation, fertilization, implantation, and decidualization (25). Increase of COX-2 expression leads to an enhanced PGE2 secretion promoting angiogenesis, inhibiting apoptosis, and stimulating proliferation and immunosuppression. COX-2-driven upregulation of different members of the prostaglandin family occurs in luteal phase endometria (4). In the non-pregnant patient group, precocious activation of the COX-pathway on the day of oocyte retrieval thus correlated with the definite secretory characteristics and altered immune cell distribution in these endometria.

Endometrial biopsies are burdensome and cannot be advocated as a routine test to assess endometrial receptivity in cycles with embryo transfer. The biological pathways emerging from the endometrial tissue in the patient populations achieving clinical pregnancy may be implemented in the future into less invasive tests, including endometrial fluid aspiration (26), to predict receptivity alterations induced by the ART procedure.

Conclusions

Hormonal conditioning of the endometrium in ART cycles involving ovarian stimulation profoundly affects endometrial development. There is substantial evidence that this process is initiated in the follicular phase. All stimulation protocols lead to precocious secretory transformation as compared to the natural cycle. Identical protocols in homogeneous patient groups induce a wide variation of endometrial maturation patterns at the time of oocyte retrieval. In cycles with embryo transfer, pregnant patients issue from endometria displaying a homogeneous morphology and gene expression pattern at the time of oocyte retrieval. Non-pregnant patients within the latter group express an increased activation of the COX-2 gene pathway. These finding may redefine many clues for endometrial receptivity applicable in less invasive endometrial exploration techniques.

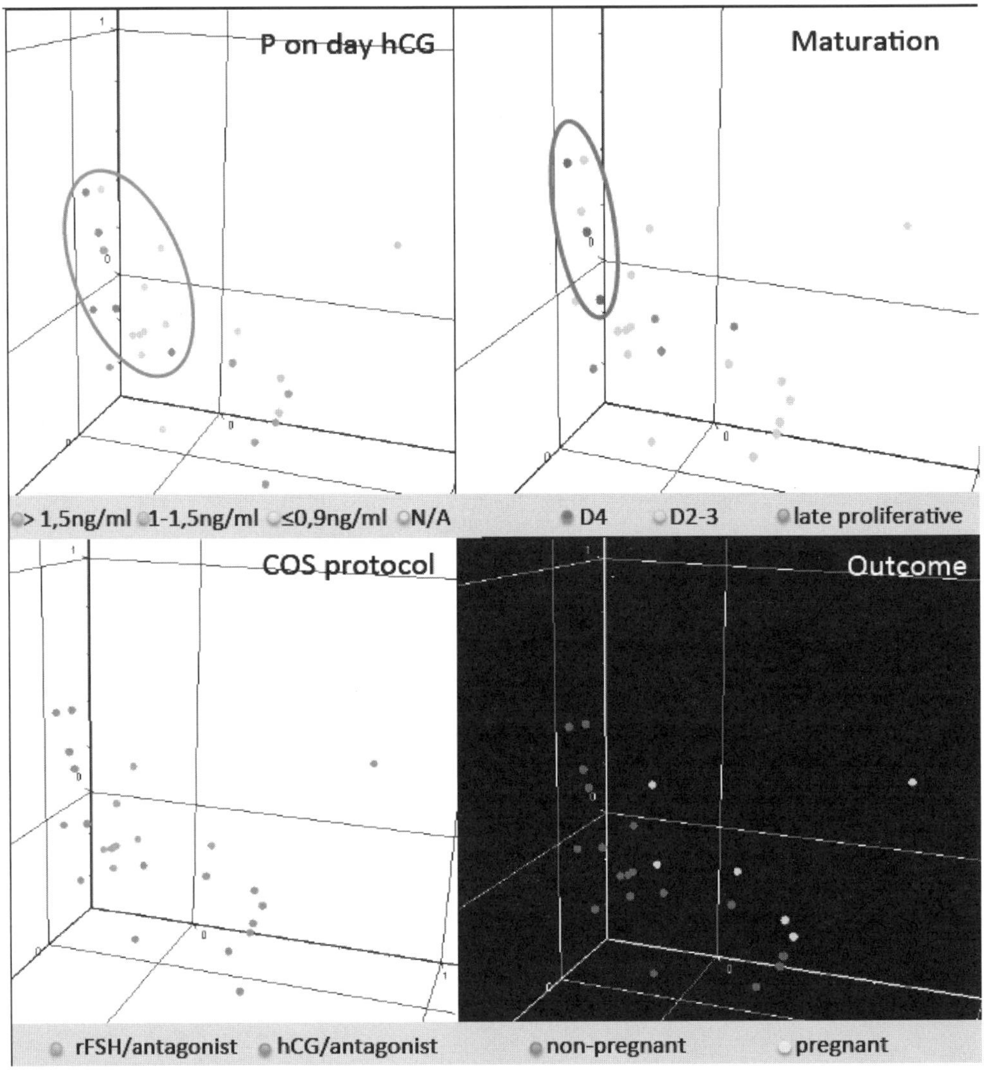

Legend to Figure 1

Gene expression performed with Affymetrix HG 133 Plus 2.0 microarray in endometria on the day of oocyte retrieval in GnRH-antagonist stimulated cycles with embryo transfer on day 3 or 5. Principal component analysis shows distinct clustering according to serum progesterone concentration on the day of hCG injection (A) and endometrial histological pattern (B), but not between two stimulation regimens (C). Gene clustering according to pregnancy outcome is shown in D (adapted from Van Vaerenbergh et al, TriCon Conference, 2011).

References

1. Coutifaris C, Myers ER, Guzick DS, Diamond MP, Carson SA, et al. Histological dating of timed endometrial biopsy tissue is not related to fertility status. Fertil Steril 2004;82: 1264–1272.
2. Murray MJ, Meyer WR, Zaino RJ, Lessey BA, Novotny DB, Ireland K, A critical analysis of the accuracy, reproducibility, and clinical utility of histologic endometrial dating in fertile women. Fertil Steril 2004; 81:1333-1343.
3. Noyes RW, Hertig AT, Rock J. Dating the endometrial biopsy. Fertil Steril 1950;1:3–25.
4. Talbi S, Hamilton AE, Vo KC, Tulac S, Overgaard MT, Dosiou C, et al. Molecular phenotyping of human endometrium distinguishes menstrual cycle phases and underlying biological processes in normo-ovulatory women. Endocrinology 2006;147:1097–1121.
5. King AE, Critchley HO. Oestrogen and progesterone regulation of the inflammatory processes in the human endometrium. J Steroid Biochem Mol Biol. 2010; 31: 116-26
6. Lessey BA . Assessment of endometrial receptivity. Fertil Steril 2011; 96: 522–529.
7. Bourgain C, Devroey P. The endometrium in stimulated cycles for IVF. Hum Reprod Update 2003;9: 515–522.
8. Lass A, Peat D, Avery S, Brinsden P. Histological evaluation of endometrium on the day of oocyte retrieval after gonadotrophin-releasing hormone agonist-follicle stimulating hormone ovulation induction for in-vitro fertilization. Hum Reprod 1998; 13:3203-3205.
9. Marchini M, Fedele L, Bianchi S, Losa GA, Ghisletta M, Candiani GB. Endometrial patterns during danazol and cyproterone acetate treatment for endometriosis: structural and ultrastructural study. Eur J Obstet Gynecol Reprod Biol 1991; 40:137-143
10. Ubaldi F, Bourgain C, Tournaye H, Smitz J, Van Steirteghem A, et al. Endometrial evaluation by aspiration biopsy on the day of oocyte retrieval in the embryo transfer cycles in patients with serum progesterone rise during the follicular phase. Fertil Steril 1997; 67: 521–526.
11. Kolibianakis EM, Bourgain C, Platteau P, Albano C, Van Steirteghem AC, et al. Abnormal endometrial development occurs during the luteal phase of nonsupplemented donor cycles treated with recombinant follicle-stimulating hormone and gonadotropin-releasing hormone antagonists. Fertil Steril 2003;80: 464–466.
12. Blockeel C, Van Vaerenbergh I, Fatemi HM, Van Lommel L, Devroey P et al, Gene expression profile in the endometrium on the day of oocyte retrieval after ovarian stimulation with low-dose hCG in the follicular phase. Mol Hum Reprod 2011: 17; 33-41
13. Evans J, Hannan N, Hincks C, Rombouts L, Salamonsen L. Defective soil for a fertile seed? Altered endometrial development is detrimental to pregnancy success. PLoS One. 2012;7:e53098. doi: 10.1371/journal.pone.0053098. Epub 2012 Dec 31
14. Van Vaerenbergh I, Van Lommel L, Ghislain V, In't Veld P, Schuit F, Fatemi HM, et al. In GnRH antagonist/rec-FSH stimulated cycles, advanced endometrial maturation on the day of oocyte retrieval correlates with altered gene expression. Hum Reprod 2009; 24:1085–91.
15. Kolibianakis EM, Bourgain C, Papanikolaou EG, Camus M, Tournaye H, et al. Prolongation of follicular phase by delaying hCG administration results in a higher incidence of endometrial advancement on the day of oocyte retrieval in GnRH antagonist cycles. Hum Reprod 2005; 20: 2453–2456.
16. Papanikolaou EG, Bourgain C, Kolibianakis E, Tournaye H, Devroey P. Steroid receptor expression in late follicular phase endometrium in GnRH antagonist IVF cycles is already altered, indicating initiation of early luteal phase transformation in the absence of secretory changes. Hum Reprod 2005; 20: 1541–1547.

17. Bourgain C, Ubaldi F, Tavaniotou A, Smitz J, Van Steirteghem AC, Devroey P. Endometrial hormone receptors and proliferation index in the periovulatory phase of stimulated embryo transfer cycles in comparison with natural cycles and relation to clinical pregnancy outcome. Fertil Steril. 2002; 78: 237-244.
18. Ochsenkühn R, Arzberger A, von Schönfeldt V, Gallwas J, Rogenhofer N, et al, Subtle progesterone rise on the day of human chorionic gonadotropin administration is associated with lower live birth rates in women undergoing assisted reproductive technology: a retrospective study with 2,555 fresh embryo transfers. Fertil Steril 2012: 98; 347-345
19. Van Vaerenbergh I, Fatemi HM, Blockeel C, Van Lommel L, In't Veld P, et al, Progesterone rise on HCG day in GnRH antagonist/rFSH stimulated cycles affects endometrial gene expression. Reprod Biomed Online 2011:22; 263-271.
20. Evans J, Salamonsen LA. Too much of a good thing? Experimental evidence suggests prolonged exposure to hCG is detrimental to endometrial receptivity. Hum Reprod. 2013 Mar 20. [Epub ahead of print]
21. Blockeel C, De Vos M, Verpoest W, Stoop D, Haentjens P et al. Can 200 IU of hCG replace recombinant FSH in the late follicular phase in a GnRH-antagonist cycle? A pilot study. Hum Reprod 2009: 24: 2910-2916
22. van der Linden M, Buckingham K, Farquhar C, Kremer JA, Metwally M. Luteal phase support for assisted reproduction cycles. Cochrane Database Syst Rev. 2011;(10): CD009154.
23. Humaidan P, Van Vaerenbergh I, Bourgain C, Alsbjerg B, Blockeel C, Schuit F et al. Endometrial gene expression in the early luteal phase is impacted by mode of triggering final oocyte maturation in recFSH stimulated and GnRH antagonist co-treated IVF cycles. Hum Reprod 2012; 27:3259-3272.
24. Van Vaerenbergh I, Blockeel C, Van Lommel L, Ghislain V, In'tVeld P et al. (2010) Cyclooxygenase-2 network as predictive molecular marker for clinical pregnancy in in-vitro fertilization. Fertil Steril 95: 448-51
25. Langenbach R, Loftin C, Lee C, Tiano H. Cyclooxygenase knockout mice: models for elucidating isoform-specific functions. Biochem Pharmacol. 1999; 15:1237-46.
26. Boomsma CM, Kavelaars A, Eijkemans MJ, Lentjes EG, Fauser BC, et al. Endometrial secretion analysis identifies a cytokine profile predictive of pregnancy in IVF. Hum Reprod 2009; 24: 1427–1435.

Trilogy 7. IFFS/WHO Trilogy: Assisted reproductive technology in the developing world

Access to reproductive medicine in the developing world

Willem Ombelet

Genk Institute for Fertility Technology, Genk, Belgium

Introduction

Infertility is a neglected health care issue in developing countries (DC), despite affecting more than 180 million couples (Rutstein and Iqbal 2004). Negative psychosocial, sociocultural, and economic consequences of childlessness are more pronounced in DC compared to Western societies. Childless women are frequently stigmatized, resulting in isolation, neglect, domestic violence, and polygamy (Dyer et al., 2002; Gerrits and Shaw 2010; Van Balen and Bos 2009; Umezulike and Efetie 2004). In DC most societies are organized so that children are necessary for care and maintenance of older parents. Moreover, in the absence of social security systems, older people are economically completely dependent on their children. Consequently, the inability to bear children is a tragedy, and childlessness can be considered as one of the most important and underappreciated reproductive health problems in DC (Ombelet et al., 2008).

The most common underlying cause for infertility in developing countries, especially in the sub-Saharan region, is severe male infertility and bilateral tubal occlusion caused by sexually transmitted infections (STIs), unsafe abortions, and postpartum infections. Bilateral tubal block can only be treated with in vitro fertilization (IVF), a treatment that is currently unavailable or too costly for most affected couples in DC (Nachtigall 2006; Ombelet et al., 2008). Reduced fecundity in human immunodeficiency virus (HIV)-infected individuals has been described and marital instability secondary to infertility may in turn increase the spread of HIV-1 infection. HIV is three times more prevalent in infertile couples when compared to fertile controls in the same population (Nabaitu et al., 1994; Dhont 2011). HIV and infertility share the same determinant of high-risk sexual behavior. Both conditions are more common in resource-poor countries, may lead to stigmatization and isolation, and are strongly influenced by socio-cultural and economic conditions.

Although IVF and related procedures get all the public attention, infertility care cannot be reduced to assisted reproductive techniques alone. Other options are equally important, such as a listening ear and psychological support for infertile couples, the availability of basic diagnostic procedures, intrauterine insemination, reproductive surgery, etc. The aim of this paper is to describe the pros and cons of infertility care in developing countries, with special attention to new and innovative simplified low-cost IVF methods that will be available in the near future.

Arguments against infertility care in DC

The two key arguments against treatment of infertility in DC are overpopulation and limited resources. The argument of **overpopulation** suggests that in countries where overpopulation poses a demographic problem, infertility management should not be supported by the government.

It is well known that the world population is expected to increase from 6.7 billion inhabitants in 2005 to 9.2 billion in 2050 (United Nations 2007). By 2050, the population of the developing world would be adding 35 million annually, 22 million of whom would be absorbed by the least-developed countries. Therefore, national and international health strategies have always focused on reducing total fertility rates (number of children per woman) while infertility care has received little or no attention at all. But even if infertility treatment could be made more accessible in DC it would probably account for less than 1% of all deliveries; increasing efforts on family planning and reproductive health education can readily overcome this small contribution to the fertility rate. United Nations data not only show that the majority of developing countries already succeeded in dropping their global fertility rate below 2.5, the data also show that the expected population growth in DC is mainly due to an improved life expectancy and not to high fertility rates (United Nations 2007).

According to the **'limited resources'** argument it is not justified to use expensive IVF techniques in countries where poverty is still an important issue and where health care systems still struggle with a huge problem of infectious diseases such as malaria, tuberculosis, and HIV. In most developing countries the reduction of maternal mortality and the promotion of contraception are considered to be the only reproductive health priorities (Aboulghar 2005). But, even with better education and preventative care programs, involuntary childlessness will remain an important problem for millions of couples.

Arguments supporting infertility care in DC

Reproductive autonomy is the main argument in favor of the provision of infertility treatment in developing countries. "Men and woman of full age, without any limitation due to race, nationality or religion, have the right to marry and to raise a family." This statement was adopted 60 years ago at the 1948 United Nations Universal Declaration of Human Rights and can't be misunderstood; it implies the right to access to fertility treatments when couples are unable to have children. At the United Nations International Conference on Population and Development in Cairo (1994) the following statement was made: "Reproductive health therefore implies that people have the capability to reproduce and the freedom to decide if, when and how often to do so … and to have the information and the means to do so …" In 2004 the World Health Assembly proposed five core statements, including "the provision of high-quality services for family-planning, including infertility services." In 2003, the International Federation of Obstetricians and Gynaecologists (FIGO) stated that "women and men have the right to the highest available standard of health care for all aspects of their sexual and reproductive health" (FIGO 2003).

From an **ethical and sociocultural** point of view, we have to ask ourselves whether we can justify withholding infertility treatment, including assisted reproductive technology (ART), in those cases where prevention has failed. Believing that the arguments of overpopulation and limited resources are strong enough for not helping infertile couples in developing countries doesn't take into account the human rights in general and the reproductive rights in particular (Vayena et al., 2002; Fathalla et al., 2006). Efforts should be made to reduce the excessive social reactions to infertility inspired by pronatalism. Therefore, infertility treatment should be part of an integrated reproductive care program including family planning and contraception, mother care, and reproductive health (Pennings et al., 2009). Education, empowerment of women, and economic prosperity are the most effective solutions to most problems related to both population growth and infertility. Simultaneously, investments in low-cost interventions are justified and urgently needed (Pennings et al., 2009). Reproductive autonomy, justice, and equity support our efforts to make ART available and accessible worldwide subject to political stability and a basic level of medical infrastructure.

Accessible infertility care: new developments

If we want to **implement accessible fertility services** in developing countries, the first objective is to simplify the diagnostic procedures (Malpani and Malpani, 2002). This can easily be organized in one-day clinics. The suggested work-up is very simple, reliable, and comparatively inexpensive. Moreover, all of these procedures can be performed by a small team of health care providers within a short period of time in an inexpensive setting (Ombelet and Campo 2007). Implementing low cost ART is only possible if we succeed in simplifying the methods of treatment in such a way that they remain effective and safe, but affordable. The number of scientific papers on simplification of ART procedures is growing every year.

For the recruitment of oocytes in an IVF program, we should avoid the use of high doses of expensive ovarian stimulation medication such as gonadotropins, gonadotropin-releasing hormone (GnRH) agonists, and GnRH antagonists, if possible. The use of clomiphene citrate has been proven in many studies to be an optimal alternative with acceptable results, minimal side effects, and a very low complication rate (Verberg et al., 2009; Kato et al., 2012).

Lowering the costs associated with laboratory procedures, namely fertilization and culture of eggs and embryos, represents another challenge. Intravaginal fertilization and culturing can be used as an inexpensive method for low cost IVF, with reasonable results (Frydman and Ranoux 2008). In our center we examined the value of a closed IVF laboratory system designed specifically for low-resource settings (see Van Blerkom). By the end of December 2012, 5 healthy babies were born as a result of this method with an embryo implantation rate of 35%, comparable with the results obtained after regular high-tech IVF.

Our method obviates the need for a complex laboratory and attendant infrastructure. Because there is no need for expensive CO^2 incubators, medical gas supply, or air purification systems, we calculated that the laboratory costs (direct and indirect costs) are between 10% and 15% of the current costs in a regular IVF setting. The running cost per IVF cycle turned out to be less than 200 .

The future

Infertility care has to be an essential part of a more comprehensive reproductive health care program including infertility and HIV prevention, family planning and safe mother care, a combination of prevention and treatment programs. The implementation of new reproductive technologies will require well-organized education and training programs. Regular audits and systems of accreditation and registration should be implemented in order to maintain appropriate standards of care in all centers involved. The need for funding is crucial and is likely to require input and collaboration from various role players.

Conclusion

During more than 30 years of IVF almost 4.5 million babies have been born. This would be a great success story if a large part of the world population could benefit from these new technologies, which is not the case. The time has come to give equitable access to effective and safe infertility care in resource-poor countries as well. The immense problem of childlessness in developing countries requires greater attention at national and international levels for reasons of social justice and equity (Fathalla 2006; Vayena et al., 2009; Ombelet 2011). Keystones in the successful implementation of infertility care in low-resource settings include simplification of ART procedures in order to establish accessible good-quality infertility services at low cost. The success and sustainability of ART in resource-poor settings will depend to a large extent on our ability to optimize these techniques in terms of availability, affordability, and effectiveness. Our preliminary outcome results clearly show that when IVF is the only solution, this simplified system may make advanced infertility treatment in DC practical, affordable, and, with respect to outcome, similar to rates reported in the developed world.

To conclude, I believe that global access to infertility care in developing countries can only be achieved when good-quality but affordable infertility care is linked to more effective family planning and safe motherhood programs. Only a global project with respect to sociocultural, ethical, economical, and political differences will be successful for millions of childless women in developing countries.

References

Aboulghar MA. The importance of fertility treatment in the developing world. BJOG 2005; 112:1174-1176.

Dhont N. Clinical, epidemiological and socio-cultural aspects of infertility in resource-poor settings', FV&V in ObGyn 2011;3:77-88. www.fvvo.eu

Dyer SJ, Abrahams N, Hoffman M, van der Spuy ZM. Men leave me as I cannot have children': women's experiences with involuntary childlessness. Hum Reprod 2002;17:1663-1668.

Fathalla MF, Sinding SW, Rosenfield A, Fathalla MMF. Sexual and reproductive health for all: a call for action. Lancet 2006;368:2095-2100.

FIGO. Resolution on Professional and Ethical Responsibilities Concerning Sexual and Reproductive Rights. 2003;www.figo.org/projects/ethical_responsibility

Frydman R, Ranoux C (2008) 'INVO: a simple, low cost effective assisted reproductive technology', Hum Reprod, ESHRE Monographs 2008;85-89.

Gerrits T, Shaw M. Biomedical infertility care in sub-Saharan Africa: a social science review of current practices, experiences and view points. FV&V in ObGyn 2010;2:194-207. www.fvvo.eu

Kato K, Takehara Y, Segawa T, Kawachiya S, Okuno T, Kobayashi T, et al. Minimal ovarian stimulation combined with elective single embryo transfer policy: age-specific results of a large, single-centre, Japanese cohort. Reprod Biol Endocrinol 2012;10:35. doi: 10.1186/1477-7827-10-35.

Malpani A, Malpani A. Simplifying assisted conception techniques to make them universally available--a view from India. Hum Reprod 2002;7:49-50.

Nabaitu J, Bachengana C, Seeley J. Marital instability in a rural population in south-west Uganda: implications for the spread of HIV-1 infection. Africa (London) 1994;64: 243-251.

Nachtigall RD. International disparities in access to infertility services. Fertil Steril 2006;85:871-875.

Ombelet W, Campo R. Affordable IVF for developing countries. Reprod Biomed Online 2007;15:257-265.

Ombelet W, Cooke I, Dyer S, Serour G, Devroey P. Infertility and the provision of infertility medical services in developing countries. Hum Reprod Update 2008;14:605-621.

Ombelet W. Reproductive healthcare systems should include accessible infertility diagnosis and treatment: An important challenge for resource-poor countries. Int J Gynaecol Obstet 2009;106:168-171.

Ombelet W. Global access to infertility care in developing countries: a case of human rights, equity and social justice. FV&V in ObGyn 2011;3:257-266. www.fvvo.eu

Pennings G, de Wert G, Shenfield F, Cohen J, Tarlatzis B, Devroey P. ESHRE Task Force

on Ethics and Law. Providing infertility treatment in resource-poor countries. Hum Reprod 2009;24:1008-1011.
Rutstein SO, Iqbal HS. Infecundity, Infertility, and Childlessness in Developing Countries. DHS Comparative Reports, WHO, 2004, p 24.
Umezulike AC, Efetie ER. The psychological trauma of infertility in Nigeria. Int J Gynaecol Obstet 2004;84:178-180.
United Nations International Conference on Population and Development, Cairo 2004, www.un.org/esa/population/cpd/cpd2004/CPD37_Res2004-2.
United Nations (2006) Department of Economic and Social Affairs, population Division (2007). World Population Prospects: The 2006 Revision, Highlights, Working Paper No ESA/P/WP.202.
Van Balen F, Bos HMW. The social and cultural consequences of being childless in poor-resource areas. FV&V in ObGyn 2009;1:106-121. www.fvvo.eu
Van Balen F, Gerrits T. Quality of infertility care in poor-resource areas and the introduction of new reproductive technologies. Hum Reprod 2001;16:215-219.
Vayena E, Peterson HB, Adamson D, Nygren KG. Assisted reproductive technologies in developing countries: are we caring yet? Fertil Steril 2009;92:413-416.
Vayena E, Rowe JP, Peterson HB. Assisted reproductive technology in developing countries: why should we care? Fertil Steril 2002;78:13-15.
Verberg MF, Macklon NS, Nargund G, Frydman R, Devroey P, Broekmans FJ, et al. 'Mild ovarian stimulation for IVF', Hum Reprod Update 2009;15:13-29.
World Health Assembly 2004, www.who.int/mediacentre/releases/2004

Cost-effective protocol in in vitro fertilization

Korula George

Bangalore Baptist Hospital, Karnataka, India

Infertility is a worldwide problem affecting almost 10% of the population (1). With advancements in reproductive medicine, most infertility issues can be treated successfully. However, treatment is expensive and hence only a small proportion of infertile couples will actually be able to make use of the treatment facilities. Although infertility has been classified as a disease by the World Health Organization (WHO), acceptance is still restricted, resulting in limited attention to the problem by health care policy makers (2). The availability of public funding or health insurance facilities differs all over the world. In lower-income countries overpopulation is an important factor and the focus is on family planning programs or other major health problems like infectious diseases or maternal mortality (3). With limited financial resources the necessity of making available infertility services is neglected.

In the developing world marriage is almost universal, with the aspiration of having children a major prerogative. The social stigma associated with infertility is difficult to accept and infertile couples are often ostracized and isolated from the community (4). Pressure from within the family is the most traumatizing. Inability to conceive is almost always perceived as the women's fault, leading to instability in the marriage relationship. Women are often subjected to physical assault or threatened with the possibility of divorce. Familial pressure often results in the husband opting for a second marriage. In these nations tubal disorders are common and are usually due to sexually transmitted diseases, postpartum infections, or post-abortion complications (5). Although focus on prevention is important, provision of treatment options also is important. The ability to access infertility services is essential and critical for the couple. Infertility needs to be considered a public health problem of high priority and provision of affordable medical facilities is vital.

Although treatment facilities are available, most couples are unable to utilize the treatment facilities due to the high cost of assisted reproductive technology (ART). Development of an affordable ART system is important. However, in order to achieve reasonable outcomes one cannot compromise on laboratory quality. A laboratory environment conforming to in vitro fertilization (IVF) standards together with the availability of standard IVF/intracytoplasmic sperm injection (ICSI) equipment is essential. One then needs to consider innovative options to reduce costs, such as: proper patient selection, limiting investigations to essential requirements, establishing alternative stimulation protocols, and altering laboratory practices (6).

The first IVF baby, Louise Brown, was born following a natural cycle IVF. The Norfolk group in the United States introduced the concept of ovarian stimulation in 1981 (7). Either oral ovulation induction agents like clomiphene citrate or urinary gonadotropins was used with the intention of marginally increasing oocyte availability. The introduction of gonadotropin-releasing hormone (GnRH) agonists resulted in an increase in the dosage required for stimulation. The thought of transferring multiple embryos to improve pregnancy rates together with the introduction of cryopreservation resulted in the concept of obtaining a large number of oocytes, causing a substantial increase in dose of the stimulation drugs and overall treatment costs. Although use of an antagonist protocol does reduce the gonadotropin requirement, the overall drug cost is not significantly reduced due to antagonist pricing (8). Overstimulation with recovery of many oocytes is associated with several detrimental factors: oocyte immaturity, oocyte aneuploidy, and endometrial defects due to high hormone levels (9). Multiple pregnancies due to transfer of many embryos make matters worse, especially in a low-resource setting. An increasing incidence of ovarian hyperstimulation together with the complications and cost factor of higher order pregnancies has resulted in the concept of a less aggressive ovarian stimulation approach (10).

In the traditional IVF stimulation protocol, high doses of gonadotropins ensure follicle-stimulating hormone (FSH) levels above the threshold level with prolongation of the FSH window time period, resulting in the production of a large number of follicles. The principle of a mild stimulation protocol is to transiently prolong the FSH window period in the midfollicular phase, thus allowing production of a few more follicles than the conventional single dominant follicle seen in a natural cycle. The introduction of the antagonist protocol supports minimal stimulation regimens by preventing an LH surge (11). The advantage of mild stimulation protocols is two-fold: create a more patient friendly protocol as well as a reduction in costs (10, 11).

Although natural cycle IVF is less demanding and inexpensive, the overall results are unacceptably low (7.2%) with a high cancellation rate (12). The modified natural cycle protocol using a GnRH antagonist and minimal stimulation with gonadotropins improves outcomes, but low efficacy has restricted widespread use (10). Clomiphene citrate was originally used in IVF for ovarian stimulation prior to being replaced by gonadotropins. Combined use with gonadotropins reduces the amount of gonadotropins required. Use of the GnRH antagonist protocol will also prevent the LH surge. Randomized trials comparing a combination of clomiphene citrate and gonadotropins with traditional protocols are contentious, as differing results have been obtained (13). Nevertheless, it certainly has a place in cost-effective mild stimulation regimens.

An uncommon protocol that uses clomiphene citrate continuously in combination with gonadotropins has been reported to be effective with acceptable pregnancy rates (14). Continuous use of clomiphene citrate from day 1/2 of the cycle until oocyte retrieval blocks the estrogen receptors in the hypothalamus and pituitary. Acting like a GnRH agonist it thus prevents an LH surge that is usually initiated by rising levels of estrogen, a result of follicular development. When used in combination with gonadotropins it results in development of a reasonable number of oocytes. The benefit of such a protocol is reduction in cost due to the nonrequirement of a GnRH analogue (6). The anti-estrogen effects of clomiphene citrate on the endometrium could affect implantation rates. However, Kawachiya et al. have reported ongoing pregnancy rates of 26.8% per embryo transfer using the said protocol (14).

Patient selection and monitoring during IVF are important in ensuring an optimal outcome. Women less than 35 years of age with a BMI less than 25 are more likely to benefit from a mild stimulation protocol. Basic investigations such as hemoglobin, viral screen, or thyroid evaluation, if indicated, will limit costs. Monitoring during IVF can be done entirely by ultrasound (15). With experienced clinicians, biochemical monitoring is not required. In the IVF laboratory, limiting the number of oocytes retrieved does reduce the usage of disposables and media. ICSI needs to be considered only for pure male factor disorders and not done on a routine basis. With reduction in the number of oocytes, embryo transfer can be planned for day 2 and the facility for cryopreservation is not likely to be required.

Using a simplified laboratory has been advocated to limit expenditure. Use of alternatives to laminar flow and incubators have been suggested such as humidicrib, warm bath, and INVOcell® (16, 17). Implementation of these innovative ideas could be of economic benefit in certain low-cost zones. However, if one wants to ensure reasonably good results one cannot compromise on the laboratory environment or equipment.

When evaluating IVF costs, several aspects need to be considered. In addition to direct costs, one does encounter indirect and downstream costs (18). Indirect costs are attributed to the patient's involvement in the procedure and include matters such as loss of pay or cost of stay or transport. Downstream costs involve expenditure due to complications, such as multiple pregnancy or premature delivery. When looking at direct costs, one can divide them into actual costs and dispensable costs. Actual costs include the actual expenditure incurred during each

IVF cycle by both the patient and the hospital. This would include expenditure for items such as drugs, culture media, and disposables like oocyte aspiration needles or plastic ware. Hospital charges, which aim to retrieve the investment made in the IVF laboratory or for payment of personnel like medical, nursing, or scientific staff, can be labeled as dispensable charges. When trying to provide IVF services for an underprivileged community, one has to look at costs with a different perspective. Excluding dispensable costs and taking measures to reduce the direct cost will ensure availability of the services for needy couples

In the developing world most IVF centers are within the private sector, being run by individuals or corporate hospitals, with a focus on providing IVF services for the affordable minority. The public field such as medical schools and government hospitals has limited facilities for infertility services. To initiate a low-cost IVF program is not going to be easy as most governments in the developing world are engaged in providing basic health care services. Motivation of successful IVF centers in the private sector to develop a social/moral obligation to provide IVF services at a reasonable cost would be endearing.

The potential of a private-public sector partnership is enormous. Government-run primary/secondary-level fertility units can be established with the intention of providing infertility treatment facilities. These facilities will not be expensive to set up and can cater to the problems of a large majority of infertile couples. A government-sponsored insurance program in collaboration with established IVF units using a low-cost approach would provide IVF services for the needy. In many European countries and in Australia, government funding for ART treatment is available, although guidelines for eligibility exist and do differ amongst countries (19). In the United States there are no subsidies, and the cost of treatment is very expensive. Hence, infertility care will not be accessible for low-income groups even in the developed world and there is a need for availability of affordable care worldwide.

Over the past decade the provision of affordable fertility facilities has been a popular subject matter. In 2001 the World Health Organization recommended that infertility should be considered as a global health problem and suggested development of a low-cost approach for low-resource settings. Universal access to reproductive health is also one of the United Nations Millennium Development Goals to be achieved by 2015 (20). The European Society of Human Reproduction and Embryology (ESHRE) set up a task force on infertility in developing countries that has assessed the problems and made innovative suggestions (2). A non-profit, low-cost IVF foundation was set up in 2007 with the aim of providing IVF services for less than 200 euro. The Walking Egg foundation, established in 2010, and the Friends of the Low-cost IVF Foundation, established in 2011, also aim to provide high-quality infertility resources in low-income settings. However, actual implementation of these suggestions does not appear to be prevalent or in evidence.

In 2011 the author's group, from an established university IVF set-up, initiated an affordable IVF program with the intention of providing IVF facilities for those unable to undergo traditional IVF (6). Utilizing an unconventional stimulation protocol (continuous use of clomiphene citrate together with gonadotropins) together with cost-limiting initiatives achieved a live birth rate and clinical pregnancy rate per transfer of 19% and 22%, respectively. The multiple pregnancy rate was 26% with no reported case of ovarian hyperstimulation. The direct cost for an IVF cycle was US $675 while ICSI cost US $725. This is probably the only available data on an actual implementation of a low-cost ART program.

Conclusion

The provision of ART facilities at an affordable cost is important. Modifications of traditional protocols and monitoring systems will help in reducing costs. In order to obtain acceptable outcomes, there can be no compromise on the laboratory quality or facilities. Health policy makers need to strategically plan an integrated approach to provide infertility services globally.

References

1. Boivin J, Bunting L, Collins AJ, Nygren GK. International estimates of infertility prevalence and infertility treatment seeking: potential need and demand for infertility medical care. Hum Reprod 2007; 22(6):1506-1512.
2. Vayena E, Rowe P, Griffin PD. Current practices and controversies in assisted reproduction: Report of a World Health Organization meeting. Geneva: World Health Organization; 2002.
3. Ombelet W, Campo R. Affordable IVF for developing coutries. Reprod Biomed Online 2007; 15(3):257-265.
4. Van Balen F, Bos HMW. The social and cultural consequences of being childless in poor resource areas. FV &V in ObGyn 2009; 1:106-121.
5. Ombelet W. Reproductive healthcare systems should include accessible infertility diagnosis and treatment: An important challenge for resource poor countries. Int J Gynaecol Obstet 2009;106:168-171.
6. Aleyamma TK, Kamath MS, Muthukumar K, Mangalaraj AM, George K. Affordable ART: a different perspective. Hum Reprod 2011;26(12):3312-8.
7. Ferraretti AP, Garcia JE, Acosta AA, Jones GS. Serum lutienizing hormone during ovulation induction with human menopausal gonadotrophin for invitro fertilitzation in normally menstruating women. Fertil Steril 1983;40:742-7.
8. Al-Inany HG, Youssef MA, Aboulghar M, Broeakmans F,Sterrenburg M, Smit J, Abou-Setta AM. Gonadotrophin-releasing hormone antagonists for assisted reproductive technology. Cochrane Database Syst Rev 2011;(5): CD001750.
9. Baart EB, Martini E, Eijkemans MJ, Van Opstal D, Beckers NG, Verhoeff A, Macklon NS, Fauser BC. Milder ovarian stimulation for in-vitro fertilization reduces aneuploidy in the human preimplantation embryo: a randomized controlled trial. Hum Reprod 2007;22(4):980-8.
10. Fauser BCJM, Nargund G, Andersen AN, Norman R, Tarlatzis B, Boivin J, Ledger W. Mild ovarian stimulation for IVF: 10 years later. Hum Reprod 2010; 25:2678-2684.
11. Figueiredo JB, Nastri CO, Vieira AD, Martins WP. Clomiphene combined with gonadotropins and GnRH antagonist versus conventional controlled ovarian hyperstimulation without clomiphene in women undergoing assisted reproductive techniques: systematic review and meta-analysis. Arch Gynecol Obstet 2013;287(4):779-90.
12. Nargund G, Waterstone J, Bland J, Philips Z, Parsons J, Campbell S. Cumulative conception and live birth rates in natural (unstimulated) IVF cycles. Hum Reprod. 2001 Feb;16(2):259-62.
13. Gibreel A, Maheshwari A, Bhattacharya S. Clomiphene citrate in combination with gonadotropins for controlled ovarian stimulation in women undergoing in vitro fertilization. Cochrane Database Syst Rev 2012;11:CD008528.

14. Kawachiya S, Segawa T, Kato K, Takehara Y, Teramoto S, Kato O. The effectiveness of clomiphene citrate in suppressing the LH surge in the minimal stimulation IVF protocol. Fertil Steril 2006; 86(Suppl. 2):S412.
15. Golan A, Herman A, Soffer Y, Bukovsky I, Ron-El R. Ultrasonic control without hormone determination for ovulation induction in in-vitro fertilization/embryo transfer with gonadotrophin-releasing hormone analogue and human menopausal gonadotrophin. Hum Reprod 1994; 9:1631-1633.
16. Frydman R, Ranoux C. INVO: a simple, low cost effective assisted reproductive technology. Hum Reprod ESHRE Monographs 2008; 85-89.
17. Hovatta O, Cooke I. Cost-effective approaches to in vitro fertilization: means to improve access. Int J Gynaecol Obstet 2006; 94:287-291.
18. Collins J. An international survey of the health economics of IVF and ICSI. Hum Reprod Update 2002; 8:265-277.
19. Chambers GM, Sullivan EA, Ishihara O, Chapman MG, Adamson GD. The economic impact of assisted reproductive technology: a review of selected developed countries. Fertil Steril 2009;91:2281-2294.
20. United Nations Development Program, Human Development Report 2003, Millennium Development Goals: A Compact among Nations to End Human Poverty (New York: Oxford University Press, 2003).

Towards universal infertility care: An in vitro fertilization system designed for low settings in the developing world

Jonathan Van Blerkom

University of Colorado, Boulder. United States

The state of IVF in the developed world

Contemporary infertility treatments have a range of assisted reproductive technologies (ART) available, including in vitro fertilization (IVF), which can be tailored to the specific circumstances of the patients. Indeed, infertility treatment is not only commonplace and widely accessible in the developed world, but is often considered a 'reproductive right.' More recently, the ART enterprise in the developed world has experienced new avenues of growth by means of the commercialization of oocyte cryobanking or of social cryopreservation, the autologous cryopreservation of oocytes for young women who want to put off having children until later years for career or other personal reasons. The medical necessity of oocyte cryopreservation has become most evident for women facing chemo/radiation therapy, the nascent area of 'onco-fertility.' In this regard, the field of medically assisted conception is continually evolving as new methods are introduced and new uses for existing procedures are embraced, such as those described above. Some methods may or have already improved outcome. In this respect, IVF has progressed markedly from its original indication as the primary treatment for tubal occlusions and subnormal sperm counts (but with largely normal morphology and motility) to encompass more complex and challenging male and female factor etiologies of infertility.

Today, IVF, intracytoplasmic sperm injection (ICSI), and oocyte and embryo vitrification are the mainstays of ART treatment in the developed world after pharmaceutical intervention and intrauterine insemination (IUI) have failed. For IVF, additional improvements in outcome have resulted from a better understanding of morphological and performance characteristics that are competence-related. These characteristics have been described as positive or negative indicators of developmental potential and have recently been standardized for selective purposes to facilitate the identification of oocytes to inseminate (by ICSI) or embryos to transfer or cryopreserve (1). An important aspect of using a standardized, time-dependent morphology or performance criteria is that it provides a common selection paradigm and descriptive language that can be used by any trained operator. Time-lapse systems, recently introduced into the clinical IVF laboratory for assessment and selective purposes, continuously document time-related morphokinetic features during the preimplantation stages that are developmentally significant and could be missed by static imaging schemes unless specifically and consistently timed (2). It is likely that further enhancements will include artificial intelligence and image matching algorithms based on large multi-center databases of morphological and morphokinetic characteristics that have been associated with outcome (3). It is worth noting that in the high-resource, high-complexity IVF centers in the developed world, advances in competence assessment such as these can be essential to improving outcome and, it should also be noted, have the real potential to eliminate the operator from the observational and assessment aspect entirely. Indeed, this could come to pass if some of the more recent microanalytical methods designed to assess culture medium containing mature oocytes and preimplantation stage embryos for metabolic activity levels (e.g., oxygen, pyruvate, glucose uptake, or changes in concentration of certain amino acids) can be definitively shown to be biomarkers of competence (4).

On the male factor side, new methods of image analysis and enhancement that have been suggested to be effective in sperm selection for ICSI are based on the ability to visually deselect sperm with certain nuclear/head abnormalities and defects (intracytoplasmic morphologically selected sperm injection [IMSI]), defects that may not be fully eliminated by conventional density gradient preparation. While there are clear benefits to eliminate such sperm for ICSI if not readily detected at the lower magnification available from conventional light microscopic optics (e.g., differential interference contrast), current outcome findings are controversial and it remains to be determined whether this technology will so improve outcome as to justify the considerable costs for equipment and additional operator time and effort (5, 6). Viewing the oocyte meiotic spindle under polarizing optics (e.g., PolScope) was a similar and costly image enhancement system for the clinical IVF laboratory that was intended to identify the location and morphology of the metaphase II (MII) spindle for ICSI. Here, the benefit was to deselect oocytes without a detectable or normally configured spindle, and to avoid 'hitting' the spindle with the ICSI pipette that, it was thought, could disrupt chromosomal attachment and result in iatrogenic aneuploidy. In both cases, the location and morphodynamic nature of the spindle during maturation turned out to be less consequential with respect to outcome than originally thought.

Although clinical pregnancy rates have nearly doubled from those reported by some of the more experienced programs soon after IVF became a 'first-line' treatment, there does appear to be a ceiling with respect to the 'take home baby rate' with each cycle, especially with single embryo transfers (SET). In large measure, this is explained by one of the most important but not necessarily unexpected findings to come from years of clinical IVF: namely, the human oocyte has an inherently high frequency of simple and complex aneuploidies detectable at MII that negatively impact outcome. Aneuploidy is seen in morphologically normal-appearing MII oocytes of young women and increase progressively and markedly in frequency at each decade of reproductive age until menopause. Unfortunately, the presence of numerical or structural chromosomal abnormalities in oocytes does not preclude their ability to be fertilized but, depending upon the specific defect, does influence the developmental ability of the embryo during the pre- and postimplantation stages.

The issue of chromosomal normality becomes especially relevant when current protocols of ovarian hyperstimulation promote the preovulatory maturation of large numbers of oocytes, some of which may not have developed the capacity to progress normally though preovulatory resumption of arrested meiosis or to properly segregate chromosomes. Mitotic errors after fertilization are also evident from cytogenetic analyses that show aneuploidies ranging from monosomies and trisomies to chaotic numerical chromosomal mosaicisms between blastomeres that will also add to the high rate of embryonic wastage, a phenomenon long known to be a natural feature of human reproductive biology. Fortunately, advances in molecular biology methodology and the development of remarkably powerful DNA amplification and sequencing instrumentation has changed the paradigm of preimplantation genetic diagnosis from fluorescence in situ hybridization (FISH) to techniques using comparative genomic hybridization (CGH). These techniques are rapid and can profile the entire genome rather than detecting specific chromosomes(s). CGH is used for preimplantation-stage embryos with single cell biopsies during cleavage or small fragments of trophectoderm during the blastocyst stage. This technology has been applied to the chromosomal analysis of the first or second polar bodies (PB), or both, which enables detection of aneuploidies at the completion of the first and second metaphases, leading to the elimination of affected oocytes or fertilized eggs for insemination or transfer, respectively (7, 8).

The state of the ART of IVF in the developing world

It is evident that the state of the art of infertility treatment in high resource settings in general, and the so-called developed world in particular, is one of increasing complexity on several fronts, all directed to improving success by reducing the risk of early developmental failure (i.e., frequency of wastage for transferred embryos) with normal, healthy babies the expected outcome. All of the goals, technical advancements, and essential expertise that define a modern clinical IVF laboratory come at increased financial costs, which for those fortunate to live in the developed world are usually borne by some form of private or state insurance, or the patients, or both. In this context, ART and IVF, including the various derivatives discussed above, are largely accessible and successful, which account for the hundreds of thousands of cycles performed worldwide in such settings each year.

A large majority of the 180 million couples affected by infertility worldwide reside in developing countries where IVF technology is not available, and if accessible, unaffordable to only the wealthy few (9, 10). The notion that infertility treatments, including an affordable mechanism for IVF, could bring procedures common in the developed world to low resource settings where it is equally needed, would seem to be a foolish endeavor given an infrastructure that is inconsistent with how IVF is routinely and most effectively performed. The idea of establishing numerous, small, self-sufficient centers that can perform IVF tends to run contrary to philanthropic mission of large philanthropic foundations, where contraception and birth control are the primary focus for funding. Likewise, a not atypical view from a developed world perspective is that advanced infertility treatment as part of an overall attempt to address issues of women's health in general and reproductive health in particular, while well-intentioned, is nevertheless misguided and doomed to failure without the support structure that enables Western-style IVF centers to operate effectively and efficiently.

The issue of why failure might be an inevitable outcome of such an effort is not an unreasonable response. By the very definition of a low-resource setting, the infrastructure found in developed counties and essential for IVF to work and to work successfully is lacking, problematic to maintain reliably or consistently, or too great a challenge to set up. If such an infrastructure were to function effectively, it would only be in large cities where, indeed, some Western-style private IVF program(s) do exist but are geared to and affordable by only a small fraction of the infertile population who tend to be the wealthiest. According to this view, it should be self-evident that multiple small centers would be difficult if not impossible to establish, and the costs inherent in setting up and maintaining a laboratory and associated services so dear as to preclude from treatment the target population a program of this type was intended to serve. Why, then, bother at all?

In this sense, skeptics and critics are correct, if the system is intended and designed to largely duplicate the typical IVF unit in a developed or Western country. It is true that (i) a reliable source of clean electricity can be a challenge and voltage fluxes or current spikes can damage or destroy sensitive electronics and microprocessors that control temperature and atmosphere in modern tissue culture incubators; (ii) the availability of certified medical grade gases used for IVF (nitrogen, carbon dioxide, and oxygen) can be problematic or effectively unavailable when the supplier is distant from the site of use and delivery and actual purity is uncertain; (iii) ultra-sterile conditions and highly filtered air commonplace in modern IVF units in developed countries may be difficult to establish or maintain; and (iv) that 'down time' due to equipment failure may close a center with patients awaiting treatment because replacement parts or technicians needed to effect repair or service cannot arrive in a timely manner. In this regard, setting up an affordable IVF center in a low-resource setting by exactly duplicating a high resource program with donated but used equipment, such as modern tissue culture incubators, can be counterproductive if a similar support structure is also a major issue.

Towards a universal IVF system for low resource, developing countries: The walking egg project

In the companion presentation to this trilogy, Dr. Willem Ombelet describes the origin, intent, and current status of the Walking Egg Project, a program designed to meet the goals of providing advanced and affordable reproductive services in the developing world. For IVF in particular, an entirely new paradigm of how IVF could be provided, which takes into account the problems and challenges noted above, was needed. The basic goal for offering IVF was that it had to be truly affordable by most in the target population and effective with respect to outcome, given that it needed to be specifically designed from the ground up for low-resource settings rather than as a 'stripped down' version of a high-resource program using donated equipment. A second feature was that procedures essential to the actual IVF process had to be simplified and largely self-sufficient, especially during the fertilization, culture, and transfer phases. In this regard, the system had to be as independent from a high-resource infrastructure as possible, such that all operations from insemination to removal for transfer precluded direct environmental exposure (including competence assessment for selection) and minimized any disruption to the culture system that could negatively affect normal development. Furthermore, the IVF system needed to be clinically tested first in a high-resource setting to show that its operation was simple, cost-effective, and safe and, with respect to outcome, produced results similar to young women treated by IVF for tubal occlusion infertility at IVF centers in the developed world. For the initial application of this IVF system for the Walking Egg Project in developing countries, the most common cause of infertility that would be seen is tubal occlusions resulting from sexually transmitted diseases and pregnancy-related infections (9, 10).

The full details of how an effective, simplified, and affordable IVF for low-resource settings was 'conceived' as part of the Walking Egg Project are described in Dr. Ombelet's presentation and elsewhere (11). However, the essence of the system is that clinical IVF can be done with essentially off-the-shelf materials made on site or inexpensively pre-packaged, depending upon location and available expertise. For this purpose, all that is needed are (i) two standard, uncoated glass vacutainers (Becton-Dickson), (ii) tubing and needles to connect them, (ii) one of any of the several commercially available complex human IVF culture media if development is to be continued to the blastocyst stage, or simpler media for up to day 3 transfers, (iii) any dark environment that can provide 37°C, and (iv) a dissecting microscope. A small sterile surround that can accommodate all operations and the microscope is desirable.

The problems inherent in designing any IVF system, whether for high- or low-resource settings, are incubation, culture conditions (pH and atmospherics), and minimization of disruption of these conditions during fertilization and preimplantation development. To achieve culture conditions typically used in clinical IVF, we took advantage of a simple and old method of carbon dioxide generation (used by the present author many years ago for transporting oocytes and embryos from certain animals over long distances for experimental purposes), namely, the mixture of weak acids and bases that in the present instance is citric acid and sodium bicarbonate, although other reagents work as well (11). During the clinical trial phase described below, we found that a similar approach using a common effervescent antacid (Alka-Seltzer) had also been used for mouse embryo culture (12), but without the precise quantification of atmosphere or culture conditions that were deemed absolutely critical in order to assure clinicians in developing countries that this simplified and largely autonomous IVF system was functionally equivalent to any used in a high-resource setting.

Accordingly, systematic titration of reagent concentration and water volume produced CO2 in one vacutainer that when connected to a second one containing about 1 mL of culture medium (Fig. A) for a specific period of time, created conditions in the culture tube that were consistent with human IVF and similar to those found in high complexity tissue culture incubators using medical grade gases (11). By quantitating the kinetics of changes in medium pH and carbon dioxide and oxygen with highly sensitive microelectrodes, a constant pH between 7.35 and 7.37 in a stable atmosphere of 12.5% O_2 and 6.4% CO_2 is created within a few hours in Global T, the primary medium used for these pilot studies. However, slight changes in citric acid or sodium bicarbonate concentrations and adjusting the time the two vacutainers are connected can increase or decrease pH by small increments, which may be suitable or needed for other medium formulations (11). Once prepared, the conditions in the enclosed tube containing equilibrated medium are stable for prolonged periods. In our experience, medium stored at this way at 5°C for at least 4 weeks fully supports human embryonic development to the hatched blastocyst stage (see below). Incubation can occur in any environment that maintains 37°C. We have used small heating blocks, battery operated portable incubators, and, as shown in Figure B, a simple water bath for incubation. If a water bath is used, one that can be tightly covered and has the ability for rotary motion is preferred because culture is in a dark environment and the rotary movement within the culture tube may be of some developmental benefit.

IVF in an equilibrated medium tube is simple. One or more cumulus oocyte complexes (COCs) are drawn into a 1 mL standard tuberculin syringe in an 18 g needle in about 50 μL of equilibrated medium (from another tube) and slowly injected onto the side of the tube so that the passage of the COCs into the medium can be visualized. During microscopic inspection at this stage, holding the tube at an angle slightly less than 45 degrees often displaces a fully expanded cumulus oophorus as it slowly slides down, allowing visualization of the oocyte and, not infrequently, confirmation of nuclear maturation status (GV [germinal vesicle] or if PB1, MII). Insemination is done with prepared sperm in the same manner. We have found that <~1,000 normally motile sperm/mL is sufficient for monospermic fertilization. Higher concentrations of up to 5,000 motile sperm/mL can be used, but with an attendant risk of dispermy. The volume containing sperm injected into the tube some hours after deposition of the COCs is at most 50 μL (11).

From this point onward, the IVF steps are the same as would be done in a high-resource setting, with one exception; because the COCs are inseminated in a closed system, cumulus and corona denudation to confirm fertilization (by pronuclear inspection) cannot be done by mechanical stripping, if the system is to remain undisturbed. While mechanical denudation can be done if the COCs are removed from the insemination tube and after stripping returned to a fresh tube of equilibrated medium, we have found that gentle vortexing of the intact culture is sufficient in most instances to remove cumulus and coronal cells at levels that permit determination of pronuclear number without disturbing the culture environment. A further enhancement for this stage is facilitated by the addition of ~15 IU of hyaluronidase in the final volume of sperm added, followed by gentle vortexing at the time of the fertilization inspection. Despite the uncoated nature of the vacutainer glass, some fertilized eggs with a small remnant of cumulus may adhere to the surface after inspection. Most of these cells will be displaced from the zona at the cleavage inspection (2-cell stage, typically) or attached in such a manner that the embryo is fixed in position but clearly visible for assessment purposes, which is a benefit for this system as it makes assessments relatively rapid. Assessments are made at predetermined times from day 2 to 6 (1), depending upon when transfer is anticipated. An important advantage this system affords is that the developmental normality of the embryo from fertilization through the preimplantation stages can be visually determined prior to transfer.

Representative examples of human embryo development obtained in this system, and observed and photographed through the glass vacutainer from day 3 to day 6, are shown in Figures 1C-F. Figures 1G and H are two blastocyst-stage embryos shown in 1F that were removed from the culture tube as if for transfer, but in this instance, for higher resolution imaging. One interesting feature of human embryo culture from the pronuclear through the blastocyst stages in this simplified system was the scarcity of fragmentation and uniformity of cell divisions during cleavage as reflected in these images. Likewise, the process of emergence from the zona pellucida was appropriate with respect to time and morphokinetics.

As discussed elsewhere (11), the IVF system was quantified and tested first in the mouse system with IVF and culture to the hatched blastocyst stage. The rates of fertilization and development to the hatched blastocyst were similar to those in conventional mouse microdrop culture (>87%), as were rates of trophectodermal outgrowth (>90% of hatched), which also occurred in the tube system. Comparative studies were undertaken with thawed bipronucleate and fresh tripronucleate human embryos with similar rates of development though the cleavage and blastocyst stages observed between the simplified and routine culture systems (open and microdrop under oil).

Dr. Ombelet and his team performed the first clinical trial of the system in Genk, Belgium, in March of 2012. The approved protocol for this trial called for day 3 transfers and single embryo transfer (SET), the former in accordance with protocol at their center and the latter with Belgian law. The trial involved 25 women with a history of failed IUIs and IVFs and partners with a count of at least 1 million normally motile sperm/mL (11). Superfluous cleavage-stage embryos were cryopreserved. Up to December 2012, the embryo implantation rate from this small cohort of comparatively low-prognosis patients was 35% with 3 healthy, full-term, vaginally delivered babies born. In January of 2013, the first baby from a cryopreserved embryo was born. Dr. Ombelet will present additional details and outcomes in his companion presentation, which will also be described elsewhere (11).

Our initial results show that a simplified culture system designed specifically for developing countries can offer affordable and successful opportunities for treatment where IVF is the only solution for a common etiology of infertility, tubal occlusions. If combined with SET and low-stimulation protocols, the total cost/IVF cycle has been estimated to be about $300. The Walking Egg Project envisages that most IVF cycles will use conventional insemination in small, free-standing centers. If our present results with low sperm counts that have relatively normal morphology and motility are confirmed, patients who may be automatically classified as needing ICSI may well benefit from conventional IVF using this system. The second phase envisaged for the Walking Egg Project would have more advanced methods such as ICSI occurring in fewer but more centralized units. While these procedures would likely entail higher cost, the culture methodology would remain the same with costs estimated to be between 10% and 15% of those at high-resource programs.

In summary, we suggest that the initial outcome findings are highly encouraging with respect to the goal of providing affordable and effective IVF solutions, first for the most common form of infertility seen in low-resource settings. We suggest that these early findings may represent the first step towards truly universal infertility care.

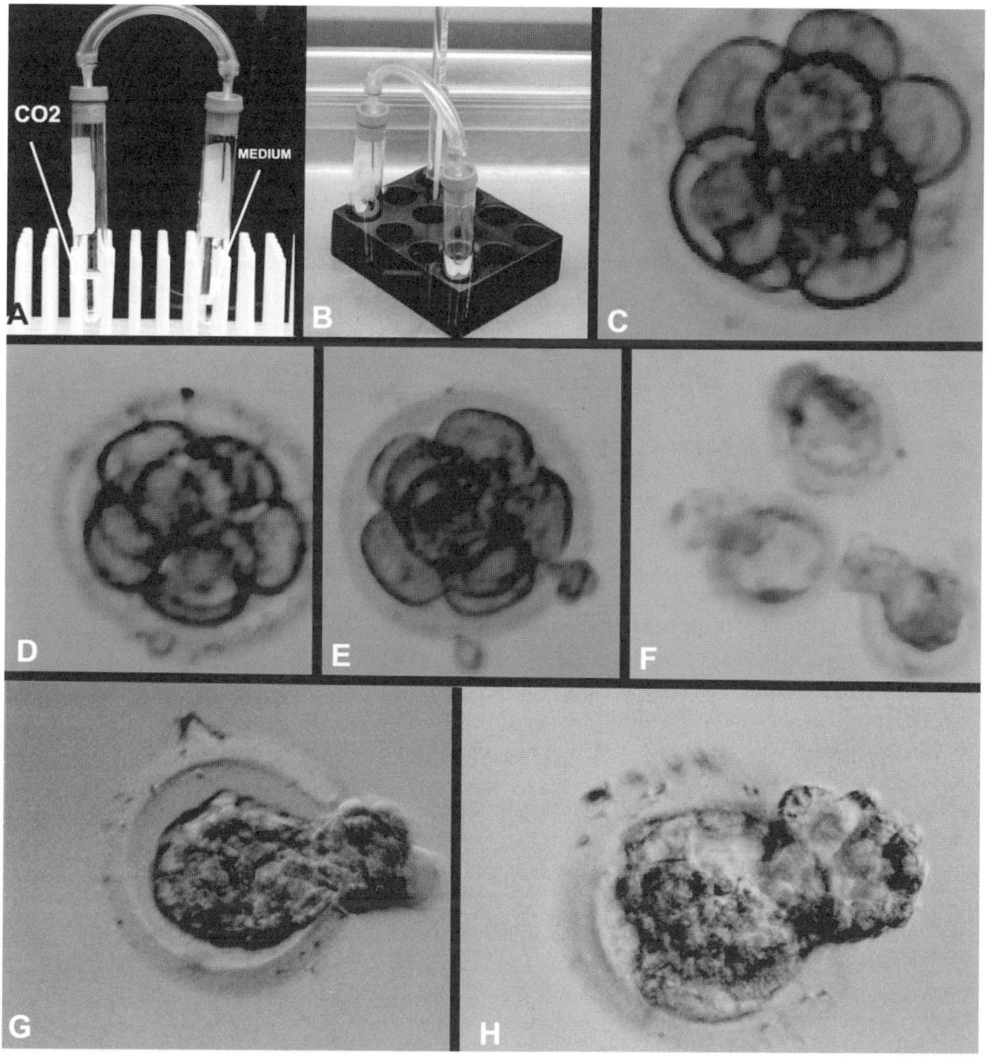

Figure legends:

A. An early prototype of the two-vacutainer system for IVF in which the tube on the left generates carbon dioxide from citric acid, sodium bicarbonate, and water, which when equilibrated with the medium containing tube on the right, creates a stable pH and atmosphere that is consistent with human IVF and normal embryo development to the hatched blastocyst stage. Precise quantification of the kinetics of pH and atmospheric formation show atmospheric and culture conditions similar to those in routine use in high resource IVF programs using triple gas, tissue culture incubators, or certified premixed gas mixtures.

B. IVF and embryo culture are performed in a closed system that is not opened until transfer. Any darkened environment providing a constant 37°C throughout the length of the culture tube is sufficient. Here, embryo culture to day 6 was done in water bath with a gently rotating platform with the tubes covered with water to near the top of the stopper.

C-F. Brightfield images taken through the vacutainer glass wall on days 3 and 6 of preimplantation embryogenesis in the simplified IVF system. While the images are shown after magnifications up to 500x, a clear indication of stage, cell number, and morphology during cleavage, and during blastocyst formation and hatching (F), can be seen through the glass.

G-H. Figures G and H are higher resolution differential interference contrast (DIC) images of two of the blastocysts shown in F after removal from the culture tube and transfer to a standard tissue culture dish. The photographs in F-H show that hatching can be readily observed while the embryos are still in their glass culture tubes, and for transfer, selection with higher resolution optics can be made after transfer to a culture dish for pickup.

References

1. Alpha Scientists in Reproductive Medicine and ESHRE Special Interest Group of Embryology: The Istanbul consensus workshop on embryo assessment: proceedings of an expert meeting. Hum Reprod 26 (2011): 1273–1283.
2. Wong C, Loewke K, Bossert N, Behr B, J De Jonge C, Baer T, Reijo Pera. Non-invasive imaging of human embryos before embryonic genome activation predicts development to the blastocyst stage Nature Biotech 28 (2011):1115–1121.
3. Manna C, Nanni L, Lumini A, Pappalardo S. Artificial intelligence techniques for embryo and oocyte classification. Reprod BioMed Online (2013) 26:42-49.
4. Hemmings D, Maruthini S, Vvjaanth S, Hogg J, Balen B, Campbell B, Leese H, Picton H. Amino acid turnover by human oocytes is influenced by gamete developmental competence, patient characteristics and gonadotrophin treatment Hum Reprod (2013) 28:1031-1044.
5. Knez K, Zorn B, Tomazevic T, Vrticnil-Bokal E, Virant-Klum I. The IMSI procedure improves poor embryo development in the same infertile couples with poor semen quality: A comparative prospective randomized study. Reprod Biol Endocrinol (2011) 9:123-127.
6. Oliveira J, Cavagna M, Petersen C, Mauri A, Massaro F, Silva L, et al. Pregnancy outcomes in women with repeated implantation failures after intracytoplasmic morphologically selected serm injection (IMSI). Reprod Biol Endocrinol (2011) 9:99-105.
7. Gutiérrez-Mateo C, Colls P, Sánchez-García J, Escudero T, Prates R, Ketterson K, Wells D, Munné S. Validation of microarray comparative genomic hybridization for comprehensive chromosome analysis of embryos. Fertil Steril (2011) 95:953-958.
8. Fragouli E, Wells, D Thornhill A, Serhal P, Faed M, Harper J, Delhanty A. Comparative genomic hybridization analysis of human oocytes and polar bodies. Hum Reprod (2006) 21:2319-2328.
9. Ombelet W, Cooke I, Dyer S, Serour G, Devroey P. Infertility and the provision of infertility medical services in developing countries. Hum Reprod Update (2008) 14, 605-621.
10. Ombelet W. Reproductive healthcare systems should include accessible infertility diagnosis and treatment: An important challenge for resource-poor countries. Int J Gynaecol Obstet (2009) 106, 168-171.
11. Van Blerkom J, Ombelet W, Klerkx E, Janssen M, Nargund Dhont, Campo R. First births with a simplified IVF procedure designed for low resource settings/developing countries: a crucial step towards universal infertility care (submitted).
12. Swain J. A self-contained culture platform using carbon dioxide produced from a chemical reaction supports mouse blastocyst development. In Vitro J Reprod Dev (2011) 57, 551-555.

Trilogy 8. Premature ovarian failure and perimenopause

Genetics of premature ovarian failure (POF)

Joe Leigh Simpson

March of Dimes, White Plains, United States

Introduction

Genetic control of ovarian development is not in doubt, to be assumed like determination and differentiation of any organ system. Failures of ovarian and oocyte development are not uncommon clinical occurrences, either complete failure (primary amenorrhea) or partial failure (secondary amenorrhea). The latter is termed premature ovarian failure (POF), or primary ovarian insufficiency (POI) as preferred by some.

Molecular genetic technology over the past decade now allows specific genes causing POF and disorders of sex development to be identified (1). This communication will survey potential causative genes in human POF. These genes have been selected on the basis of having known roles as hormones or growth factors, or being orthologues of genes that produce a POF phenotype in murine knockout models.

I. Chromosomal deletions and genes on the X short arm (Xp)

Until the molecular era, considerable effort was devoted to phenotypic–karyotypic correlations in hopes of clinical utility (prognosis) and gene localization. Terminal deletions or other rearrangements were observed to occur on the X short arm (Xp) and X long arm (Xq), often causing ovarian failure. Approximately half of individuals deleted for most of the X short arm [46,X,del(Xp)(p11)] show primary amenorrhea; most of the others have secondary amenorrhea. Women who have more distal Xp deletions [del(X)(p21.1 to 22.1.22)] retain more of the X genome and menstruate more often than 45,X or 46,X,del (X) (p11) women; however, many are still infertile or have secondary amenorrhea. See Simpson for further details (1).

Of candidate genes on Xp, only 1 has been studied in detail. Located on Xp11.2, Bone Morphogenetic Protein 15(BMP15) is a member of the transforming growth factor-beta (TGFβ) superfamily. TGF genes direct many developmental pathways through binding and activating transmembrane serine/threonine kinase receptors. BMP15 is specifically involved in folliculogenesis. Female mice in which BMP is deleted (knock out) are subfertile and show decreased ovulation rates and reduced litter size and litters per lifetime (2). BMP15 was first associated with POF by Di Pasquale and coworkers (3), who reported a heterozygous Y235C missense mutation in the second exon of the BMP15 gene in each of 2 sisters having ovarian failure. The proband had streak gonads and elevated follicle-stimulating hormone (FSH); the younger sibling had only a single episode of vaginal spotting. The mother was homozygous normal, Y235C being transmitted from the father. In vitro evidence existed for a dominant-negative effect. In subsequent studies, the frequency of BMP variants was higher in POF than controls; however, control women often showed the same perturbations as POF, albeit in lower frequency.

Sequencing of the entire BMP15 gene is now being pursued. Excluding 1 variant that did not alter protein structure, Rosetti et al. (4) observed mutations in 11 of 300 cases. Wang et al. (5) found 1 perturbation in 100 Chinese. Lakhal et al. (6) reported a heterozygous Ser5Arg in 1 of 30 French cases, all having a positive family history. On the other hand, in 92 Chinese POF cases Zhang et al. (7) found no perturbations, and in a European sample Tiotiu et al. (8) failed to find a plausible mutation in 50 patients.

In conclusion, some heterozygous BMP15 mutations plausibly result in POF, probably acting by dimerization with other TGFβ proteins. However, not all mutations alter the secondary protein structure, some only polymorphisms.

II. X chromosome long arm (Xq)

Chromosomal deletions involving the X long arm mirror the topography of the X short arm. Absence of most of the X long arm [del(Xq13)] is invariably characterized by primary amenorrhea. Lack of only the telomeric region [del(X)(q27)] is characterized by secondary amenorrhea or no abnormalities at all. Deletions occurring between the two extremes [Xq21 or Xq13] display intermediate phenotypes. The long arm contains several genes of interest.

XIST – Xq13 contains the X-inactivation center, which acts through the gene product XIST. That loss of germ cells is almost universal in del (Xq13) cases may or may not be the direct result of perturbation of XIST. Disturbances of X-inactivation per se may itself lead to ovarian failure.

DIAPH2 (Diaphanous) – Located in the Xq21-24 region, DIAPH2 is the homolog of Drosphilia melanogaster diaphanous (dia). In Drosphilia, dia is a member of a family of proteins that help establish cell polarity, govern cytokinesis, and reorganize the actin cytoskeleton. In Drosphilia, mutations cause sterility in both male and female subjects (9). Xq21/autosome translocation was disrupted in the last intron of DIAPH2 in a woman having POF (10).

XPNPEP2 – Disruptions involving XPNPEP2 (11) occurred as result of an X autosomal translocation in a woman with POF. The gene acts as an aminopeptidase.

Angiotensor II (Type 2) (ATZ) Receptor- ATZ is located on Xq22-23. Atretic rodent granulosa cells express this gene product, and a plausible relationship exists to human POF. Katsuya (12) studied 2 families in each of which siblings had POF; no ATZ mutation was found.

Progesterone Receptor Membrane Component 1 (PRMC1) – This gene was interrogated in 67 POF cases by Mansouri et al. (13), who found 1 heterozygous mutation (H165R). The change occurred in a domain necessary for nontranscriptional regulation of cytochrome P450, potentially exerting a functional effect.

Familial Mental Retardation 1 (FMR1) – Fragile X syndrome is the most common cause of X-linked mental retardation. The molecular basis involves repetition of the triplet repeat CGG of the FMR1 gene, located on Xq27. If more than 200 repeats exist, transcriptional silencing of an RNA-binding protein occurs. The normal number of CGG repeats is 29 or 30; heterozygous women having 55-199 repeats are said to have a premutation (14). During female meiosis, the number of triplet repeats may increase (expand), the result being affected offspring (fragile X syndrome) if the number of CGG repeats is greater than 200. Mental retardation, characteristic facial features, and large testes are present in males.

Of relevance here is that female premutation carriers are at risk for POF (15). An international collaborative survey by Allingham-Hawkins and coworkers (16) analyzed 1,268 controls, 50 familial POF cases, and 244 sporadic POF cases. Sixteen percent (63 of 395) of premutation carriers experienced menopause before 40 years of age; frequency in controls was 0.4%. Sullivan and colleagues (14) found 12.9% of premutation carriers to have POF, compared to 1.3% (2/157) controls. Risk for POF is highest with 80-99 repeats, and there is no further increase after >100 repeats; women having the full mutation (>200 CGG) do not show POF (16). From another perspective, 1%-5% of sporadic POF cases have a premutation (15). If another family member also has POF, the likelihood of a premutation rises up to 15% (15).

III. Autosomal genes exerting direct endocrine effects

A. *FSH β* – FSH β is located on chromosome 2. Mutations in FSH-β are rare but when occurring are invariably associated with primary amenorrhea. Matthews and colleagues (17) described a homozygous 2 base pair (bp) deletion in exon 3. In 1998 Layman and coworkers (18) reported a compound heterozygote (Val61X/Cysb9Gly), showing a functional effect in vitro. In a recent review, only 4 additional cases were found (19).

B. *FSHR (Inactivating FSH Receptor)* – Mutations of FSHR, located on chromosome 2, are common in Finland but rare elsewhere. In 1995 Aittomaki and colleagues (20, 21) identified 75 women in Finland having 46,XX primary or secondary amenorrhea, confirmed by FSH > 40 MIU/mL. A missense mutation in exon 7 (Ala566Val) was found in 6 families. This mutation lies in the extracellular portion of this G-protein. Heterozygous women are normal. The Ala566 Val mutation is uncommon outside Finland. No mutations were found in North American women having either 46,XX hypergonadotropic hypogonadism or POF (22). Similar findings were reported from Brazil (23) and Mexico (24). Population studies by Jiang (25) showed population frequencies not exceeding 0.1% outside Finland: 1 in 1200 Switzerland, 0 of 540 Singapore and 0 of 1,140 Denmark. A review of all missense mutations was recently tabulated by Siegel et al. (19).

C. *LH Receptor LHR* - LHR mutations have been recognized in 46,XX women having primary amenorrhea, but only in family cases in which a 46,XY sibling had 46,XY Leydig cell hypoplasia and XY sex reversal (26, 27). Most LHR mutations have been detected in the transmembrane domain of this G-protein receptor. For example, Latronico et al. (28) observed homozygous Ala593Pro. 46,XX women with LHR mutations show oligomenorrhea; ovulation does not occur, even though gametogenesis proceeds until the preovulatory stage (29).

D. *Inhibin A (INHA)* - Inhibins (INHs) exert negative feedback inhibition on FSH and are opposed by activins, which enhance FSH secretion. Perturbation of INHA could thus plausibly cause ovarian failure. Shelling and colleagues (30) reported missense G769A in 3 of 43 New Zealand POF patients (7%) but in only 1 of 150 controls (0.7%). However, the mother of 1 of the 3 G769A individuals had the same perturbation and was clinically normal. Marozzi and coworkers (31) found G769A in 7 of 157 Italian POF individuals, 3 of 12 primary amenorrhea cases, and 0 of 36 early menopausal (40-45 years) women. Dixit and colleagues (32) found G769A in 9 of 80 Indian POF cases. Also in India, Prakash et al. (33) found heterozygous G769A in 3 of 30 cases with primary amenorrhea, 3 of 20 with secondary amenorrhea, and 2 of 50 controls. In conclusion, association exists between G769A and POF, but G769A does not obligatorily confer ovarian failure.

E. *17α* - Hydroxylase/17,20 Desmolase Deficiency (CYP17) - 46,XX individuals with a CYP17 mutation may present with primary amenorrhea or premature ovarian failure (34). Ovaries are hypoplastic and may have a streak-like appearance; oocytes fail to exceed diameters more than 2.5 mm (35).

F. *Aromatase Mutations (CYP19)* - Women with 46,XX aromatase deficiency (CYP19), encoded on 15q21.1, may present with primary amenorrhea. Ito and coworkers (36) reported CYP19 mutation in a 46,XX 18-year-old Japanese woman having primary amenorrhea and cystic ovaries. Compound heterozygosity existed, 2 different point mutations in exon 10. Conte and colleagues (37) reported aromatase deficiency in a 46,XX woman presenting with primary amenorrhea, elevated gonadotropins, and ovarian cysts. Compound heterozygosity was observed for 2 exon 10 mutations.

G. *NR5A1(SF1)* - This gene encodes a nuclear protein that serves as a master transcriptional regulator of multiple endocrine genes: STAR, CYP11A1, CYP19A1, AMH, INHA, and LHB. NR5A1 is expressed predominantly in ovarian somatic cells, namely granulosa cells, theca cells, interstitial cells, and corpus lutea. Granulosa cell-specific NR5A1 knockout mice exhibit infertility, hypoplastic ovaries with decreased follicles, and absent corpora lutea. Genetic pathways involving NR5A1 are complex because mutations are also found in 46,XY disorders of sex development (DSD), producing widely diverse phenotypes that include adrenal insufficiency, hypospadias, cryptorchidism, anorchidia, and male infertility (38-41). Lourenco et al. (42) initially described 4 families in which family members showed both 46,XY and 46,XX POF. In 25 additional sporadic POF cases, 2 had a NR5A1 mutation. Janse et al. (43) found heterozygous variants in 5 of 356 Dutch cases. Philibert et al. (44) observed a mutation in 1 of 26 French cases, and Lakhal et al. (45) found 0 novel variants in 55 Tunisian POF cases. The unusual expressivity and penetrance of NR5A1 means clinically that different individuals with the same mutation may present with premature ovarian failure, early menopause, or diminished ovarian reserve (46, 47).

IV. Autosomal genes causing nonsyndromic POF

In this section we shall review autosomal genes that cause nonsyndromic POF, that is, POF as the only major phenotypic abnormality. These genes might exert their effects during embryonic differentiation – formation of genital ridge, germ cell migration, differentiation of the bipotential gonad, ovulation, or oogenesis. These genes act mechanistically in multiple ways: DNA binding, transcription, RNA binding or cellular actions of protein gene product.

A. *Forkhead Transcription Factor 2 (FOXL2)* - FOXL2 plays the pivotal role in ovarian development. Encoded on 3q21-24, FOXL2 protein maintains suppression of SRY during embryogenesis and, hence, allows ovarian determination and differentiation to proceed. FOXL2 and other forkhead DNA-binding proteins are crucial in signal induction. The importance of FOXL2 in humans was first recognized through the human blepharophimosis-ptosis-epicanthus (BPE) syndrome, an autosomal dominant disorder. FOXL2 is expressed in eyelids and ovaries (48), consistent with the BPE phenotype. In each of 4 families, FOXL2 mutations co-segregated with BPE and POF (48, 49). Observed mutations include nonsense mutations, stop codons, and a 17-bp duplication that resulted in a frameshift and truncated protein. FOXL2 mutations are also in about 1% of nonsyndromic POF, specifically POF lacking eyelid abnormalities. De Baere and colleagues (49) found no FOXL2 mutations in 30 POF cases, Harris et al. (50) 2 in 70 cases, and Gersak et al. (51) 1 in 70 cases.

B. *Newborn Ovary Homeobox (NOBOX)* - NOBOX is a homeobox gene, binding DNA and functioning as a transcription factor. NOBOX is oocyte specific, expressed from the primordial follicle through metaphase II. Female murine knockouts model show ovarian failure, whereas males are normal. Qin et al. (52) found 2 novel missense mutations (Arg355His and Arg360Gin) among 96 Caucasian POF cases. Arg355His was present in a conserved region, and electrophoretic mobility shift arrays showed disrupted binding of the NOBOX homeodomain to DNA; thus, capacity exists for a dominant negative effect.

C. *LIM DNA-Binding Proteins (LHX8)* - LIM homeobox genes encode DNA binding proteins and are characterized by tandemly repeated domains composed of cysteine rich, double zinc-finger motifs. Lhx8 transcripts localize to mouse oocytes, germ cells through antral follicles; null mice lack germ cells (53). Qin et al. (54) sequenced LHX8 in 95 Caucasian women with POF, and found no novel SNPs.

D. *Forkhead Transcription (FOX01A)* - Watkins et al. (55) found a single conservative change (P84L) in FOX01A among 90 POF cases. The woman with P84L was Slovenian.

E. *Forkhead Transcription 3A (FOX03A)* - FOX03A regulates G1/S transition in granulosa cells. Of 60 POF cases (30 New Zealand, 30 Slovenia), 2 showed potentially significant FOX03A mutations; no abnormalities were present in controls (55). One of the mutations was a single heterozygous mutation in a Slovenian woman characterized by a non-conservative amino acid charge (Ser421Leu), potentially capable of inducing a conformational protein change. The other mutation was Arg506His, found in a New Zealand woman.

F. *Factor in Germline Alpha (FIGLA)* - This gene on 2p13.3 encodes a germ cell specific basic helix-loop-helix transcription factor. FIGLA regulates expression of zona pellucida genes and is expressed in the embryonal ovary. In Figla knockout mice, primordial follicles are either not formed or lost soon after birth. Zhao et al. (56) studied 100 Han Chinese with POF and found 2 variants in 10 women. In 2 cases a missense mutation was found, one a 15-36 deletion (p.G6fsX66) that resulted in haploinsufficiency and the other a 419-421 del (140 del N). Functional studies of the latter (140delN) demonstrated that FIGLA binding to the TCF3 helix-loop helix was impeded. Wang et al. (57) considered 5 novel heterozygous variants in 114 Chinese POF cases to be significant, compared to 0 in 100 controls.

G. *POU5F1* - This transcription factor gene, located on 6p21.31, is significantly down-regulated in Nobox knockout mice, who lack ovaries. POU5F1 is thus a candidate gene for a downstream target of NOBOX. Wang et al. (58) sequenced 175 Chinese POF cases and found 1 non-synonymous variant (Pro13Thr), a heterozygous hydrophobic to hydrophilic substitution.

H. *NANOS3* - NANOS3 is a RNA-binding protein. Female and male knockout mice are infertile; female mice show no other phenotypic effect (59). Qin at al. (60) studied 80 Chinese and 88 American Caucasians with POF. The only variant found was a synonymous nucleotide substitution known already to be present in the general population (60).

I. *G Protein and G Protein Receptors (GPR3)* - GPs are regulatory proteins that serve as ligands for hormone-specific cell surface G-protein receptors, which in turn lead to intracellular signal transduction. The oocyte-specific G-stimulating protein-coupled receptor GPR3 is known to have a role in maintaining meiotic arrest in the mouse oocyte. Female mice lacking GPR3 develop premature ovarian aging and oocyte attrition as result of spontaneous resumption of meiosis in antral follicles, independent of the LH surge (61). Kovanchi et al. (62) interrogated GPR3 in 82 Caucasian women with premature ovarian failure (POF), finding no perturbations of significance. One heterozygous mutation was found (c.51C>A), but this substitution does not alter the amino acid sequence and is registered in the general population database. GPR3 mutations cannot yet be shown to be a common explanation for POF.

J. *RET Finger Protein-Like 4 (RFPL4)* - RING finger-like protein (RFPL4) is expressed in oocytes and in mice exclusively found there. RFPL4 encodes an E3 ubiquitin protein ligase, which regulates protein degradation. Human RFLP4 (19q13.4) interacts with oocyte proteins of the ubiquitin-protease degradation pathway (63). Suzumori et al. (64) stated that no mutations were found in Japanese with POF.

K. *KIT* - KIT is an autosomal (4q12) gene that encodes the tyrosine kinase transmembrane regulator for mast/stem cell growth factor (65). Both c-kit receptor and its ligand (KL) constitute 2 murine loci known before the molecular era to be characterized by decreased germ cells: white spotting (W) and steel (L). Human KIT is thus a candidate gene for POF. Shibanuma et al. (66) sequenced coding regions in 40 women with POF and found only 1 synonymous mutation not considered of plausible causation.

L. *Growth Differentiation Factor 9 (GDF9)* - A member of the TGFβ family, GDF9 is expressed in oocytes and can form dimers with BMP15. That a dominant negative effect could be conferred by a heterozygous mutation is thus plausible. Various GDF9 heterozygous mutations have been detected in European and Asian samples (67-70) but not in all (5, 71, 72). If heterozygous missense mutations causing hydrophobic to hydrophilic amino acid alterations were causative, GDF9 perturbations could account for a substantial number of POF cases.

M. Bone Morphogenetic Protein Receptor 1B (BMPR1B) - Homozygous deletion (del 359-366) of BMPR1B, a receptor in the TGFβ superfamily, was reported by Demirhan et al. (73). A 16-year-old female had ovarian failure and acromesomelic chondrodystrophy. Murine knockouts are infertile (74), but heterozygous mutations of the BMPR1B homolog in sheep conversely leads to increased fertility (gain of function) (75).

N. *Transforming Growth Factor B Receptor 3 (TGRBR3)* - Qin et al. (76) sequenced 112 Chinese POF cases and found 2 heterozygous missense variants (E459G;P825L).

O. *ADAMTS* - ADAMTS is a metalloprotease that proteolytically cleaves transmembrane proteins to release extracellular domains. Located on 5q, ADAMTS was associated with POF in the discovery set in a Dutch genome-wide association study (GWAS) involving 99 POF cases and 181 controls (77). However, findings were negative in their replicate. Thus, the role of ADAMTS might play in POF remains unclear.

V. Pleiotropic Mendelian disorders with POF

Many single gene disorders are pleiotropic, affecting multiple organ systems. Sometimes the organ system involves ovaries and, hence, may result in POF. These pleiotropic genes are informative because their mechanism of action can point to novel pathways not immediately evident to the reproductive medicine investigator. Several genes have already been mentioned above.

A. *FOXL2* - The pivotal role FOXL2 plays in ovarian development has already received comment and was recognized initially through the pleiotropic gene causing blepharophimosis-ptosis-epicanthus (BPE) syndrome.

B. *Galactosemia* - Galactosemia is caused by deficiency of galactose 1-phosphate uridyl transferase (GALT) deficiency. Ovarian failure was described by Kaufman and coworkers (78), who observed POF in 12 of 18 galactosemic women. Waggoner and colleagues (79) reported ovarian failure in 8 of 47 (17%) women with galactosemia. Pathogenesis involves galactose toxicity after birth, given that elevated levels of toxic metabolites in the fetus are cleared rapidly during pregnancy by maternal enzymes. Indeed, one neonate with galactosemia showed normal ovarian histology (80).

C. *Carbohydrate-Deficient Glycoprotein (Phosphomannomutase Deficiency, PMM2)* - In type 1 carbohydrate-deficient-glycoprotein (CDG) deficiency, mannose-6-phosphate cannot be converted to mannose-1-phosphate. This lipid-linked oligosaccharide is necessary for secretory glycoproteins. Neurologic abnormalities (81) and ovarian failure occur (82, 83). Located on 16p13, PMM2 is typically caused by a missense mutation (84).

D. *Autoimmune Regulation/Autoimmune Polyendocrinopathy-Candidiasis-Ectodermal Dystrophy (APECED)* - The AIRE gene (21q22.3) can if perturbed lead to multi-system abnormalities: alopecia, vitiligo, keratopathy, malabsorption, hepatitis, and mucocutaneous candidiasis. Ovarian hypoplasia often occurs (55%), usually in the third decade (85). Many different AIRE perturbations have been found in this autosomal dominant disorder, not only nonsense mutations but frame shifts (85). No particular mutation leads to ovarian failure as distinct from other autoimmune phenomena. AIRE mutations have not yet been sought in women with isolated POF (nonsyndromic).

E. *Ovarian Leukodystrophy (Eukaryotic Translation Initiation Factor EIF2B)* – "Vanishing white matter" leads to variable but progressive neurological degeneration. Ovarian failure may coexist (86,87). That the causative gene (EIF2B) allows denatured stress-related proteins to accumulate makes plausible relevance to oogenesis, given ongoing oocyte degeneration. Fogli et al. (88) found variants in EIF2B2, EIF2B4, and EIF2B5 in POF cases with neurologic abnormalities, but in nonsyndromic POF none (0) of 93 (89).

F. *Symphalangism and Noggin (NOG)* - Noggin (NOG) is located on 17q22 and is responsible for the autosomal dominant disorder proximal symphalangism (SYM1). Characteristic features include ankylosis of the proximal interphalangeal joints, carpal-tarsal fusion, brachydactyly, and deafness. NOG is expressed in the ovary and is antagonistic to Bone Morphogenic Proteins 4 and 7 (90), members of the TGF family. One SYM1 case has shown POF and a NOG mutation (91).

G. *Perrault Syndrome* - XX gonadal dysgenesis with neurosensory deafness is termed Perrault syndrome (91), an autosomal recessive disorder (92-94). Causative genes seem likely to emerge from the connexin family, but no example is yet evident. Mutations in the connexin gene family are responsible for many forms of congenital deafness in humans. Mice null for connexin 37 show gonadal failure due to arrest at the antral stage of oogenesis (95).

H. *DNA Mismatch (MSH4, MSN5, SPO11) and Recombinant Genes (DMC1)* - DNA mismatch genes are pivotal in repairing DNA damage. In 41 POF women Mandon-Pepin et al. (96) sought mutations in MSH4, MSH5, and SPO11. One heterozygous mutation (P295) for MSH5 was found. Another (M200V) was found for DMC1, a gene pivotal for meiotic recombination and without which orderly chromosome disjunction cannot occur.

I. *Mitochondrial Genes: Progressive External Ophthalmoplegia (PEO)* - Mitochondrial DNA mutations (mtDNA) usually affect muscular and neurological systems. Perturbations of mitochondrial genes are good candidates for POF because the mature oocyte has the greatest number of DNA copies of any human cell. In progressive external ophthalmoplegia (PEO) clinical features are proximal myopathy, sensory ataxia, and parkinsonism. The causative mutation lies in polymerase gamma. In 3 of 7 families studied by Luoma et al. (97), POF cosegregated with PEO. A Y955C mutation was found in 2 of these 3 families. Y995 (tyrosine to cytosine) affects a highly conserved region, rendering functional plausibility. Compound heterozygosity (N468D/A1105T) was observed by Pagnamenta et al. (98) in another 3-generation family in which multiple family members were affected with both PEO and POF.

VI. Genome-wide studies and potential regulatory regions

In the future, candidate gene studies will increasingly be subsumed by whole genome approaches. Thus, of great significance is the single large-scale GWAS study performed. Qin et al. (99) performed a landmark study involving 800 Han Chinese cases and like controls, including 2 replication cohorts. The most significant "hit" was 8q22.3. That 8q22.3 is a "gene desert" region implies a role in regulation of gene expression. Possibly 8q22.3 in females is analogous to a 17q region in males, the region upstream of human 17q pivotal for testicular differentiation. If perturbed, sex reversal results even if both the Y regulatory SRY and autosomal male determinant SOX9 are intact.

VII. Summary: Genetic causation and clinical relevance

Genetic investigations into premature ovarian failure (POF) are revealing the genes that govern ovarian development and oogenesis. A potentially important regulatory region (8q22.3) has been identified, as well as over two dozen genes whose perturbations explain forms of nonsyndromic POF. The deleterious effects for some of these gene perturbations is clinically predictable (e.g., FSH, FSHR), whereas for others it was not prior to studies that showed effects in murine knockout models. Pleiotropic genes may in addition result in POF along with various structural anomalies. Overall, a molecular (genetic) explanation can be found in only 15% of cases. Only FMR1 premutation and FSHR mutations in Finland are perturbed in more than 1%-2% of POF cases in any given ethnic group. Considerable genetic heterogeneity in POF thus exists.

The clinical goal of elucidating POF genes is to improve clinical outcomes. Screening for causative genes one could identify women destined to develop POF at an earlier age than would otherwise occur. This could be facilitated in the future by an interrogation using an ovarian gene DNA "chip" that contains sequences for known ovarian genes. Early child-bearing could be encouraged for these women. Ovarian slices or oocytes could be cryopreserved. Identification of these women by these strategies would offer reproductive options prior to ovarian failure.

References

1. Simpson JL. Disorders of the gonads, genital tract and genitalia. In: Rimoin DLC, J.M.; Pyertiz, R.E.; Korf, B.R., ed. Principles and Practice of Medical Genetics. New York, N.Y. : Churchill-Livingstone, 2012:in press
2. Dube JL, Wang P, Elvin J, Lyons KM, Celeste AJ, Matzuk MM. The bone morphogenetic protein 15 gene is X-linked and expressed in oocytes. Mol Endocrinol 1998;12:1809-17.
3. Di Pasquale E, Beck-Peccoz P, Persani L. Hypergonadotropic ovarian failure associated with an inherited mutation of human bone morphogenetic protein-15 (BMP15) gene. Am J Hum Genet 2004;75:106-11.

4. Rossetti R, Di Pasquale E, Marozzi A, Bione S, Toniolo D, Grammatico P et al. BMP15 mutations associated with primary ovarian insufficiency cause a defective production of bioactive protein. Hum Mutat 2009;30:804-10.
5. Wang B, Wen Q, Ni F, Zhou S, Wang J, Cao Y et al. Analyses of growth differentiation factor 9 (GDF9) and bone morphogenetic protein 15 (BMP15) mutation in Chinese women with premature ovarian failure. Clin Endocrinol (Oxf) 2010;72:135-6.
6. Lakhal B, Laissue P, Braham R, Elghezal H, Saad A, Fellous M et al. A novel BMP15 variant, potentially affecting the signal peptide, in a familial case of premature ovarian failure. Clin Endocrinol (Oxf) 2009;71:752-3.
7. Zhang P, Shi YH, Wang LC, Chen ZJ. Sequence variants in exons of the BMP-15 gene in Chinese patients with premature ovarian failure. Acta Obstet Gynecol Scand 2007;86:585-9.
8. Tiotiu D, Alvaro Mercadal B, Imbert R, Verbist J, Demeestere I, De Leener A et al. Variants of the BMP15 gene in a cohort of patients with premature ovarian failure. Hum Reprod 2010;25:1581-7.
9. Castrillon DH, Wasserman SA. Diaphanous is required for cytokinesis in Drosophila and shares domains of similarity with the products of the limb deformity gene. Development 1994;120:3367-77.
10. Bione S, Sala C, Manzini C, Arrigo G, Zuffardi O, Banfi S et al. A human homologue of the Drosophila melanogaster diaphanous gene is disrupted in a patient with premature ovarian failure: evidence for conserved function in oogenesis and implications for human sterility. Am J Hum Genet 1998;62:533-41.
11. Prueitt RL, Ross JL, Zinn AR. Physical mapping of nine Xq translocation breakpoints and identification of XPNPEP2 as a premature ovarian failure candidate gene. Cytogenet Cell Genet 2000;89:44-50.
12. Katsuya T, Horiuchi M, Minami S, Koike G, Santoro NF, Hsueh AJ et al. Genomic organization and polymorphism of human angiotensin II type 2 receptor: no evidence for its gene mutation in two families of human premature ovarian failure syndrome. Mol Cell Endocrinol 1997;127:221-8.
13. Mansouri MR, Schuster J, Badhai J, Stattin EL, Losel R, Wehling M et al. Alterations in the expression, structure and function of progesterone receptor membrane component-1 (PGRMC1) in premature ovarian failure. Hum Mol Genet 2008;17:3776-83.
14. Sullivan AK, Marcus M, Epstein MP, Allen EG, Anido AE, Paquin JJ et al. Association of FMR1 repeat size with ovarian dysfunction. Hum Reprod 2005;20:402-12.
15. Wittenberger MD, Hagerman RJ, Sherman SL, McConkie-Rosell A, Welt CK, Rebar RW et al. The FMR1 premutation and reproduction. Fertil Steril 2007;87:456-65.
16. Allingham-Hawkins DJ, Babul-Hirji R, Chitayat D, Holden JJ, Yang KT, Lee C et al. Fragile X premutation is a significant risk factor for premature ovarian failure: the International Collaborative POF in Fragile X study--preliminary data. Am J Med Genet 1999;83:322-5.
17. Matthews CH, Borgato S, Beck-Peccoz P, Adams M, Tone Y, Gambino G et al. Primary amenorrhoea and infertility due to a mutation in the beta-subunit of follicle-stimulating hormone. Nat Genet 1993;5:83-6.
18. Layman LC, Amde S, Cohen DP, Jin M, Xie J. The Finnish follicle-stimulating hormone receptor gene mutation is rare in North American women with 46,XX ovarian failure. Fertil Steril 1998;69:300-2.
19. Siegel ET, Kim HG, Nishimoto HK, Layman LC. The molecular basis of impaired follicle-stimulating hormone action: evidence from human mutations and mouse models. Reprod Sci 2013;20:211-33.

20. Aittomaki K. The genetics of XX gonadal dysgenesis. Am J Hum Genet 1994;54:844-51.
21. Aittomaki K, Lucena JL, Pakarinen P, Sistonen P, Tapanainen J, Gromoll J et al. Mutation in the follicle-stimulating hormone receptor gene causes hereditary hypergonadotropic ovarian failure. Cell 1995;82:959-68.
22. Liu JY, Gromoll J, Cedars MI, La Barbera AR. Identification of allelic variants in the follicle-stimulating hormone receptor genes of females with or without hypergonadotropic amenorrhea. Fertil Steril 1998;70:326-31.
23. da Fonte Kohek MB, Batista MC, Russell AJ, Vass K, Giacaglia LR, Mendonca BB et al. No evidence of the inactivating mutation (C566T) in the follicle-stimulating hormone receptor gene in Brazilian women with premature ovarian failure. Fertil Steril 1998;70:565-7.
24. de la Chesnaye E, Canto P, Ulloa-Aguirre A, Mendez JP. No evidence of mutations in the follicle-stimulating hormone receptor gene in Mexican women with 46,XX pure gonadal dysgenesis. Am J Med Genet 2001;98:125-8.
25. Jiang M, Aittomaki K, Nilsson C, Pakarinen P, Iitia A, Torresani T et al. The frequency of an inactivating point mutation (566C-->T) of the human follicle-stimulating hormone receptor gene in four populations using allele-specific hybridization and time-resolved fluorometry. J Clin Endocrinol Metab 1998;83:4338-43.
26. Latronico AC, Abell AN, Arnhold IJ, Liu X, Lins TS, Brito VN et al. A unique constitutively activating mutation in third transmembrane helix of luteinizing hormone receptor causes sporadic male gonadotropin-independent precocious puberty. J Clin Endocrinol Metab 1998;83:2435-40.
27. Sultan C, Lumbroso S. LH receptor defects. In: Kempers RD, Cohen J, Haney AF, Younger JB, eds. Fertility and Reproductive Medicine - Proceedings of the XVI World Congress on Fertility and Sterility San Francisco: Elsevier Science, 1998.
28. Latronico AC, Chai Y, Arnhold IJ, Liu X, Mendonca BB, Segaloff DL. A homozygous microdeletion in helix 7 of the luteinizing hormone receptor associated with familial testicular and ovarian resistance is due to both decreased cell surface expression and impaired effector activation by the cell surface receptor. Mol Endocrinol 1998;12:442-50.
29. Matzuk MM, Lamb DJ. Genetic dissection of mammalian fertility pathways. Nat Cell Biol 2002;4 Suppl:s41-9.
30. Shelling AN, Burton KA, Chand AL, van Ee CC, France JT, Farquhar CM et al. Inhibin: a candidate gene for premature ovarian failure. Hum Reprod 2000;15:2644-9.
31. Marozzi A, Porta C, Vegetti W, Crosignani PG, Tibiletti MG, Dalpra L et al. Mutation analysis of the inhibin alpha gene in a cohort of Italian women affected by ovarian failure. Hum Reprod 2002;17:1741-5.
32. Dixit H, Deendayal M, Singh L. Mutational analysis of the mature peptide region of inhibin genes in Indian women with ovarian failure. Hum Reprod 2004;19:1760-4.
33. Prakash GJ, Ravi Kanth VV, Shelling AN, Rozati R, Sujatha M. Mutational analysis of inhibin alpha gene revealed three novel variations in Indian women with premature ovarian failure. Fertil Steril 2010;94:90-8.
34. Simsek E, Ozdemir I, Lin L, Achermann JC. Isolated 17,20-lyase (desmolase) deficiency in a 46,XX female presenting with delayed puberty. Fertil Steril 2005;83:1548-51.
35. Araki S, Chikazawa K, Sekiguchi I, Yamauchi H, Motoyama M, Tamada T. Arrest of follicular development in a patient with 17 alpha-hydroxylase deficiency: folliculogenesis in association with a lack of estrogen synthesis in the ovaries. Fertil Steril 1987;47:169-72.
36. Ito Y, Fisher CR, Conte FA, Grumbach MM, Simpson ER. Molecular basis of aromatase deficiency in an adult female with sexual infantilism and polycystic ovaries. Proc Natl Acad Sci U S A 1993;90:11673-7.

37. Conte FA, Grumbach MM, Ito Y, Fisher CR, Simpson ER. A syndrome of female pseudohermaphrodism, hypergonadotropic hypogonadism, and multicystic ovaries associated with missense mutations in the gene encoding aromatase (P450arom). J Clin Endocrinol Metab 1994;78:1287-92.
38. Bashamboo A, Ferraz-de-Souza B, Lourenco D, Lin L, Sebire NJ, Montjean D et al. Human male infertility associated with mutations in NR5A1 encoding steroidogenic factor 1. Am J Hum Genet 2010;87:505-12.
39. Kohler B, Lin L, Mazen I, Cetindag C, Biebermann H, Akkurt I et al. The spectrum of phenotypes associated with mutations in steroidogenic factor 1 (SF-1, NR5A1, Ad4BP) includes severe penoscrotal hypospadias in 46,XY males without adrenal insufficiency. Eur J Endocrinol 2009;161:237-42.
40. Lin L, Achermann JC. Steroidogenic factor-1 (SF-1, Ad4BP, NR5A1) and disorders of testis development. Sex Dev 2008;2:200-9.
41. Philibert P, Zenaty D, Lin L, Soskin S, Audran F, Leger J et al. Mutational analysis of steroidogenic factor 1 (NR5a1) in 24 boys with bilateral anorchia: a French collaborative study. Hum Reprod 2007;22:3255-61.
42. Lourenco D, Brauner R, Lin L, De Perdigo A, Weryha G, Muresan M et al. Mutations in NR5A1 associated with ovarian insufficiency. N Engl J Med 2009;360:1200-10.
43. Janse F, de With LM, Duran KJ, Kloosterman WP, Goverde AJ, Lambalk CB et al. Limited contribution of NR5A1 (SF-1) mutations in women with primary ovarian insufficiency (POI). Fertil Steril 2012;97:141-6 e2.
44. Philibert P, Paris F, Lakhal B, Audran F, Gaspari L, Saad A et al. NR5A1 (SF-1) gene variants in a group of 26 young women with XX primary ovarian insufficiency. Fertil Steril 2013;99:484-9.
45. Lakhal B, Ben-Hadj-Khalifa S, Bouali N, Philipert P, Audran F, Braham R et al. Mutational screening of SF1 and WNT4 in Tunisian women with premature ovarian failure. Gene 2012;509:298-301.
46. Ciaccio M, Costanzo M, Guercio G, De Dona V, Marino R, Ramirez PC et al. Preserved fertility in a patient with a 46,XY disorder of sex development due to a new heterozygous mutation in the NR5A1/SF-1 gene: evidence of 46,XY and 46,XX gonadal dysgenesis phenotype variability in multiple members of an affected kindred. Horm Res Paediatr 2012;78:119-26.
47. Warman DM, Costanzo M, Marino R, Berensztein E, Galeano J, Ramirez PC et al. Three new SF-1 (NR5A1) gene mutations in two unrelated families with multiple affected members: within-family variability in 46,XY subjects and low ovarian reserve in fertile 46,XX subjects. Horm Res Paediatr 2011;75:70-7.
48. Crisponi L, Deiana M, Loi A, Chiappe F, Uda M, Amati P et al. The putative forkhead transcription factor FOXL2 is mutated in blepharophimosis/ptosis/epicanthus inversus syndrome. Nat Genet 2001;27:159-66.
49. De Baere E, Dixon MJ, Small KW, Jabs EW, Leroy BP, Devriendt K et al. Spectrum of FOXL2 gene mutations in blepharophimosis-ptosis-epicanthus inversus (BPES) families demonstrates a genotype--phenotype correlation. Hum Mol Genet 2001;10:1591-600.
50. Harris SE, Chand AL, Winship IM, Gersak K, Aittomaki K, Shelling AN. Identification of novel mutations in FOXL2 associated with premature ovarian failure. Mol Hum Reprod 2002;8:729-33.
51. Gersak K, Harris SE, Smale WJ, Shelling AN. A novel 30 bp deletion in the FOXL2 gene in a phenotypically normal woman with primary amenorrhoea: case report. Hum Reprod 2004;19:2767-70.

52. Qin Y, Choi Y, Zhao H, Simpson JL, Chen ZJ, Rajkovic A. NOBOX homeobox mutation causes premature ovarian failure. Am J Hum Genet 2007;81:576-81.
53. Pangas SA, Choi Y, Ballow DJ, Zhao Y, Westphal H, Matzuk MM et al. Oogenesis requires germ cell-specific transcriptional regulators Sohlh1 and Lhx8. Proc Natl Acad Sci U S A 2006;103:8090-5.
54. Qin Y, Zhao H, Kovanci E, Simpson JL, Chen ZJ, Rajkovic A. Analysis of LHX8 mutation in premature ovarian failure. Fertil Steril 2008;89:1012-4.
55. Watkins WJ, Umbers AJ, Woad KJ, Harris SE, Winship IM, Gersak K et al. Mutational screening of FOXO3A and FOXO1A in women with premature ovarian failure. Fertil Steril 2006;86:1518-21.
56. Zhao H, Chen ZJ, Qin Y, Shi Y, Wang S, Choi Y et al. Transcription factor FIGLA is mutated in patients with premature ovarian failure. Am J Hum Genet 2008;82:1342-8.
57. Wang B, Mu Y, Ni F, Zhou S, Wang J, Cao Y et al. Analysis of FOXO3 mutation in 114 Chinese women with premature ovarian failure. Reprod Biomed Online 2010;20:499-503.
58. Wang J, Wang B, Song J, Suo P, Ni F, Chen B et al. New candidate gene POU5F1 associated with premature ovarian failure in Chinese patients. Reprod Biomed Online 2011;22:312-6.
59. Tsuda M, Sasaoka Y, Kiso M, Abe K, Haraguchi S, Kobayashi S et al. Conserved role of nanos proteins in germ cell development. Science 2003;301:1239-41.
60. Qin Y, Zhao H, Kovanci E, Simpson JL, Chen ZJ, Rajkovic A. Mutation analysis of NANOS3 in 80 Chinese and 88 Caucasian women with premature ovarian failure. Fertil Steril 2007;88:1465-7.
61. Mehlmann LM, Saeki Y, Tanaka S, Brennan TJ, Evsikov AV, Pendola FL et al. The Gs-linked receptor GPR3 maintains meiotic arrest in mammalian oocytes. Science 2004;306:1947-50.
62. Kovanci E, Simpson JL, Amato P, Rohozinski J, Heard MJ, Bishop CE et al. Oocyte-specific G-protein-coupled receptor 3 (GPR3): no perturbations found in 82 women with premature ovarian failure (first report). Fertil Steril 2008;90:1269-71.
63. Suzumori N, Burns KH, Yan W, Matzuk MM. RFPL4 interacts with oocyte proteins of the ubiquitin-proteasome degradation pathway. Proc Natl Acad Sci U S A 2003;100:550-5.
64. Suzumori N, Pangas SA, Rajkovic A. Candidate genes for premature ovarian failure. Curr Med Chem 2007;14:353-7.
65. Richards KA, Fukai K, Oiso N, Paller AS. A novel KIT mutation results in piebaldism with progressive depigmentation. J Am Acad Dermatol 2001;44:288-92.
66. Shibanuma K, Tong ZB, Vanderhoof VH, Vanevski K, Nelson LM. Investigation of KIT gene mutations in women with 46,XX spontaneous premature ovarian failure. BMC Womens Health 2002;2:8.
67. Zhao H, Qin Y, Kovanci E, Simpson JL, Chen ZJ, Rajkovic A. Analyses of GDF9 mutation in 100 Chinese women with premature ovarian failure. Fertil Steril 2007;88:1474-6.
68. Dixit H, Rao LK, Padmalatha V, Kanakavalli M, Deenadayal M, Gupta N et al. Mutational screening of the coding region of growth differentiation factor 9 gene in Indian women with ovarian failure. Menopause 2005;12:749-54.
69. Kovanci E, Rohozinski J, Simpson JL, Heard MJ, Bishop CE, Carson SA. Growth differentiating factor-9 mutations may be associated with premature ovarian failure. Fertil Steril 2007;87:143-6.
70. Laissue P, Christin-Maitre S, Touraine P, Kuttenn F, Ritvos O, Aittomaki K et al. Mutations and sequence variants in GDF9 and BMP15 in patients with premature ovarian failure. Eur J Endocrinol 2006;154:739-44.
71. Chand AL, Ponnampalam AP, Harris SE, Winship IM, Shelling AN. Mutational analysis of BMP15 and GDF9 as candidate genes for premature ovarian failure. Fertil Steril 2006;86:1009-12.

72. Takebayashi K, Takakura K, Wang H, Kimura F, Kasahara K, Noda Y. Mutation analysis of the growth differentiation factor-9 and -9B genes in patients with premature ovarian failure and polycystic ovary syndrome. Fertil Steril 2000;74:976-9.
73. Demirhan O, Turkmen S, Schwabe GC, Soyupak S, Akgul E, Tastemir D et al. A homozygous BMPR1B mutation causes a new subtype of acromesomelic chondrodysplasia with genital anomalies. J Med Genet 2005;42:314-7.
74. Yi SE, LaPolt PS, Yoon BS, Chen JY, Lu JK, Lyons KM. The type I BMP receptor BmprIB is essential for female reproductive function. Proc Natl Acad Sci U S A 2001;98:7994-9.
75. Wilson T, Wu XY, Juengel JL, Ross IK, Lumsden JM, Lord EA et al. Highly prolific Booroola sheep have a mutation in the intracellular kinase domain of bone morphogenetic protein IB receptor (ALK-6) that is expressed in both oocytes and granulosa cells. Biol Reprod 2001;64:1225-35.
76. Qin CR, Chen SL, Yao JL, Wu WQ, Xie JS. Identification of novel missense mutations of the TGFBR3 gene in Chinese women with premature ovarian failure. Reprod Biomed Online 2011;23:697-703.
77. Knauff EA, Franke L, van Es MA, van den Berg LH, van der Schouw YT, Laven JS et al. Genome-wide association study in premature ovarian failure patients suggests ADAMTS19 as a possible candidate gene. Hum Reprod 2009;24:2372-8.
78. Kaufman FR, Kogut MD, Donnell GN, Goebelsmann U, March C, Koch R. Hypergonadotropic hypogonadism in female patients with galactosemia. N Engl J Med 1981;304:994-8.
79. Waggoner DD, Buist NR, Donnell GN. Long-term prognosis in galactosaemia: results of a survey of 350 cases. J Inherit Metab Dis 1990;13:802-18.
80. Levy HL, Driscoll SG, Porensky RS, Wender DF. Ovarian failure in galactosemia. N Engl J Med 1984;310:50.
81. Matthijs G, Schollen E, Pardon E, Veiga-Da-Cunha M, Jaeken J, Cassiman JJ et al. Mutations in PMM2, a phosphomannomutase gene on chromosome 16p13, in carbohydrate-deficient glycoprotein type I syndrome (Jaeken syndrome). Nat Genet 1997;16:88-92.
82. de Zegher F, Jaeken J. Endocrinology of the carbohydrate-deficient glycoprotein syndrome type 1 from birth through adolescence. Pediatr Res 1995;37:395-401.
83. Kristiansson B, Stibler H, Wide L. Gonadal function and glycoprotein hormones in the carbohydrate-deficient glycoprotein (CDG) syndrome. Acta Paediatr 1995;84:655-9.
84. Bjursell C, Stibler H, Wahlstrom J, Kristiansson B, Skovby F, Stromme P et al. Fine mapping of the gene for carbohydrate-deficient glycoprotein syndrome, type I (CDG1): linkage disequilibrium and founder effect in Scandinavian families. Genomics 1997;39:247-53.
85. Wang CY, Davoodi-Semiromi A, Huang W, Connor E, Shi JD, She JX. Characterization of mutations in patients with autoimmune polyglandular syndrome type 1 (APS1). Hum Genet 1998;103:681-5.
86. Boltshauser E, Barth PG, Troost D, Martin E, Stallmach T. "Vanishing white matter" and ovarian dysgenesis in an infant with cerebro-oculo-facio-skeletal phenotype. Neuropediatrics 2002;33:57-62.
87. Schiffmann R, Tedeschi G, Kinkel RP, Trapp BD, Frank JA, Kaneski CR et al. Leukodystrophy in patients with ovarian dysgenesis. Ann Neurol 1997;41:654-61.
88. Fogli A, Rodriguez D, Eymard-Pierre E, Bouhour F, Labauge P, Meaney BF et al. Ovarian failure related to eukaryotic initiation factor 2B mutations. Am J Hum Genet 2003;72:1544-50.
89. Fogli A, Gauthier-Barichard F, Schiffmann R, Vanderhoof VH, Bakalov VK, Nelson LM et al. Screening for known mutations in EIF2B genes in a large panel of patients with premature ovarian failure. BMC Womens Health 2004;4:8.

90. Groppe J, Greenwald J, Wiater E, Rodriguez-Leon J, Economides AN, Kwiatkowski W et al. Structural basis of BMP signalling inhibition by the cystine knot protein Noggin. Nature 2002;420:636-42.
91. Perrault M, Klotz P, Housset E. Deux cas de syndrome de Turner avec surdi-mutite dans une meme fratrie. . Bull Mem Soc Med Hop Paris 1951;67:79-84.
92. Josso N, de Grouchy J, Frezal J, al. e. Le syndrome de Turner familial etude de deux families avec caryotypes XO er XX. . Ann Pediatr 1963;10:163-7.
93. Nishi Y, Hamamoto K, Kajiyama M, Kawamura I. The Perrault syndrome: clinical report and review. Am J Med Genet 1988;31:623-9.
94. Pallister PD, Opitz JM. The Perrault syndrome: autosomal recessive ovarian dysgenesis with facultative, non-sex-limited sensorineural deafness. Am J Med Genet 1979;4:239-46.
95. Simon AM, Goodenough DA, Li E, Paul DL. Female infertility in mice lacking connexin 37. Nature 1997;385:525-9.
96. Mandon-Pepin B, Touraine P, Kuttenn F, Derbois C, Rouxel A, Matsuda F et al. Genetic investigation of four meiotic genes in women with premature ovarian failure. Eur J Endocrinol 2008;158:107-15.
97. Luoma P, Melberg A, Rinne JO, Kaukonen JA, Nupponen NN, Chalmers RM et al. Parkinsonism, premature menopause, and mitochondrial DNA polymerase gamma mutations: clinical and molecular genetic study. Lancet 2004;364:875-82.
98. Pagnamenta AT, Taanman JW, Wilson CJ, Anderson NE, Marotta R, Duncan AJ et al. Dominant inheritance of premature ovarian failure associated with mutant mitochondrial DNA polymerase gamma. Hum Reprod 2006;21:2467-73.
99. Qin Y, Zhao H, Xu J, Shi Y, Li Z, Qiao J et al. Association of 8q22.3 locus in Chinese Han with idiopathic premature ovarian failure (POF). Hum Mol Genet 2012;21:430-6.

Female health implications of premature ovarian insufficiency

Bart C. Fauser

University Medical Center, Utrecht, The Netherlands

Ovarian insufficiency results in absent ovarian production of estrogen and progesterone. However, the postmenopausal ovary continues to produce some androgens. We have recently shown in a meta-analysis in ovarian insufficiency that next to estrogens androgen levels also are significantly reduced. Gonadal steroids not only are important for healthy functioning of the reproductive tract, but also for women's general health issues such as elasticity of the skin, muscle strength, sexuality, maintenance of bone mass, the cardiovascular system, cognition, and, finally, well-being and quality of life. This short review is based on a seminar published in the Lancet (DeVos, Lancet, 2010, vol 376, page 911).

Very few long-term follow-up studies have been performed to investigate the general health implications of primary ovarian insufficiency. Moreover, many women with the disorder are advised to use steroid hormone replacement therapy for many years up to the normal age of menopause. This generally accepted strategy, however, is not based on proper scientific evidence. In addition, effects of hormone replacement used at a young age on breast cancer risk also remain uncertain. The only proven effects are on bone density. Moreover, much attention is focused towards androgen replacement in androgen-deficient women. Again, evidence supporting its beneficial effects remains unconvincing.

In case of premature menopause, effects of a persistent state of severe steroid depletion should be seriously considered. However, only indirect information can be obtained from specific conditions such as gonadal failure after cancer treatment or for women who underwent oophorectomy. Quality of life and general health in survivors of cancer may not necessarily be related to ovarian insufficiency per se. Moreover, potential implications of chemotherapy, radiotherapy, surgery, or differences in androgen levels (ovarian insufficiency vs. removal of ovaries) cannot be ignored. Increasing amounts of evidence come from the comparison of women presenting with early or late menopause in relation to general health issues. All of these issues should be taken into consideration and discussed with the women. Clinical evidence suggests that many women diagnosed with early menopause do not start with hormone replacement therapy or stop within 3-6 months after initiation. This should also be viewed in the context of infertility, because this is often when diagnosis of premature menopause is made. It feels counter-intuitive to use hormones, when women still hope for the miracle to happen.

Estrogens are important for bone remodeling. Consequently, estrogen deficiency results in an imbalance between osteoclast and osteoblast activity and a progressive loss of trabecular bone. Osteoporosis can be diagnosed by the assessment of bone density, with a reasonable ability to predict fracture risk. Decreased bone density can be noted within 3-6 months of the start of profound suppression of ovarian steroids by administering gonadotropin-releasing hormone agonists for steroid-dependent disease. Increased bone fragility leads to a 50% lifetime risk of fracture and a 15% risk of hip fracture—a major cause of disability and death—in white women with a normal age of menopause. There are no systematic follow-up studies regarding fracture risk in women diagnosed with primary ovarian insufficiency, with or without hormone replacement therapy.

Menopause adversely affects long-term cognitive function, and surgical menopause has been associated with distinct impairment of cognitive function and memory. In 100 women diagnosed with ovarian insufficiency, substantial changes in social anxiety, depression, and self-esteem have been described. Increased risks of minor cognitive impairment or dementia, depressive and anxiety symptoms, parkinsonism, and increased mortality from neurological and mental events have been noted in women who underwent unilateral or bilateral oophorectomy. Many reports also associate cardiovascular disease risk and mortality with age of menopause (i.e., age of menopause within the normal range, premature, or following oophorectomy). We have shown subtle abnormalities in the lipid profile in relatively young women with premature menopause as compared to age and body weight-matched controls. Age at menopause is associated with carotid atherosclerosis as assessed with ultrasonography. The postmenopausal use of estradiol seems to reduce progression of this disorder, although studies regarding postmenopausal hormone therapy and cardiovascular risk are inconclusive. The risk of cardiovascular mortality was significantly higher for women with natural early compared with late menopause (age-adjusted hazard ratio [HR] 0.98, 95% confidence interval [CI] 0.97–0.99, P=0.01 for every year menopause is delayed) in a cohort of 12,000 postmenopausal women. A meta-analysis demonstrated a clear association between postmenopausal hormonal status and cardiovascular disease in women with an induced menopause (age-adjusted HR 2.62, 95% CI 2.05–3.35) due to bilateral oophorectomy. A small but significant inverse correlation between age of natural menopause and all-cause mortality was established in both a 37-year follow-up in almost 20,000 women from Norway and a 20-year follow-up in 68,000 US women.

Increased cardiovascular mortality was also noted after bilateral oophorectomy before 45 years of age (HR 1.67, 95% CI 1.16–2.40, P=0.006) with increased overall mortality in women not using estrogen therapy until they were aged 45 years or more (1.84, 1.27–2.68, P=0.001). A 24-year follow-up of more than 16,000 women who had a hysterectomy with or without bilateral oophorectomy (as part of the Nurses' Health Study) showed a hazard ratio of 1.12 (95% CI 1.03–1.21) for total mortality.

Reproductive aging and fertility therapy

Marcelle I. Cedars

University of California, San Francisco, United States

Introduction

Women are unique in the universal loss of reproductive function at an age before other vital systems fail. The peak of germ cell endowment is reached at 6 months in utero with 5-7 million oocytes. Almost concomitantly with the cessation of germ cell mitosis, apoptosis and atresia begin so that at birth ~1-2 million oocytes remain. This normal process of atresia continues, unabated, so that at puberty ~500,000 remain, declining to ~25,000 in the late 30s and to <1000 at 51-52 years when menopause ensues.[1] Yet, age at natural menopause varies between <40-60 years,[2] while the median age at menopause ranges between 49-52.[3] This loss of ovarian germ and somatic cell function has a profound impact on women in terms of declining fertility. The investigation of ovarian aging, and its potential relation to markers of fertility, has been limited by inadequacies in measuring "ovarian age." Gross determinations of pre-, peri-, and post-menopausal status have been determined by staging methods that incorporate menstrual cycle and hormonal characteristics.[4,5] However, these criteria, even with the inclusion of follicle-stimulating hormone (FSH), were late in the reproductive spectrum and did not add much to the study of ovarian aging and its impact on fertility. Newer methods to assess ovarian aging focus on estimates of follicular reserve that can be assessed in women of all ages, including antral follicle count (AFC), the number of follicles visible by transvaginal ultrasound,[6-8] and antimüllerian hormone (AMH), a biochemical marker of ovarian reserve.[9-12] Currently, AFC and AMH are viewed as potentially valuable markers for the early stages of ovarian aging but they lack standardization[5] and good correlation with natural fecundability. However, while debate continues regarding superiority of one over the other,[13-16] both measures have been shown to aid in the assessment of ovarian stimulation potential.

Validation of AFC as an index of ovarian aging is based on studies showing AFC to co-vary with chronological age,[8,17,18] to correlate with ovarian response in treatments using assisted reproductive technology (ART),[19-21] and, in statistical models, to predict menopause onset.[7,22,23] AFC is stable across consecutive menstrual cycles and across follicular and luteal phases of the menstrual cycle,[18,24-27] but varies widely among women at any given age.[8] AMH also co-varies with chronological age, AFC, and ovarian response in ART and has many of the same measurement advantages of AFC, including relative stability within and across menstrual cycles.[9] Additionally, AMH correlated with onset of menopause in a recent prospective longitudinal study of women of late-reproductive age.[28] Both AFC and AMH have a high correlation (>70%) with the number of non-growing follicles.[29] Age related-normograms for AMH[30,31] and AFC[32,33] have been published, but the cohorts are cross-sectional and/or represent only infertile populations. Furthermore, these "ovarian reserve" tests are static, reflecting a single point-in-time, but ovarian aging is an ongoing process. The longitudinal assessment of AFC and AMH is required to provide a window into a woman's reproductive aging trajectory, allow modifiable risk factors to be examined, and provide new opportunities to examine ovarian aging in relation to early markers of fertility decline.

Biomarkers of ovarian age and fertility

There is a well-known gradual decline in fertility with increasing age.[34-36] It has been proposed that the intervals between reproductive events (decline in fertility, end of reproduction and menopause) are fixed, with the variable being the age at menopause.[37] This hypothesis would imply quantity and "quality" decline in parallel,[38,39] and may explain the considerable variation in reproductive potential among women of the same chronological age. Most studies of "ovarian reserve" (FSH, AFC, AMH) have focused on the infertile population, where biomarkers correlate with ovarian response to exogenous stimulation and pregnancy outcomes.[40-42] However, some investigators suggest ovarian reserve reflects primarily **quantity and not the quality** of remaining oocytes. In support, several studies suggested ovarian reserve testing is poorly predictive of achieving pregnancy or miscarriage after ART.[42-44] Even the recent study evaluating AMH as a predictor of response and pregnancy outcome in gonadotropin-releasing hormone (GnRH) antagonist cycles in good responders found AMH a predictor of pregnancy outcome through oocyte yield and not directly on blastocyst quality.[15] In contrast, studies in subfertile women suggest high FSH is associated with a decline in pregnancy rate and longer time to spontaneous pregnancy regardless of age, and earlier age of menopause is associated with infertility and pregnancy loss.[36] Trisomic pregnancies were noted to be more common in women near menopause, with low oocyte recovery, and a prior history of ovarian surgery independent of age.[45] The limited studies of ovarian aging in the general population have focused on whether ovarian reserve markers are associated with aneuploid pregnancies. While earlier studies suggested elevated FSH was associated with trisomies, a prospective study failed to find an association between FSH and pregnancy outcome.[46-49] Consistent with these findings, no difference was found in levels of FSH, inhibin B, or AFC between women who had trisomic spontaneous abortions (n=54) and those with chromosomally normal abortions or live birth.[50] The only study exploring the impact of AMH on natural fecundability is a small pilot study,[51] while ours was the first to begin evaluating the association between ovarian reserve, by AFC, and fertility in the general population.[52] Our study found a significantly lower AFC in women who had experienced difficulties conceiving, independent of chronologic age.

As women have entered the workforce in growing numbers, there has been a delay in childbearing, increased infertility, and pregnancy loss. Limited factors have been shown to influence time to pregnancy (prior contraceptive usage, cigarette smoking, alcohol usage, increased body mass index [BMI], caffeine, and SES [socioeconomic status]). The factors known to specifically influence ovarian aging are even more limited. This continues to be an active area of investigation. However, the tools available now (biomarkers as above) may still help us directly in counseling and managing our patients.

Evaluating patients prior to treatment

Ovarian aging is best reflected by AMH and AFC as discussed above, but even the patient's history may yield valuable information regarding ovarian aging and fertility potential. Menopause is a retrospective marker for the reproductive capacity of the preceding years. Numerous family studies have demonstrated strong associations between mothers' and daughters' age of menopause,[53-55] as well as increased frequency of early menopause in sisters and grandmothers of women with early menopause.[56] Genetic risk accounts for approximately 40%-50% of the individual variability in age at menopause that is seen in the population.[54] Given this strong heritability of age at menopause, mother's age at menopause has been shown to correlate with a daughter's FSH,[57] AFC,[58] and AMH.[59] Thus, this may be a key component in the patient's history. Additionally, shortened inter-menstrual interval has been associated with lowered pregnancy rates[60-62] suggesting this may be one of the earliest "symptoms" of ovarian aging. Lowered luteal phase progesterone[63,64] is also an early finding in normally cycling older women and may be suggested by a history of pre-cycle spotting.

Once the history is completed, assessment of ovarian "age" by AMH or AFC should be undertaken. While the "battle" remains regarding superiority of one over the other,[13,14] both, in skilled hands, predict ovarian response. Thus, for patients actively undergoing treatment, the knowledge of expected response may dictate prognostication regarding response and individualization of stimulation dosing. The usefulness in predicting future fertility in a patient not actively trying to conceive (see below) may be less secure.

Getting older women pregnant

Spontaneous conception

The earliest study to evaluate ovarian reserve markers and spontaneous conception[65] found no additive benefit of assessing either AMH or AFC compared to assessment of age with respect to predicting spontaneous pregnancy in a group of patients with unexplained infertility or mild male factor. However, only 52 couples were included in the observational phase of this study. Lowered levels of both AMH[51] and AFC[52] have been associated with increased time to conception in fecundability studies. While not an absolute factor, "subfertility" was noted in an age-controlled evaluation. Despite limited data to support a correlation between markers of ovarian age and oocyte "quality" in assisted reproduction, in spontaneous conceptions, where only a single follicle is produced monthly and thus "response" (oocyte number) does not play a role, the fertilization and implantation of a single oocyte – hence "quality" – seems to be reflected by known markers of oocyte quantity suggesting a correlation between quantity and quality.

Intrauterine insemination (IUI)

There have been only a few studies evaluating ovarian reserve markers in IUI cycles. While limited in numbers, the study by van Rooij[66] found no additive benefit, over age, of assessing AMH or AFC. More recent data fail to find consensus. The only other study to evaluate the role of AFC in predicting IUI outcome evaluated a heterogeneous group including male factor infertility, and found that pregnancy rates were higher with higher AFC.[67] For AMH, while one study[68] suggested AMH was predictive of success rate with IUI, this study did not control for age in the assessment of AMH. In the same year, a study evaluating age-controlled quartiles of AMH[69] found no association between AMH and IUI outcome. It is not clear if stimulation with IUI may overcome some of the "subfertility" noted in spontaneous conception, with lowered markers of ovarian reserve, since the number of follicles produced during stimulation has been shown in all studies to correlate with successful pregnancy.

The impact of age, alone, appears to be high for IUI success perhaps more so than for other treatments. A retrospective study of over 4,000 cycles[70] suggested rates drop to 5% for women 41 and 42 while they drop further to 1% for women over 42. However, this study involved only stimulation with clomiphene citrate. It is not clear, given the importance of oocyte number (due to high aneuploidy risk) in older women, that stimulation with gonadotropins might not have increased this low success rate in the older women. Studies to address this question have been small and increasing; the recommendation is to move directly to in vitro fertilization (IVF) for older patients (although it should be remembered for many of the same reasons – decreased oocyte quantity and quality – success rates with IVF are also low in women > 42 years of age utilizing their own eggs).

Assisted reproductive technology (ART)

Most of the available data regarding the usefulness of ovarian reserve markers have come from ART cycles. As above, controversy continues regarding "which" marker may be superior, but consistently, AFC and AMH have been shown to be predictive of the number of follicles developed, estradiol levels, and the number of oocytes retrieved. Thus, AMH and AFC serve a primary role in determining stimulation protocols. While this has been applied most to limit risk of "over" stimulation – they may equally be applied to women with expected lowered response. This is helpful both in terms of counseling regarding expectations for oocyte number but also ultimate pregnancy success – especially as women age and a higher percentage of retrieved oocytes are genetically compromised.

As discussed above, age impacts both quantity and quality of oocytes. And while there is intrinsic variability in the quantity of oocytes/follicles for any given age, evidence suggests that age is still the strongest predictor of live birth in ART.[71] While this study suggested both AFC and AMH (equally) predicted poor response, neither added to the prediction of pregnancy over age alone. Studies that have suggested either AMH[72] or AFC[73,74] predict not only ovarian response to stimulation but also pregnancy rate are flawed by not fully controlling for age in their analyses despite showing a strong association between these markers of ovarian reserve and age. Models that include age and ovarian reserve markers have also been developed. A recent validation study of 822 subjects suggested the independent prediction of age and AMH.[75] However, the confidence intervals were large and the ability to predict outcome for any individual woman was low. This problem was exacerbated by the small numbers in some of the pre-selected groups, especially young women with low counts.

As previously discussed, with increasing age there is an increasing percentage of genetically abnormal oocytes. Thus, it would potentially take more oocytes to "identify" one that is normal and capable of healthy development and delivery. Thus, it is not illogical to think that, especially with increasing age, the number of oocytes retrievable would play a much greater role in ultimate pregnancy outcome. And, as both AMH and AFC predict oocyte number, there is an additive benefit to age alone, particularly in older women.

Perhaps the greatest role for markers of ovarian reserve in ART is to determine the starting stimulation type and dosing.[76] We have previously shown a very tight correlation between the AFC and the number of oocytes retrieved. Thus, it could be argued, identifying the "poor responder" need not await a prior failed/cancelled cycle. The ability to predict the number of oocytes retrievable very clearly allows prospective stimulation selection. This is particularly important for the expected high responder, to avoid ovarian hyperstimulation syndrome, but also for the poor responder to avoid cycle cancellation and to help predict prognosis (see above). Some groups have developed nomograms to assist in this process.[77,78] But while this may be a step forward in prospective, active management of patients, not knowing the "best" of the poor responder protocols still compromises patient care and represents a critical clinical need.

Additional effects of increased maternal age

Regardless of how conception occurs, the increasing risk for aneuploidy with increasing age increases the risk for spontaneous pregnancy loss.[79,80] These rates approach 65% in the oldest women, even with ART.[81] Older women are also at increased maternal and neonatal risk including stillbirth, gestational diabetes, preterm delivery, and operative delivery.[82-85]

Additional effects of paternal age

While many earlier studies of paternal age did not control for maternal age, recently there has been a renewed interest in the independent impact of paternal age on pregnancy and childhood health. While not all studies have been consistent, many do suggest an increased risk for spontaneous loss and Down syndrome with increasing paternal age.[86-90] Paternal age has been associated with an increased risk of schizophrenia in multiple populations.[91-93] Additionally, there has been an increasing awareness of an increased risk for Autism and Autism Spectrum Disorder (ASD).[94-98]

Summary

Increasing maternal age (and perhaps paternal age) makes chances for conception lower and risk of pregnancy loss higher. This decline in fertility efficiency is largely due to the increased risk for oocyte aneuploidy. Biomarkers of ovarian aging are increasingly being utilized in fertility care and now in the evaluation of normal cycling women prior to conception attempts. While data are strong that these markers reflect well the primordial pool, the data are less strong with respect to chances for pregnancy success. This is due largely to the fact that these biomarkers do not correlate well with aneuploidy risk, the strongest ultimate driver of success. The exception may be for women with increasing age, where the known increased aneuploidy risk may be overcome in the face of high follicle numbers. A recent evidence-based review, from the Society of Obstetricians and Gynaecologists of Canada,[99] has presented recommendations for the older patient. Much is included about the need to adequately counsel women regarding chances for success and increased risk for pregnancy loss. Additionally, they discuss the limited expected success rate with ovulation induction and IUI for the woman over 40, suggesting these treatments should be utilized sparingly (most pregnancies in the first 2 cycles) and then women should progress to IVF. They do point out, however, the highest success rate for older women occurs with oocyte donation. While this recommendation may be sound, as clinicians, we frequently find ourselves faced with counseling and caring for women who are not yet ready for this choice. We must continue to improve our ability to identify women at risk for accelerated ovarian aging and to counsel them appropriately. Whether our abilities to identify these women prospectively and the new availability for oocyte cryopreservation will "level the playing field," as recently stated in a Wall Street Journal article, and whether this is the direction we should be moving, remain to be decided.

References

1. Moore KL, Persaud TVN. Before we are born: essentials of embryology and birth defects. Fifth ed. Philadelphia, PA: W.B. Saunders Company; 1998. 13-35 p.
2. Treloar AE. Menstrual cyclicity and the pre-menopause. Maturitas. 1981;3(3-4):249-64. Epub 1981/12/01. PubMed PMID: 7334935.
3. Morabia A, Costanza MC, Neoplasia WHOCS. International variability in ages at menarche, first livebirth, and menopause. Am J Epidemiol. 1998;148(12):1195-205. PubMed PMID: ISI:000077613000012.
4. Soules MR, Sherman S, Parrott E, Rebar R, Santoro N, Utian W, et al. Stages of Reproductive Aging Workshop (STRAW). J Womens Health Gend Based Med. 2001;10(9):843-8. PubMed PMID: 11747678.

5. Harlow SD, Gass M, Hall JE, Lobo R, Maki P, Rebar RW, et al. Executive summary of the Stages of Reproductive Aging Workshop +10: addressing the unfinished agenda of staging reproductive aging. Climacteric. 2012. Epub 2012/02/18. doi: 10.3109/13697137.2011.650656. PubMed PMID: 22338612.
6. Hansen K, Massey J, Craig, L. Antral follicle counts obtained by transvaginal ultrasound and histological examination are correlated with ovarian non-growing follicle number. Fertil Steril. 2007(88):S79-80.
7. Hansen KR, Knowlton NS, Thyer AC, Charleston JS, Soules MR, Klein NA. A new model of reproductive aging: the decline in ovarian non-growing follicle number from birth to menopause. Hum Reprod. 2008;23(3):699-708. Epub 2008/01/15. doi: dem408 [pii]10.1093/humrep/dem408. PubMed PMID: 18192670.
8. Rosen MP, Sternfeld B, Schuh-Huerta SM, Reijo Pera RA, McCulloch CE, Cedars MI. Antral follicle count: absence of significant midlife decline. Fertil Steril. 2010;94(6):2182-5. Epub 2010/02/13. doi: S0015-0282(09)04294-0 [pii]10.1016/j.fertnstert.2009.12.045. PubMed PMID: 20149366.
9. Ledger WL. Clinical utility of measurement of anti-mullerian hormone in reproductive endocrinology. J Clin Endocrinol Metab. 2010;95(12):5144-54. Epub 2010/12/07. doi: 95/12/5144 [pii] 10.1210/jc.2010-0701. PubMed PMID: 21131535.
10. La Marca A, Sighinolfi G, Radi D, Argento C, Baraldi E, Artenisio AC, et al. Anti-Mullerian hormone (AMH) as a predictive marker in assisted reproductive technology (ART). Hum Reprod Update. 2010;16(2):113-30. Epub 2009/10/02. doi: dmp036 [pii]10.1093/humupd/dmp036. PubMed PMID: 19793843.
11. Majumder K, Gelbaya TA, Laing I, Nardo LG. The use of anti-Mullerian hormone and antral follicle count to predict the potential of oocytes and embryos. Eur J Obstet Gynecol Reprod Biol. 2010;150(2):166-70. Epub 2010/03/13. doi: S0301-2115(10)00095-3 [pii]10.1016/j.ejogrb.2010.02.029. PubMed PMID: 20223579.
12. Rosen MP, Johnstone E, McCulloch CE, Schuh-Huerta SM, Sternfeld B, Reijo-Pera RA, et al. A characterization of the relationship of ovarian reserve markers with age. Fertil Steril. 2012;97(1):238-43. Epub 2011/12/02. doi: S0015-0282(11)02716-6 [pii] 10.1016/j.fertnstert.2011.10.031. PubMed PMID: 22130324.
13. Loh JS, Maheshwari A. Anti-Mullerian hormone--is it a crystal ball for predicting ovarian ageing? Hum Reprod. 2011;26(11):2925-32. Epub 2011/08/19. doi: 10.1093/humrep/der271. PubMed PMID: 21849297.
14. Nelson SM, Anderson RA, Broekmans FJ, Raine-Fenning N, Fleming R, La Marca A. Anti-Mullerian hormone: clairvoyance or crystal clear? Hum Reprod. 2012;27(3):631-6. Epub 2012/01/13. doi: 10.1093/humrep/der446. PubMed PMID: 22238112.
15. Arce JC, La Marca A, Mirner Klein B, Nyboe Andersen A, Fleming R. Antimullerian hormone in gonadotropin releasing-hormone antagonist cycles: prediction of ovarian response and cumulative treatment outcome in good-prognosis patients. Fertil Steril. 2013;99(6):1644-53 e1. Epub 2013/02/12. doi: 10.1016/j.fertnstert.2012.12.048. PubMed PMID: 23394782.
16. Nelson SM. Biomarkers of ovarian response: current and future applications. Fertil Steril. 2013;99(4):963-9. Epub 2013/01/15. doi: 10.1016/j.fertnstert.2012.11.051. PubMed PMID: 23312225.
17. Reuss ML, Kline J, Santos R, Levin B, Timor-Tritsch I. Age and the ovarian follicle pool assessed with transvaginal ultrasonography. Am J Obstet Gynecol. 1996;174(2):624-7. PubMed PMID: 8623796.
18. Scheffer GJ, Broekmans FJ, Dorland M, Habbema JD, Looman CW, te Velde ER. Antral follicle counts by transvaginal ultrasonography are related to age in women with proven natural fertility. Fertil Steril. 1999;72(5):845-51. Epub 1999/11/24. doi: S0015-0282(99)00396-9 [pii]. PubMed PMID: 10560988.

19. Aflatoonian A, Oskouian H, Ahmadi S, Oskouian L. Prediction of high ovarian response to controlled ovarian hyperstimulation: anti-Mullerian hormone versus small antral follicle count (2-6 mm). J Assist Reprod Genet. 2009;26(6):319-25. Epub 2009/06/23. doi: 10.1007/s10815-009-9319-5. PubMed PMID: 19543966; PubMed Central PMCID: PMCPMC2729857.
20. Frattarelli JL, Levi AJ, Miller BT, Segars JH. A prospective assessment of the predictive value of basal antral follicles in in vitro fertilization cycles. Fertil Steril. 2003;80(2):350-5. Epub 2003/08/12. doi: S0015028203006642 [pii]. PubMed PMID: 12909498.
21. Klinkert ER, Broekmans FJ, Looman CW, Habbema JD, te Velde ER. The antral follicle count is a better marker than basal follicle-stimulating hormone for the selection of older patients with acceptable pregnancy prospects after in vitro fertilization. Fertil Steril. 2005;83(3):811-4. Epub 2005/03/08. doi: S0015-0282(04)03005-5 [pii] 10.1016/j.fertnstert.2004.11.005. PubMed PMID: 15749527.
22. Broekmans FJ, Faddy MJ, Scheffer G, te Velde ER. Antral follicle counts are related to age at natural fertility loss and age at menopause. Menopause. 2004;11(6 Pt 1):607-14. Epub 2004/11/17. doi: 00042192-200411060-00007 [pii]. PubMed PMID: 15545788.
23. Giacobbe M, Mendes Pinto-Neto A, Simoes Costa-Paiva LH, Martinez EZ. The usefulness of ovarian volume, antral follicle count and age as predictors of menopausal status. Climacteric. 2004;7(3):255-60. Epub 2005/01/27. PubMed PMID: 15669549.
24. Pache TD, Wladimiroff JW, de Jong FH, Hop WC, Fauser BC. Growth patterns of nondominant ovarian follicles during the normal menstrual cycle. Fertil Steril. 1990;54(4):638-42. Epub 1990/10/01. PubMed PMID: 2209884.
25. Scheffer GJ, Broekmans FJ, Bancsi LF, Habbema JD, Looman CW, Te Velde ER. Quantitative transvaginal two- and three-dimensional sonography of the ovaries: reproducibility of antral follicle counts. Ultrasound Obstet Gynecol. 2002;20(3):270-5. Epub 2002/09/17. doi: 10.1046/j.1469-0705.2002.00787.x [pii] 10.1046/j.1469-0705.2002.00787.x. PubMed PMID: 12230451.
26. van Disseldorp J, Lambalk CB, Kwee J, Looman CW, Eijkemans MJ, Fauser BC, et al. Comparison of inter- and intra-cycle variability of anti-Mullerian hormone and antral follicle counts. Hum Reprod. 2010;25(1):221-7. Epub 2009/10/21. doi: dep366 [pii] 10.1093/humrep/dep366. PubMed PMID: 19840990.
27. Rombauts L, Onwude JL, Chew HW, Vollenhoven BJ. The predictive value of antral follicle count remains unchanged across the menstrual cycle. Fertil Steril. 2011;96(6):1514-8. Epub 2011/10/22. doi: S0015-0282(11)02504-0 [pii] 10.1016/j.fertnstert.2011.09.005. PubMed PMID: 22014878.
28. Freeman EW, Sammel MD, Lin H, Gracia CR. Anti-mullerian hormone as a predictor of time to menopause in late reproductive age women. J Clin Endocrinol Metab. 2012;97(5):1673-80. Epub 2012/03/02. doi: 10.1210/jc.2011-3032. PubMed PMID: 22378815; PubMed Central PMCID: PMC3339896.
29. Hansen KR, Hodnett GM, Knowlton N, Craig LB. Correlation of ovarian reserve tests with histologically determined primordial follicle number. Fertil Steril. 2011;95(1):170-5. Epub 2010/06/05. doi: S0015-0282(10)00603-5 [pii] 10.1016/j.fertnstert.2010.04.006. PubMed PMID: 20522327.
30. Almog B, Shehata F, Suissa S, Holzer H, Shalom-Paz E, La Marca A, et al. Age-related normograms of serum antimullerian hormone levels in a population of infertile women: a multicenter study. Fertil Steril. 2011;95(7):2359-63, 63 e1. Epub 2011/04/05. doi: S0015-0282(11)00370-0 [pii] 10.1016/j.fertnstert.2011.02.057. PubMed PMID: 21457958.
31. Shebl O, Ebner T, Sir A, Schreier-Lechner E, Mayer RB, Tews G, et al. Age-related distribution of basal serum AMH level in women of reproductive age and a presumably healthy cohort. Fertil Steril. 2011;95(2):832-4. Epub 2010/10/26. doi: S0015-0282(10)02542-2 [pii] 10.1016/j.fertnstert.2010.09.012. PubMed PMID: 20970126.

32. La Marca A, Spada E, Sighinolfi G, Argento C, Tirelli A, Giulini S, et al. Age-specific nomogram for the decline in antral follicle count throughout the reproductive period. Fertil Steril. 2011;95(2):684-8. Epub 2010/08/28. doi: S0015-0282(10)02195-3 [pii] 10.1016/j.fertnstert.2010.07.1069. PubMed PMID: 20797717.
33. Almog B, Shehata F, Shalom-Paz E, Tan SL, Tulandi T. Age-related normogram for antral follicle count: McGill reference guide. Fertil Steril. 2011;95(2):663-6. Epub 2010/09/28. doi: S0015-0282(10)02461-1 [pii] 10.1016/j.fertnstert.2010.08.047. PubMed PMID: 20869703.
34. Menken J, Trussell J, Larsen U. Age and infertility. Science. 1986;233(4771):1389-94. Epub 1986/09/26. PubMed PMID: 3755843.
35. Evers JL. Female subfertility. Lancet. 2002;360(9327):151-9. Epub 2002/07/20. doi: S0140-6736(02)09417-5 [pii] 10.1016/S0140-6736(02)09417-5. PubMed PMID: 12126838.
36. Kok HS, van Asselt KM, van der Schouw YT, Grobbee DE, te Velde ER, Pearson PL, et al. Subfertility reflects accelerated ovarian ageing. Hum Reprod. 2003;18(3):644-8. Epub 2003/03/05. PubMed PMID: 12615839.
37. Broekmans F. Female reproductive ageing: current knowledge and future trends. Trends Endocrinol Metab. 2007;18(2):58-65.
38. Zheng CJ, Byers B. Oocyte selection: a new model for the maternal-age dependence of Down syndrome. Hum Genet. 1992;90(1-2):1-6. Epub 1992/09/01. PubMed PMID: 1427764.
39. Warburton D. Biological aging and the etiology of aneuploidy. Cytogenet Genome Res. 2005;111(3-4):266-72. Epub 2005/09/30. doi: CGR20051113_4266 [pii] 10.1159/000086899. PubMed PMID: 16192704.
40. Lee TH, Liu CH, Huang CC, Hsieh KC, Lin PM, Lee MS. Impact of female age and male infertility on ovarian reserve markers to predict outcome of assisted reproduction technology cycles. Reprod Biol Endocrinol. 2009;7:100. Epub 2009/09/19. doi: 1477-7827-7-100 [pii] 10.1186/1477-7827-7-100. PubMed PMID: 19761617; PubMed Central PMCID: PMCPMC2754482.
41. Nardo LG, Gelbaya TA, Wilkinson H, Roberts SA, Yates A, Pemberton P, et al. Circulating basal anti-Mullerian hormone levels as predictor of ovarian response in women undergoing ovarian stimulation for in vitro fertilization. Fertil Steril. 2009;92(5):1586-93. Epub 2008/10/22. doi: S0015-0282(08)03837-5 [pii] 10.1016/j.fertnstert.2008.08.127. PubMed PMID: 18930213.
42. Broekmans FJ, Kwee J, Hendriks DJ, Mol BW, Lambalk CB. A systematic review of tests predicting ovarian reserve and IVF outcome. Hum Reprod Update. 2006;12(6):685-718. Epub 2006/08/08. doi: dml034 [pii] 10.1093/humupd/dml034. PubMed PMID: 16891297.
43. Haadsma ML, Groen H, Fidler V, Bukman A, Roeloffzen EM, Groenewoud ER, et al. The predictive value of ovarian reserve tests for spontaneous pregnancy in subfertile ovulatory women. Hum Reprod. 2008;23(8):1800-7. Epub 2008/06/24. doi: den234 [pii] 10.1093/humrep/den234. PubMed PMID: 18567901.
44. Haadsma ML, Groen H, Fidler V, Seinen LH, Broekmans FJ, Heineman MJ, et al. The predictive value of ovarian reserve tests for miscarriage in a population of subfertile ovulatory women. Hum Reprod. 2009;24(3):546-52. Epub 2008/12/09. doi: den384 [pii] 10.1093/humrep/den384. PubMed PMID: 19059944.
45. Haadsma ML, Mooij TM, Groen H, Burger CW, Lambalk CB, Broekmans FJ, et al. A reduced size of the ovarian follicle pool is associated with an increased risk of a trisomic pregnancy in IVF-treated women. Hum Reprod. 2010;25(2):552-8. Epub 2009/11/19. doi: dep404 [pii] 10.1093/humrep/dep404. PubMed PMID: 19920066.

46. van Montfrans JM, van Hooff MH, Huirne JA, Tanahatoe SJ, Sadrezadeh S, Martens F, et al. Basal FSH concentrations as a marker of ovarian ageing are not related to pregnancy outcome in a general population of women over 30 years. Hum Reprod. 2004;19(2):430-4. Epub 2004/01/30. PubMed PMID: 14747192.
47. Nasseri A. Elevated day 3 serum follicle stimulating hormone and/or estradiol may predict fetal aneuploidy. Fertil Steril. 1999;71(4):715-8.
48. van Montfrans JM, Dorland M, Oosterhuis GJ, van Vugt JM, Rekers-Mombarg LT, Lambalk CB. Increased concentrations of follicle-stimulating hormone in mothers of children with Down's syndrome. Lancet. 1999;353(9167):1853-4. Epub 1999/06/08. doi: S0140673699009368 [pii]. PubMed PMID: 10359418.
49. van Montfrans JM, van Hooff MH, Martens F, Lambalk CB. Basal FSH, estradiol and inhibin B concentrations in women with a previous Down's syndrome affected pregnancy. Hum Reprod. 2002;17(1):44-7. Epub 2002/01/05. PubMed PMID: 11756360.
50. Kline J, Kinney A, Reuss ML, Kelly A, Levin B, Ferin M, et al. Trisomic pregnancy and the oocyte pool. Hum Reprod. 2004;19(7):1633-43. Epub 2004/05/29. doi: 10.1093/humrep/deh310 deh310 [pii]. PubMed PMID: 15166127.
51. Steiner AZ, Herring AH, Kesner JS, Meadows JW, Stanczyk FZ, Hoberman S, et al. Antimullerian hormone as a predictor of natural fecundability in women aged 30-42 years. Obstet Gynecol. 2011;117(4):798-804. Epub 2011/03/23. doi: 10.1097/AOG.0b013e3182116bc8 00006250-201104000-00006 [pii]. PubMed PMID: 21422850.
52. Rosen MP, Johnstone E, Addauan-Andersen C, Cedars MI. A lower antral follicle count is associated with infertility. Fertil Steril. 2011;95(6):1950-4 e1. Epub 2011/03/08. doi: S0015-0282(11)00230-5 [pii] 10.1016/j.fertnstert.2011.01.151. PubMed PMID: 21376313.
53. Torgerson DJ, Thomas RE, Reid DM. Mothers and daughters menopausal ages: is there a link? Eur J Obstet Gynecol Reprod Biol. 1997;74(1):63-6. PubMed PMID: 9243205.
54. Van Asselt K, Kok H, Pearson PL, al. E. Heritability of menopause age in mothers and daughters. Fertil Steril. 2004;82(5):1348-51. PubMed PMID: PMID: 15533358.
55. Mishra G, Hardy R, Kuh D. Are the effects of risk factors for timing of menopause modified by age? Results from a British birth cohort study. Menopause. 2007;14(4):717-24. Epub 2007/02/07. doi: 10.1097/GME.0b013e31802f3156. PubMed PMID: 17279060.
56. Cramer DW, Xu H, Harlow BL. Family history as a predictor of early menopause. Fertil Steril. 1995;64(4):740-5. Epub 1995/10/01. PubMed PMID: 7672145.
57. Steiner AZ, Baird DD, Kesner JS. Mother's menopausal age is associated with her daughter's early follicular phase urinary follicle-stimulating hormone level. Menopause. 2008;15(5):940-4. Epub 2008/09/10. doi: 10.1097/gme.0b013e31816429e5. PubMed PMID: 18779679; PubMed Central PMCID: PMC2856641.
58. Rosen MP, Johnstone EB, Gillham SJ, Modan AE, Lipshutz AK, Reijo-Pera R, et al. Is antral follicle count a genetic trait? Menopause. 2010;17(1):109-13. Epub 2009/09/16. doi: 10.1097/gme.0b013e3181b48a88. PubMed PMID: 19752762.
59. Bentzen JG, Forman JL, Larsen EC, Pinborg A, Johannsen TH, Schmidt L, et al. Maternal menopause as a predictor of anti-Mullerian hormone level and antral follicle count in daughters during reproductive age. Hum Reprod. 2013;28(1):247-55. Epub 2012/11/09. doi: 10.1093/humrep/des356. PubMed PMID: 23136135.
60. Brodin T, Bergh T, Berglund L, Hadziosmanovic N, Holte J. Menstrual cycle length is an age-independent marker of female fertility: results from 6271 treatment cycles of in vitro fertilization. Fertil Steril. 2008;90(5):1656-61. Epub 2007/12/25. doi: 10.1016/j.fertnstert.2007.09.036. PubMed PMID: 18155201.

61. van der Steeg JW, Steures P, Eijkemans MJ, Habbema JD, Hompes PG, Michgelsen HW, et al. Predictive value of pregnancy history in subfertile couples: results from a nationwide cohort study in the Netherlands. Fertil Steril. 2008;90(3):521-7. Epub 2007/11/06. doi: 10.1016/j.fertnstert.2007.07.1301. PubMed PMID: 17980877.
62. Wise LA, Mikkelsen EM, Rothman KJ, Riis AH, Sorensen HT, Huybrechts KF, et al. A prospective cohort study of menstrual characteristics and time to pregnancy. Am J Epidemiol. 2011;174(6):701-9. Epub 2011/07/02. doi: 10.1093/aje/kwr130. PubMed PMID: 21719742; PubMed Central PMCID: PMC3166706.
63. Santoro N, Brown JR, Adel T, Skurnick JH. Characterization of reproductive hormonal dynamics in the perimenopause. J Clin Endocrinol Metab. 1996;81(4):1495-501. Epub 1996/04/01. PubMed PMID: 8636357.
64. Mersereau JE, Evans ML, Moore DH, Liu JH, Thomas MA, Rebar RW, et al. Luteal phase estrogen is decreased in regularly menstruating older women compared with a reference population of younger women. Menopause. 2008;15(3):482-6. Epub 2008/01/19. doi: 10.1097/gme.0b013e31815982cf. PubMed PMID: 18202592.
65. van Rooij IA, Broekmans FJ, Hunault CC, Scheffer GJ, Eijkemans MJ, de Jong FH, et al. Use of ovarian reserve tests for the prediction of ongoing pregnancy in couples with unexplained or mild male infertility. Reproductive biomedicine online. 2006;12(2):182-90. Epub 2006/02/16. PubMed PMID: 16478583.
66. Broer SL, Eijkemans MJ, Scheffer GJ, van Rooij IA, de Vet A, Themmen AP, et al. Anti-mullerian hormone predicts menopause: a long-term follow-up study in normoovulatory women. J Clin Endocrinol Metab. 2011;96(8):2532-9. Epub 2011/05/27. doi: 10.1210/jc.2010-2776. PubMed PMID: 21613357.
67. Erdem M, Erdem A, Guler I, Atmaca S. Role of antral follicle count in controlled ovarian hyperstimulation and intrauterine insemination cycles in patients with unexplained subfertility. Fertil Steril. 2008;90(2):360-6. Epub 2007/09/25. doi: 10.1016/j.fertnstert.2007.06.028. PubMed PMID: 17889858.
68. Lin JW, Caffrey JL, Chang MH, Lin YS. Sex, menopause, metabolic syndrome, and all-cause and cause-specific mortality cohort analysis from the Third National Health and Nutrition Examination Survey. J Clin Endocrinol Metab. 2010;95(9):4258-67. doi: 10.1210/jc.2010-0332. PubMed PMID: ISI:000281640300041.
69. Tremellen K, Kolo M. Serum anti-Mullerian hormone is a useful measure of quantitative ovarian reserve but does not predict the chances of live-birth pregnancy. The Australian & New Zealand journal of obstetrics & gynaecology. 2010;50(6):568-72. Epub 2010/12/08. doi: 10.1111/j.1479-828X.2010.01232.x. PubMed PMID: 21133869.
70. Dovey S, Sneeringer RM, Penzias AS. Clomiphene citrate and intrauterine insemination: analysis of more than 4100 cycles. Fertil Steril. 2008;90(6):2281-6. Epub 2008/01/15. doi: 10.1016/j.fertnstert.2007.10.057. PubMed PMID: 18191842.
71. Broer SL, van Disseldorp J, Broeze KA, Dolleman M, Opmeer BC, Bossuyt P, et al. Added value of ovarian reserve testing on patient characteristics in the prediction of ovarian response and ongoing pregnancy: an individual patient data approach. Hum Reprod Update. 2013;19(1):26-36. Epub 2012/11/29. doi: 10.1093/humupd/dms041. PubMed PMID: 23188168.
72. Irez T, Ocal P, Guralp O, Cetin M, Aydogan B, Sahmay S. Different serum anti-Mullerian hormone concentrations are associated with oocyte quality, embryo development parameters and IVF-ICSI outcomes. Archives of gynecology and obstetrics. 2011;284(5):1295-301. Epub 2011/07/13. doi: 10.1007/s00404-011-1979-6. PubMed PMID: 21748312.

73. Holte J, Brodin T, Berglund L, Hadziosmanovic N, Olovsson M, Bergh T. Antral follicle counts are strongly associated with live-birth rates after assisted reproduction, with superior treatment outcome in women with polycystic ovaries. Fertil Steril. 2011;96(3):594-9. Epub 2011/09/02. doi: 10.1016/j.fertnstert.2011.06.071. PubMed PMID: 21880276.
74. Jayaprakasan K, Chan Y, Islam R, Haoula Z, Hopkisson J, Coomarasamy A, et al. Prediction of in vitro fertilization outcome at different antral follicle count thresholds in a prospective cohort of 1,012 women. Fertil Steril. 2012;98(3):657-63. Epub 2012/07/04. doi: 10.1016/j.fertnstert.2012.05.042. PubMed PMID: 22749225.
75. Khader A, Lloyd SM, McConnachie A, Fleming R, Grisendi V, La Marca A, et al. External validation of anti-Mullerian hormone based prediction of live birth in assisted conception. Journal of ovarian research. 2013;6(1):3. Epub 2013/01/09. doi: 10.1186/1757-2215-6-3. PubMed PMID: 23294733; PubMed Central PMCID: PMC3546900.
76. Fleming R, Broekmans F, Calhaz-Jorge C, Dracea L, Alexander H, Nyboe Andersen A, et al. Can anti-Mullerian hormone concentrations be used to determine gonadotrophin dose and treatment protocol for ovarian stimulation? Reproductive biomedicine online. 2013;26(5):431-9. Epub 2013/03/20. doi: 10.1016/j.rbmo.2012.02.027. PubMed PMID: 23507133.
77. La Marca A, Papaleo E, Grisendi V, Argento C, Giulini S, Volpe A. Development of a nomogram based on markers of ovarian reserve for the individualisation of the follicle-stimulating hormone starting dose in in vitro fertilisation cycles. BJOG. 2012;119(10):1171-9. Epub 2012/07/19. doi: 10.1111/j.1471-0528.2012.03412.x. PubMed PMID: 22805536.
78. La Marca A, Grisendi V, Giulini S, Argento C, Tirelli A, Dondi G, et al. Individualization of the FSH starting dose in IVF/ICSI cycles using the antral follicle count. Journal of ovarian research. 2013;6(1):11. Epub 2013/02/08. doi: 10.1186/1757-2215-6-11. PubMed PMID: 23388048; PubMed Central PMCID: PMC3568720.
79. Hook EB, Cross PK, Jackson L, Pergament E, Brambati B. Maternal age-specific rates of 47,+21 and other cytogenetic abnormalities diagnosed in the first trimester of pregnancy in chorionic villus biopsy specimens: comparison with rates expected from observations at amniocentesis. Am J Hum Genet. 1988;42(6):797-807. Epub 1988/06/01. PubMed PMID: 2967030; PubMed Central PMCID: PMC1715211.
80. Hook EB. Rates of chromosome abnormalities at different maternal ages. Obstet Gynecol. 1981;58(3):282-5. PubMed PMID: 6455611.
81. Serour G, Mansour R, Serour A, Aboulghar M, Amin Y, Kamal O, et al. Analysis of 2,386 consecutive cycles of in vitro fertilization or intracytoplasmic sperm injection using autologous oocytes in women aged 40 years and above. Fertil Steril. 2010;94(5):1707-12. Epub 2009/11/10. doi: 10.1016/j.fertnstert.2009.09.044. PubMed PMID: 19896654.
82. Gilbert WM, Nesbitt TS, Danielsen B. Childbearing beyond age 40: pregnancy outcome in 24,032 cases. Obstet Gynecol. 1999;93(1):9-14. Epub 1999/01/23. PubMed PMID: 9916947.
83. Favilli A, Pericoli S, Acanfora MM, Bini V, Di Renzo GC, Gerli S. Pregnancy outcome in women aged 40 years or more. The journal of maternal-fetal & neonatal medicine : the official journal of the European Association of Perinatal Medicine, the Federation of Asia and Oceania Perinatal Societies, the International Society of Perinatal Obstet. 2012;25(8):1260-3. Epub 2011/11/30. doi: 10.3109/14767058.2011.643327. PubMed PMID: 22122237.
84. Kenny LC, Lavender T, McNamee R, O'Neill SM, Mills T, Khashan AS. Advanced maternal age and adverse pregnancy outcome: evidence from a large contemporary cohort. PloS one. 2013;8(2):e56583. Epub 2013/02/26. doi: 10.1371/journal.pone.0056583. PubMed PMID: 23437176; PubMed Central PMCID: PMC3577849.

85. Karabulut A, Ozkan S, Bozkurt AI, Karahan T, Kayan S. Perinatal outcomes and risk factors in adolescent and advanced age pregnancies: Comparison with normal reproductive age women. Journal of obstetrics and gynaecology : the journal of the Institute of Obstetrics and Gynaecology. 2013;33(4):346-50. Epub 2013/05/10. doi: 10.3109/01443615.2013.767786. PubMed PMID: 23654312.
86. Erickson JD. Paternal age and Down syndrome. Am J Hum Genet. 1979;31(4):489-97. Epub 1979/07/01. PubMed PMID: 158308; PubMed Central PMCID: PMC1685888.
87. Erickson JD, Bjerkedal TO. Down syndrome associated with father's age in Norway. J Med Genet. 1981;18(1):22-8. Epub 1981/02/01. PubMed PMID: 6454784; PubMed Central PMCID: PMC1048652.
88. Kleinhaus K, Perrin M, Friedlander Y, Paltiel O, Malaspina D, Harlap S. Paternal age and spontaneous abortion. Obstet Gynecol. 2006;108(2):369-77. Epub 2006/08/02. doi: 10.1097/01.AOG.0000224606.26514.3a. PubMed PMID: 16880308.
89. Maconochie N, Doyle P, Prior S, Simmons R. Risk factors for first trimester miscarriage--results from a UK-population-based case-control study. BJOG. 2007;114(2):170-86. Epub 2007/02/20. doi: 10.1111/j.1471-0528.2006.01195.x. PubMed PMID: 17305901.
90. Toriello HV, Meck JM. Statement on guidance for genetic counseling in advanced paternal age. Genetics in medicine : official journal of the American College of Medical Genetics. 2008;10(6):457-60. Epub 2008/05/23. doi: 10.1097/GIM.0b013e318176fabb. PubMed PMID: 18496227; PubMed Central PMCID: PMC3111019.
91. Malaspina D HSFS, et al. ADvancing paternal age and the risk of schizophrenia. Archives of General Psychiatry. 2001;58(4):361-7. doi: 10.1001/archpsyc.58.4.361.
92. Byrne M, Agerbo E, Ewald H, Eaton WW, Mortensen PB. Parental age and risk of schizophrenia: a case-control study. Arch Gen Psychiatry. 2003;60(7):673-8. Epub 2003/07/16. doi: 10.1001/archpsyc.60.7.673. PubMed PMID: 12860771.
93. Zammit S, Allebeck P, Dalman C, Lundberg I, Hemmingson T, Owen MJ, et al. Paternal age and risk for schizophrenia. The British journal of psychiatry : the journal of mental science. 2003;183:405-8. Epub 2003/11/05. PubMed PMID: 14594914.
94. Lauritsen MB, Pedersen CB, Mortensen PB. Effects of familial risk factors and place of birth on the risk of autism: a nationwide register-based study. Journal of child psychology and psychiatry, and allied disciplines. 2005;46(9):963-71. Epub 2005/08/20. doi: 10.1111/j.1469-7610.2004.00391.x. PubMed PMID: 16108999.
95. Reichenberg A, Gross R, Weiser M, Bresnahan M, Silverman J, Harlap S, et al. Advancing paternal age and autism. Arch Gen Psychiatry. 2006;63(9):1026-32. Epub 2006/09/06. doi: 10.1001/archpsyc.63.9.1026. PubMed PMID: 16953005.
96. Croen LA, Najjar DV, Fireman B, Grether JK. Maternal and paternal age and risk of autism spectrum disorders. Archives of pediatrics & adolescent medicine. 2007;161(4):334-40. Epub 2007/04/04. doi: 10.1001/archpedi.161.4.334. PubMed PMID: 17404129.
97. Ben Itzchak E, Lahat E, Zachor DA. Advanced parental ages and low birth weight in autism spectrum disorders--rates and effect on functioning. Research in developmental disabilities. 2011;32(5):1776-81. Epub 2011/04/19. doi: 10.1016/j.ridd.2011.03.004. PubMed PMID: 21498045.
98. Parner ET, Baron-Cohen S, Lauritsen MB, Jorgensen M, Schieve LA, Yeargin-Allsopp M, et al. Parental age and autism spectrum disorders. Annals of epidemiology. 2012;22(3):143-50. Epub 2012/01/27. doi: 10.1016/j.annepidem.2011.12.006. PubMed PMID: 22277122.
99. Liu K, Case A. Advanced reproductive age and fertility. Journal of obstetrics and gynaecology Canada : JOGC = Journal d'obstetrique et gynecologie du Canada : JOGC. 2011;33(11):1165-75. Epub 2011/11/16. PubMed PMID: 22082792.

Trilogy 9. Fibroids

Highlights in the basic science of uterine fibroids

Erica E. Marsh

Northwestern University, Chicago, IL

Introduction

Uterine leiomyomas are well-defined benign smooth muscle tumors of the uterus that represent a significant health care burden amongst women. These tumors are commonly known as "fibroids" due to their fibrous appearance and extensive extracellular matrix. In the United States, they are present in 30%-50% of women of reproductive age and have an overall cumulative incidence in women of ~70% by the age of 50 (1). Furthermore, leiomyomas disproportionately affect African-American women across the age spectrum (2) with epidemiological studies showing a cumulative incidence of almost 90% by the age of 50 (1). While some women with these tumors have no symptoms, many women develop heavy menstrual bleeding, pressure symptoms, pelvic pain, infertility, and recurrent pregnancy loss (3). The chronic morbidity associated with the spectrum of symptoms (menorrhagia, infertility, pelvic pain, etc.) caused by leiomyomas and the lack of long-term medical treatment options explain why they remain the leading cause of hysterectomy in the United States (4). Recent analyses estimate the costs of leiomyomata to the US health care system to be as much as $34 billion dollars annually (5). Despite their prevalence and clear public health impact, relatively little is understood about their etiology and pathogenesis. Although it is beyond the scope of this Trilogy presentation to cover all of the basic science findings in leiomyoma research, we will try to summarize the key developments and highlight future areas for advancement.

Tumor initiation

Monoclonal in origin

It is well established that these tumors are monoclonal in origin. This finding was first published in 1965. Using the sex-linked electrophoretic variants of glucose-6-phosphate dehydrogenase, Linder and Gartler reported that 27 leiomyomas had either the A or B band in contrast to the 86 myometrial tissues that, with the exception of one sample, had both bands in essentially equal amounts. Further support of a monoclonal origin of leiomyomas came from phosphoglycerokinase (PGK) gene studies. The PGK gene is located on the X chromosome and, using a polymerase chain reaction (PCR) method that targeted the methylated PGK gene allele, it was found that all leiomyoma samples contained a single inactive allele indicating a monoclonal origin (6). A similar methodology was used by Zhang et al. using the methylation status of the X-linked androgen receptor gene (7).

Karyotypic abnormalities

At one time, it was hypothesized that the initiation and progression of leiomyomas were the result of karytyopic abnormalities. While we now know that this is less likely the case, as most leiomyomas have a normal karyotype, much was learned from the genetic derangements that contribute to the pathogenesis of a subset of these tumors. The first reports of cytogenetic abnormalities in leiomyomas were published in the late 1980s (8-10). Mark et al. published data from a series of 21 leiomyomas that revealed that 51% of the tumors had abnormal karyotypes largely consisting of structural (versus numerical) anomalies most commonly involving chromosomes 1, 2, and 12 (8). In 1991, Rein et al. published data from a series of 13 leiomyomas, and clonal chromosome rearrangements were found in 54% of the tumors. The rearrangement involved 12q14-15 in 5 of the 13 samples. Later, larger studies revealed a lower prevalence of chromosomal abnormalities than the earlier smaller studies. In 1997, Brosens et al. published data from a series of 217 leiomyomas and found that of the 182 tumors that could be grown in culture, 29% were found to have cytogenetic abnormalities. Rearrangements most often involved chromosomes 6, 7, and 12 in this population. A 2003 study by Kataoka et al. examined karyotypes from 302 leiomyomas from a population of Japanese women and only 21 (6.9%) were found to have abnormal karyotypes. Chromosomes 1, 7, 12, and 14 were most highly identified in the rearrangements (11).

Single gene defects

Fumarate hydratase (FH) was one of the first genes presented as the potential etiologic factor in leiomyoma pathogenesis. However, further studies demonstrated that a FH mutation was implicated almost exclusively in patients impacted by one of two Mendelian syndromes: multiple cutaneous and uterine leiomyomatosis (MCUL1) and hereditary leiomyomatosis and renal cell cancer (HLRCC) (12, 13). The High Mobility Group proteins HMGA1 and HMGA2 have both been implicated in the pathogenesis of leiomyomas – particularly those associated with certain karyotypic derangements. Elevated HMGA1 expression has been associated with fibroids that contain the 6p21 alteration. HMGA2 was initially noted to be overexpressed in fibroids with the 12q15 chromosomal rearrangement but has subsequently been shown to be elevated, albeit to a lesser extent, in tumors without this rearrangement.

The most exciting genetic discovery in leiomyomas in recent history is the finding of the MED12 mutation. The mediator complex subunit 12 (MED12) is a subunit of the Mediator Complex, which links RNA polymerase II to gene-specific transcription factors. In 2011, using whole exome sequencing, MED12 was identified as the most frequently mutated target in 18 tumors sequenced. The finding was validated and found to be mutated in 70% of leiomyomas (n= 207) in a population of Finnish women (14). Similar findings were reported in a racially diverse population of women from the United States (15). The MED12 finding was further validated in 28 leiomyoma samples from South African women, although at a lower frequency rate of 50% (16). In 2013, Mäkinen et al. reported that MED12 exon 2 mutations vary based on leiomyoma histological type (17). They found that MED12 exon 2 mutations were present in 59% of common type leiomyomas versus 17% of leiomyoma variants (i.e., cellular, atypical, mitotically active, and leiomyomas from hereditary leiomyomatosis and renal cell cancer [HLRCC] patients). The exact role of MED12 in the pathogenesis of leiomyomas remains to be identified but the gene certainly holds promise as having a key role in the etiology of these tumors.

Stem cells

A newer focus of research in leiomyoma initiation is the role of a stem cell or side population of cells from which these tumors arise. Myometrial stem cells were identified in the mouse uterus in 2007 by Szotek et al. (18). Later that year, Ono et al. reported on a side population of cells from the human uterus that had the functional characteristics of stem cells (18). This side population was able to undergo osteogenic and adipocytic differentiation with selective media induction. Stem/progenitor cells were reported from uterine leiomyomas by Chang et al. in

2010 but were found to be fewer in number than myometrial stem cells and were found to be more terminally differentiated (19). In 2012, Ono et al. identified a side population in leiomyomas and similarly found that they represented a smaller population in leiomyomas than the side population in myometrium (1% vs. 2%) (20). This study further found that this side population contained the MED12 mutation, had lower estrogen and progesterone receptor levels, and was necessary for in vivo growth of leiomyoma xenograft tumors.

Fibroid progression

Sex steroids

Sex steroids had been known to play a significant role in the growth of leiomyomas for decades (21). The finding was initially based largely on epidemiological studies that demonstrated that leiomyomas were not seen prior to menarche, presented and became symptomatic during the reproductive years, and then regressed during menopause. These findings were confirmed with the availability of gonadotropin-releasing hormone (GnRH) agonist therapy. Both progesterone (P4) and estrogen (E2) are master gene regulators and exert their cellular effects largely via nuclear receptors (PR-A, PR-B, ER-α, and ER-β), which most studies have found to be overexpressed in leiomyoma versus myometrium.

While estradiol was initially thought to be the primary driver of fibroid growth, recent studies have shown that progesterone is the more dominant mitogen and that estradiol's main role may be to maintain the expression of PR. Specifically, progesterone has been shown to promote Bcl-2 expression, activate the Akt pathway, and regulate KLF11 expression (22-24). Aromatase (CYP19A1) synthesizes estrogens from androgens and has also been shown to be overexpressed in leiomyomas versus myometrium (25) and has further been shown to have higher expression in fibroids from African-American women versus Caucasian and Japanese women (26).

Differential genetic regulation

FIGURE 1

MicroRNA cellular pathway. The gene for the miRNA is transcribed by RNA polymerase II into a single strand of RNA. This single strand folds into a hairpin-like structure and becomes the double-stranded primary miRNA (pri-miRNA). The hairpin-like structure is subsequently cleaved in the nucleus by Drosha, forming the pre-miRNA. The pre-miRNA then enters the cytoplasm via the protein channel Exportin, where it is cleaved into a small piece of double-stranded RNA by the enzyme Dicer. The double-stranded small RNA then separates into single strands, with one strand being degraded and the other strand forming a complex with Argonaute proteins. This newly formed protein/nucleic acid complex is called an RNA-induced silencing complex (RISC). These complexes then either bind messenger RNA (mRNA) with exact complementarity, leading to cleavage of the mRNA by the RISC, or bind with partial complementarity, leading to repression of translation.

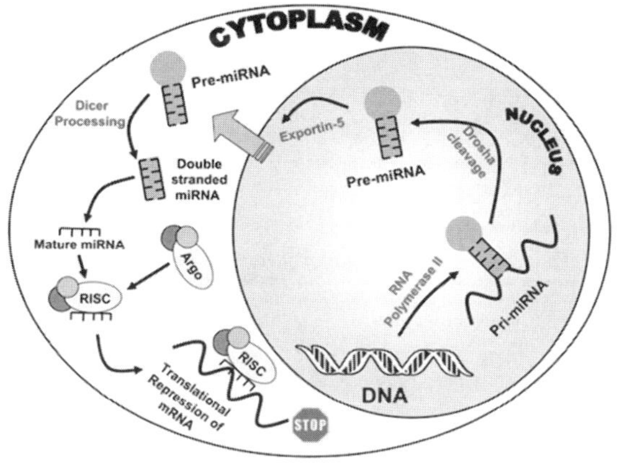

Marsh. miRNA expression in uterine leiomyomas. Fertil Steril 2008.

A number of tissue gene microarray studies have been published on leiomyomas versus normal adjacent myometrial tissue under a number of treatment conditions and across a number of patient populations (27-32). While there are some inconsistencies across studies due to the varying patient populations, cycle stages, and treatment conditions, a number of pathophysiological pathways have been identified in these microarray studies including the retinoic acid pathway, energy homeostasis pathways, insulin-like growth factor (IGGF)-signaling, extracellular matrix (ECM), and others. MicroRNAs (miRNAs) are small noncoding RNAs that negatively regulated post-transcriptional gene expression. In 2007, Marsh et al. and Wang et al. demonstrated differential miRNA expression in leiomyoma versus matched myometrial tissues (33, 34). It has also been demonstrated that several miRNAs are differentially regulated by sex steroids (35). Leet-7, which has been implicated in regulation of HMGA2 (36, 37), and miRR-21, which has been implicated in programmed cell death (38, 39), have been the miRNAs most investigated in leiomyomas at this point. DNA methylation has been implicated in cancer pathogenesis and tumorigenesis. In 2007, Yamagata et al. reported differential methylation between leiomyoma and myometrium using restriction landmark genomic scanning (40). They also found differential expression of DNA methyltransferases between leiomyoma and myometrium. Methylation studies utilizing array technology have been published recently and demonstrate a wide range of hyper- and hypomethylated gene promoter regions with a number of tumor suppressors being hypermethylated in leiomyomas (41, 42).

Extracellular matrix and TGF-β

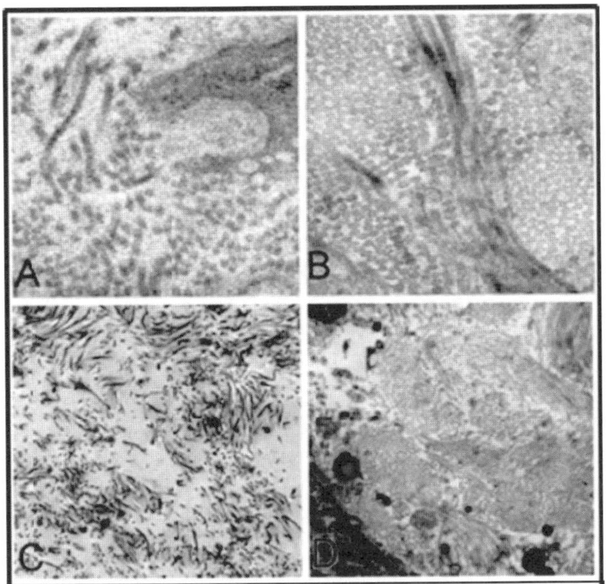

Figure 2: Electron Microscopy of leiomyoma (A&C) versus myometrium (B&D). Leppert et al 2004; Used with permission from Fertility and Sterility.

Despite being the key phenotypic distinguishing finding between myometrium and leiomyoma, the ECM is the least-investigated aspect of these tumors. What is known is that leiomyomas contain >50% more ECM than normal adjacent myometrium and that collagens, particularly the major fibrillar collagens, make up most of the ECM. The minor fibrillar collagens also have been reported to be overexpressed in leiomyoma versus myometrium. Integrins also have been shown to be differently expressed in leiomyomas (43, 44). Chen et al. recently found that integrin-β1 was significantly overexpressed in leiomyoma versus myometrium and that this overexpression leads to increased cell spreading and proliferation (44). Dermatopontin, a 22 kDa protein located in the ECM, has a number of functions including accelerating collagen fibrillogenesis and modification of newly formed collagen fibrils (45, 46). It has been shown to be down-regulated in leiomyoma similar to another fibrotic disorder – keloids (47, 48).

In addition to the composition of the matrix of these tumors, there are structural differences in the leiomyoma matrix that may play a role in the progression of these tumors. Leppert et al. demonstrated that the collagen fibrils in leiomyoma were randomly aligned and widely dispersed versus myometrium (see Figure 2) (49). Rogers et al. demonstrated that there are different levels of mechanical stress in myometrial tissues versus leiomyoma tissue (50). This differential mechanical stress leads to differential solid-state signaling in leiomyomas versus myometrium.

A number of growth factors have been implicated in leiomyoma growth including TGF-β, insulin-like growth factor (IGF), epidermal growth factor (EGF), platelet-derived growth factor (PDGF), vascular endothelial growth factor (VEGF), and fibroblast growth factor (FGF) (51). None has been shown to have a more significant role than TGF-β due to its effects on both cell proliferation and ECM production.

Future directions

While a comprehensive discussion of the basic science of uterine fibroids is beyond the scope of this Trilogy summary, we have tried to summarize key areas in the understanding of the pathophysiology of this prevalent condition. The MED12 mutation discovery holds a great amount of promise, and experiments are underway in a number of laboratories to determine the role and functional impairment (if any) of the mutation. As microRNAs have entered the arena of therapeutic intervention, they too hold a great deal of promise. The new generation of hormone modulators also holds promise for therapeutic intervention, especially in the area of selective progesterone receptor modulator (SPRMS) and aromatase inhibitors.

References

1. Baird DD, et al. High cumulative incidence of uterine leiomyoma in black and white women: ultrasound evidence. Am J Obstet Gynecol 2003. 188(1): p. 100-7.
2. Marsh EE, et al. Racial differences in fibroid prevalence and ultrasound findings in asymptomatic young women (18-30 years old): a pilot study. Fertil Steril 2013.
3. Walker CL and Stewart EA. Uterine fibroids: the elephant in the room. Science, 2005. 308(5728): p. 1589-92.
4. Carlson KJ, Nichols DH, Schiff I. Indications for hysterectomy. N Engl J Med 1993. 328(12): p. 856-60.
5. Cardozo ER, et al. The estimated annual cost of uterine leiomyomata in the United States. Am J Obstet Gynecol 2012. 206(3): p. 211 e1-9.
6. Hashimoto K, et al. Clonal determination of uterine leiomyomas by analyzing differential inactivation of the X-chromosome-linked phosphoglycerokinase gene. Gynecol Obstet Invest 1995. 40(3): p. 204-8.
7. Zhang P, et al. Use of X-chromosome inactivation pattern to determine the clonal origins of uterine leiomyoma and leiomyosarcoma. Hum Pathol 2006. 37(10): p. 1350-6.
8. Mark J, et al. Cytogenetical observations in human benign uterine leiomyomas. Anticancer Res 1988. 8(4): p. 621-6.

9. Gibas Z, Griffin CA, Emanuel BS. Clonal chromosome rearrangements in a uterine myoma. Cancer Genet Cytogenet 1988. 32(1): p. 19-24.
10. Sait SN, et al. A uterine leiomyoma showing both t(12;14) and del(7) abnormalities. Cancer Genet Cytogenet 1989. 37(2): p. 157-61.
11. Kataoka S, et al. Cytogenetic analysis of uterine leiomyoma: the size, histopathology and GnRHa-response in relation to chromosome karyotype. Eur J Obstet Gynecol Reprod Biol 2003. 110(1): p. 58-62.
12. Stewart EA, Morton CC. The genetics of uterine leiomyomata: what clinicians need to know. Obstet Gynecol 2006. 107(4): p. 917-21.
13. Aissani B, Wiener H, Zhang K. Multiple hits for the association of uterine fibroids on human chromosome 1q43. PLoS One 2013. 8(3): p. e58399.
14. Makinen N, et al. MED12, the mediator complex subunit 12 gene, is mutated at high frequency in uterine leiomyomas. Science 2011. 334(6053): p. 252-5.
15. McGuire MM, et al. Whole exome sequencing in a random sample of North American women with leiomyomas identifies MED12 mutations in majority of uterine leiomyomas. PLoS One 2012. 7(3): p. e33251.
16. Makinen N, et al. MED12 exon 2 mutations are common in uterine leiomyomas from South African patients. Oncotarget 2011. 2(12): p. 966-9.
17. Makinen N, et al. MED12 exon 2 mutations in histopathological uterine leiomyoma variants. Eur J Hum Genet 2013.
18. Szotek PP, et al. Adult mouse myometrial label-retaining cells divide in response to gonadotropin stimulation. Stem Cells 2007. 25(5): p. 1317-25.
19. Chang HL, et al. Uterine leiomyomas exhibit fewer stem/progenitor cell characteristics when compared with corresponding normal myometrium. Reprod Sci 2010. 17(2): p. 158-67.
20. Ono M, et al. Role of stem cells in human uterine leiomyoma growth. PLoS One 2012. 7(5): p. e36935.
21. Marsh EE, Bulun SE. Steroid hormones and leiomyomas. Obstet Gynecol Clin North Am 2006. 33(1): p. 59-67.
22. Yin P, et al. Progesterone receptor regulates Bcl-2 gene expression through direct binding to its promoter region in uterine leiomyoma cells. J Clin Endocrinol Metab 2007. 92(11): p. 4459-66.
23. Hoekstra AV, et al. Progestins activate the AKT pathway in leiomyoma cells and promote survival. J Clin Endocrinol Metab 2009. 94(5): p. 1768-74.
24. Yin P, et al. Transcription factor KLF11 integrates progesterone receptor signaling and proliferation in uterine leiomyoma cells. Cancer Res 2010. 70(4): p. 1722-30.
25. Bulun SE, Simpson ER, Word RA. Expression of the CYP19 gene and its product aromatase cytochrome P450 in human uterine leiomyoma tissues and cells in culture. J Clin Endocrinol Metab 1994. 78(3): p. 736-43.
26. Ishikawa H, et al. High aromatase expression in uterine leiomyoma tissues of African-American women. J Clin Endocrinol Metab 2009. 94(5): p. 1752-6.
27. Dimitrova IK, et al. Gene expression profiling of multiple leiomyomata uteri and matched normal tissue from a single patient. Fertil Steril 2009. 91(6): p. 2650-63.
28. Litovkin KV, et al. Microarray study of gene expression in uterine leiomyoma. Exp Oncol 2008. 30(2): p. 106-11.
29. Luo X, et al. Genomic and proteomic profiling II: comparative assessment of gene expression profiles in leiomyomas, keloids, and surgically-induced scars. Reprod Biol Endocrinol 2007. 5: p. 35.

30. Mihalich A, et al. Interferon-inducible genes, TNF-related apoptosis-inducing ligand (TRAIL) and interferon inducible protein 27 (IFI27) are negatively regulated in leiomyomas: implications for a role of the interferon pathway in leiomyoma development. Gynecol Endocrinol 2012. 28(3): p. 216-9.
31. Leppert PC, Catherino WH, and Segars JH. A new hypothesis about the origin of uterine fibroids based on gene expression profiling with microarrays. Am J Obstet Gynecol 2006. 195(2): p. 415-20.
32. Pan Q, Luo X, and Chegini N. Genomic and proteomic profiling I: leiomyomas in African Americans and Caucasians. Reprod Biol Endocrinol 2007. 5: p. 34.
33. Marsh EE, et al. Differential expression of microRNA species in human uterine leiomyoma versus normal myometrium. Fertil Steril 2008. 89(6): p. 1771-6.
34. Wang T, et al. A micro-RNA signature associated with race, tumor size, and target gene activity in human uterine leiomyomas. Genes Chromosomes Cancer 2007. 46(4):p. 336-47.
35. Pan Q, Luo X, Chegini N. Differential expression of microRNAs in myometrium and leiomyomas and regulation by ovarian steroids. J Cell Mol Med 2008. 12(1): p. 22740.
36. Klemke M, et al. Loss of let-7 binding sites resulting from truncations of the 3' untranslated region of HMGA2 mRNA in uterine leiomyomas. Cancer Genet Cytogenet 2010. 196(2): p. 119-23.
37. Peng Y, et al. Antiproliferative effects by Let-7 repression of high-mobility group A2 in uterine leiomyoma. Mol Cancer Res 2008. 6(4): p. 663-73.
38. Fitzgerald JB, et al. Role of microRNA-21 and programmed cell death 4 in the pathogenesis of human uterine leiomyomas. Fertil Steril 2012. 98(3): p. 726-734 e2.
39. Pan Q, Luo X, Chegini N. microRNA 21: response to hormonal therapies and regulatory function in leiomyoma, transformed leiomyoma and leiomyosarcoma cells. Mol Hum Reprod 2010. 16(3): p. 215-27.
40. Yamagata Y, et al. Aberrant DNA methylation status in human uterine leiomyoma. Mol Hum Reprod 2009. 15(4): p. 259-67.
41. Navarro A, et al. Genome-wide DNA methylation indicates silencing of tumor suppressor genes in uterine leiomyoma. PLoS One 2012. 7(3): p. e33284.
42. Maekawa R, et al. Disease-dependent differently methylated regions (D-DMRs) of DNA are enriched on the X chromosome in uterine leiomyoma. J Reprod Dev 2011. 57(5): p. 604-12.
43. Malik M, Segars J, Catherino WH. Integrin beta1 regulates leiomyoma cytoskeletal integrity and growth. Matrix Biol 2012. 31(7-8): p. 389-97.
44. Chen HM, et al. Overexpression of Integrin-beta1 in Leiomyoma Promotes Cell Spreading and Proliferation. J Clin Endocrinol Metab 2013.
45. Kato A, et al. Dermatopontin interacts with fibronectin, promotes fibronectin fibril formation, and enhances cell adhesion. J Biol Chem 2011. 286(17): p. 14861-9.
46. MacBeath JR, Shackleton DR, Hulmes DJ. Tyrosine-rich acidic matrix protein (TRAMP) accelerates collagen fibril formation in vitro. J Biol Chem 1993. 268(26): p. 19826-32.
47. Tsibris JC, et al. Insights from gene arrays on the development and growth regulation of uterine leiomyomata. Fertil Steril 2002. 78(1): p. 114-21.
48. Catherino WH, et al. Reduced dermatopontin expression is a molecular link between uterine leiomyomas and keloids. Genes Chromosomes Cancer 2004. 40(3): p. 204-17.
49. Leppert PC, et al. Comparative ultrastructure of collagen fibrils in uterine leiomyomas and normal myometrium. Fertil Steril 2004. 82 Suppl 3: p. 1182-7.
50. Rogers R, et al. Mechanical homeostasis is altered in uterine leiomyoma. Am J Obstet Gynecol 2008. 198(4): p. 474 e1-11.
51. Sozen I, Arici A. Interactions of cytokines, growth factors, and the extracellular matrix in the cellular biology of uterine leiomyomata. Fertil Steril 2002. 78(1): p. 1-12.

The natural history of fibroids

Celine Lönnerfors

Skane University Hospital, Lund, Sweden

Uterine fibroids (leiomyomas) are associated with substantial morbidity for a number of women and are the leading cause of hysterectomy in the United States. The estimated annual cost to the US health care system for the morbidity associated with uterine fibroids is as much as $34 billion dollars (1, 2).

In an unselected female population, uterine fibroids are reported to be present in between 5%-25% and increases with age during the fertile period (3). Prevalence studies using ultrasonographic screening indicate that fibroids start at a young age and increase with age until menopause in nearly all populations studied (4-6). The majority of women with fibroids are asymptomatic and to a large extent probably unaware of the condition. Most sources state that fibroids are symptomatic in approximately 25% of women (7). Fibroid sizes range from small enough to not be palpable or visible by ultrasound to bulky masses large enough to distort the woman's abdominal contour. Whether or not a fibroid causes any symptoms is related to, but not wholly dependent on, its size. The most common symptoms are heavy or abnormal uterine bleeding, pelvic pain, and pressure. In addition, fibroids might be the determining factor in 2%-3% of women with unexplained fertility and are in some women associated with recurrent pregnancy loss (8).

There are few known risk factors for uterine fibroids, other than being a woman of reproductive age. Several characteristics apart from ethnicity have consistently been found to be inversely associated with uterine fibroids: parity (9-13), age at first or last childbirth (10-13), age at menarche (9, 11, 13, 14), and menopause (9, 10, 12, 14). Conflicting data have emerged regarding the roles of oral contraceptives (9-11, 13, 15), smoking history (9, 10, 16-18), and obesity (9, 10, 14, 16, 18).

The growth patterns of uterine fibroids vary; some fibroids grow slowly, others may remain the same size or even shrink spontaneously. Peddada et al. studied 72 premenopausal women over a period of 12 months where fibroid volume was measured by up to 4 magnetic resonance imaging (MRI) scans. On average, the leiomyoma growth tended to be slow with a median of 9% change in volume over a 6 month period (19). However, leiomyoma growth and shrinkage ranged from -89% to +138% both within the same uterus and between different women (19). Growth rates also appeared to be related to race. It is well known that African American women are more likely to have fibroids. In addition, they have fibroids at a younger age and are likely to have more or larger fibroids (19-21). Peddada et al. found that white women had significantly lower leiomyoma growth rates as they approached menopause, whereas African American women's growth rates remained unchanged (19). Thus, the recommended management of similar fibroids in women may differ according to race. An African American woman is three times more likely to undergo a hysterectomy due to fibroids in comparison to a white woman (19, 21).

Fibroids are the most common benign tumors in the uterus whereas sarcomas are rare (3 to 7 per 100,000 United States population) but associated with a poor prognosis. It is important to be aware of malignancies arising in the uterus and to differentiate between benign and malignant conditions. Rapid leiomyoma growth is not associated with the risk of uterine sarcoma and this should not be the basis for recommending a hysterectomy (22). Parker et al. found the total incidence of uterine sarcoma to be 0.23% in 1,332 patients operated on for uterine leiomyoma. The incidence was 0.27% among the 371 women having surgery for rapidly growing leiomyoma (22).

Lifestyle factors may also impact fibroid development. Some studies have suggested that obese women are at higher risk of fibroids (10, 11, 14, 16, 20) while others find no increased risk (9, 18). Takeda at al. found a significantly higher body mass index (BMI), blood pressure, serum triglyceride level, and fasting plasma glucose in women who underwent hysterectomy or myomectomy for fibroids compared to women who underwent surgery for other benign indications (23), which coincides with results by Shikora et al. (24). In their Fibroid Growth Study, Peddada et al. found no correlation between fibroid growth and BMI (19). Csatlos et al. suggest that substances that help the body maintain tissues, such as insulin-like growth factor, may affect fibroid growth and Laughlin et al. propose that additional factors such as metabolic, dietary, infection and uterine injury, stress, and environmental factors may also play a role in fibroid development (25, 26). Faerstein et al. found smoking for approximately 20 years or more was associated with a 40% decreased risk of fibroids in comparison with nonsmoking, which is thought to be due to an estrogen-deficient state (20). This negative impact on fibroids by smoking is supported by other studies (9, 10, 17).

Leiomyoma development and growth has long been associated with gonadal steroid hormones (27). Fibroids contain more estrogen and progesterone receptors than do normal uterine muscle cells. Both estrogen and progesterone play important roles in leiomyoma biology, yet selective steroidal modulation produces variable clinical outcomes. Women who take oral contraceptives are generally thought to have a lower risk of fibroids and some evidence also shows that progestin-only contraceptives may decrease risk, but the evidence is contradicting (9-11, 13, 15). In addition, GnRH analogues and progesterone receptor modulators are demonstrating effectiveness and current research involves retinoic acid, pirfenidone, components of green tea, and vitamin D3 (7, 28-31). The main problem is the high risk of recurrence of disease after conservative surgery and a return to baselines once treatment with GnRH-analogues is discontinued. The progesterone receptor modulator ulipristal acetate is approved for short-term clinical use prior to surgery and has shown efficacy with a significant reduction in uterine bleeding and fibroid volume, but long-term data are unavailable (32-34).

Fertility aspects

The influence of fibroids on fertility is poorly understood. The heterogeneity of the disease makes it difficult to establish whether myomas in general are a cause of infertility or merely associated with the inability to conceive. Submucous myomas or myomas distorting the endometrial cavity impair fertility, but conflicting results exist regarding intramural and subserous myomas (8, 35, 36). The proximity to the endometrium as well as the size of the lesion seem to be important factors and myomas might be the determining factor in 2%-3% of women with unexplained infertility (37). Possible mechanisms may be deformation of the uterine contour, tubal ostia, or cervix or changed contractility of the uterine muscle interfering with sperm and ovum transport. Altered blood flow and/or growth factor expression in an abnormal endometrium overlying the myoma may also have an impact on successful implantation.

With regards to in vitro fertilization (IVF) treatment, myomas that distort the endometrial cavity have been associated with decreased pregnancy and implantation rates. Studies have shown IVF outcomes to be improved in women following myomectomy in women with myomas distorting the uterine cavity (38, 39). Sunkara et al. found in their meta-analysis on 19 observational studies comprising 6,087 IVF cycles a significant decrease in the live birth and clinical pregnancy rates in women with intramural myomas with no involvement of the endometrial cavity (40).

Pregnancy and childbirth

Pregnancy and childbirth seem to have a protective effect and may decrease the risk of developing uterine fibroids (41-45). The prevalence of myomas during pregnancy is approximately 10% (36). Prospective studies using ultrasound to follow the size throughout pregnancy have shown that 60%-78% of fibroids do not demonstrate any significant change in volume during pregnancy (41-43). One third may grow and the increase in volume happens almost exclusively in the first trimester. Most women with fibroids have uneventful pregnancies, but it is suggested that uterine fibroids are associated with an increased risk of spontaneous miscarriage, preterm labor, placental abruption, malpresentation, labor dystocia, caesarean delivery, retained placenta, intrauterine growth retardation, and postpartum hemorrhage (41).

Fibroids might affect 0.1%-3.9% of pregnancies (36, 37) and major complications seem to be related to whether the placenta and the myoma are in contact. Spontaneous shrinkage is found in nearly 80% of women within 6 months of delivery (44). Postpregnancy remodeling of the uterus may affect and decrease the risk of leiomyomas and explain the protective effect of parity (45-47).

Conclusion

Leiomyomas are a common phenotype representing many genotypes and somatic mutations leading to different symptoms and growth patterns (7). Many factors thought to have an impact on the development and/or growth of fibroids such as ethnicity, age, obesity, time and number of pregnancies, use of oral contraceptives, and other medications are an integral part of a woman's life. The natural history is complex, individual, and largely unknown. Due to the heterogeneity of the disease the knowledge and available evidence is limited and predicting the natural course of development of an individual fibroid is impossible. Understanding the diversity of disease in both pathophysiology and symptomatology will hopefully lead to targeted treatment in the short-term and prevention strategies in the long-term. With more women delaying childbearing, the high prevalence of fibroids, and the heightened risk of fibroids with increasing age, the number of women in whom fibroids will have an impact on fertility is expected to rise. Inhibiting growth or inducing regression appears to be the main opportunity for prevention.

References

1. Farquhar CM, Steiner CA. Hysterectomy rates in the United States 1990–1997. Obstet Gynecol 2002;99:229–34.
2. Cardozo ER, Clark AD, Banks NK, Henne MB, Stegmann BJ, Segars JH.The estimated annual cost of uterine leiomyomata in the United States. Am J Obstet Gynecol 2012; 206(3):211 e 1-9.
3. Payson M, Leppert P, Segars J. Epidemiology of myomas. Obstet Gynecol Clin North Am 2006;33(1):1-11.
4. Day Baird D, Dunson DB, Hill MC, Cousins D, Schectman JM. High cumulative incidence of uterine leiomyoma in black and white women: ultrasound evidence. Am J Obstet Gynecol 2003;188:100–7.
5. Laughlin SK, Baird DD, Savitz DA, Herring AH, Hartmann KE. Prevalence of uterine leiomyomas in the first trimester of pregnancy: an ultrasound-screening study. Obstet Gynecol 2009;113:630–5.

6. Eskenazi B, Warner M, Samuels S, Young J, Gerthoux PM, Needham L, et al. Serum dioxin concentrations and risk of uterine leiomyoma in the Seveso Women's Health Study. Am J Epidemiol 2007;166:79–87.
7. Laughlin SK, Stewart EA. Uterine leiomyomas: individualizing the approach to a heterogeneous condition. Obstet Gynecol 2011;117(2 Pt 1):396–403.
8. Khaund A, Lumsden MA. Impact of fibroids on reproductive function. Best Pract Res Clin Obstet Gynaecol 2008;22(4):749-60.
9. Samadi AR, Lee NC, Flanders WD, Boring JR 3rd, Parris EB. Risk factors for selfreported uterine fibroids: a case-control study. Am J Public Health 1996;86:858–62.
10. Ross KR, Pike MC, Vessey MP, Bull D, Yeates D, Casagrande JT. Risk factors for uterine fibroids: reduced risk associated with oral contraceptives. Br Med J 1986;293:359–62.
11. Lumbiganon P, Rugpao S, Phandhu-fung S, Laopaiboon M, Vudhikamraksa N, Werawatakul Y. Protective effect of depot-medroxyprogesterone acetate on surgically treated uterine leiomyomas: a multicentre case-control study.Br J Obstet Gynaecol 1996;103:909–14.
12. Parazzini F, Negri E, La Vecchia C, Chatenoud L, Ricci E, Guarnerio P. Reproductive factors and risk of uterine fibroids. Epidemiology 1996;7:440–2.
13. Marshall LM, Spiegelman D, Goldman MB, et al. A prospective study of reproductive factors and oral contraceptive use in relation to the risk of uterine leiomyomata. Fertil Steril 1998;70:432–9.
14. Parazzini F, La Vecchia C, Negri E, Cecchetti G, Fedele L. Epidemiologic characteristics of women with uterine fibroids. Obstet Gynecol 1988;72:853–7.
15. Chiaffarino F, Parazzini F, La Vecchia C, Marsico S, Surace M, Ricci E. Use of oral contraceptives and uterine fibroids: results from a case-control study. Br J Obstet Gynaecol 1999;106:857–60.
16. Marshall LM, Spiegelman D, Manson JE, Goldman MB, Barbieri RL, Stampfer MJ, Willett WC, Hunter DJ. Risk of uterine leiomyomata among premenopausal women in relation to bodysize and cigarette smoking. Epidemiology 1998;9:511–17.
17. Parazzini F, Negri E, La Vecchia C, Rabaiotti M, Luchini L, Villa A, Fedele L. Uterine myomas and smoking. J Reprod Med 1996;41:316–20.
18. Wyshak G, Frisch RE, Albright NL, Albright TE, Schiff I. Lower prevalence of benign diseases of the breast and benign tumors of the reproductive system among former college athletes compared to non-athletes. Br J Cancer 1986;54:841–5.
19. Peddada SD, Laughlin SK, Miner K, Guyon JP, Haneke K, Vahdat HL, Semelka RC, Kowalik A, Armao D, Davis B, Baird DD. Growth of uterine leiomyomata among premenopausal black and white women. Proc Natl Acad Sci U S A. 2008;105:19887–92.
20. Faerstein E, Szklo M,Rosenshein N. Risk factors for uterine leiomyoma: a practice-based case-control study. African-American heritage, reproductive history, body size, and smoking. Am J Epidemiol 2001;153(1):1-10.
21. Wilcox LS, Koonin LM, Pokras R, Strauss LT, Xia Z, Peterson HB. Hysterectomy in the United States, 1988–1990. Obstet Gynecol 1994;83:549–55.
22. Parker WH, Fu YS, Berek JS. Uterine sarcoma in patients operated on for presumed leiomyoma and rapidly growing leiomyoma. Obstet Gynecol 1994;83:414–8.
23. Takeda T, Sakata M, Isobe A, Miyake A, Nishimoto F, Ota Y, Kamiura S, Kimura T. Relationship between metabolic syndrome and uterine leiomyomas: a case-control study. Gynecol Obstet Invest 2008;66:14-17.
24. Shikora SA, Niloff JM, Bistrian BR, Forse RA, Blackburn GL. Relationship between obesity and uterine leiomyomata. Nutrition 1991;7(4):251-5.

25. Csatlos E, Rigo Jr J, Laky M, Joo JG. Gene expression patterns of insulin-like growth factor 2 in human uterine fibroid tissues: a genetic study with clinical correlations. Gynecol Obstet Invest 2013;75:185-90.
26. Laughlin DK, Schroeder JC, Baird DD. New directions in the epidemiology of uterine fibroids. Semin Reprod Med 2010;28(3):204-17.
27. Walker CL, Stewart EA. Uterine fibroids: the elephant in the room. Science 2005;308:1589–92.
28. Malik M, Webb J, Catherino WH. Retinoic acid treatment of human leiomyoma cells transformed the cell phenotype to one strongly resembling myometrial cells. Clin Endocrinol (Oxf) 2008;69:462–70.
29. Lee BS, Margolin SB, Nowak RA. Pirfenidone: a novel pharmacological agent that inhibits leiomyoma cell proliferation and collagen production. J Clin Endocrinol Metab 1998;83:219–23.
30. Zhang D, Al-Hendy M, Richard-Davis G, Montgomery-Rice V, Sharan C, Rajaratnam V, Khurana A, Al-Hendy A. Green tea extract inhibits proliferation of uterine leiomyoma cells in vitro and in nude mice. Am J Obstet Gynecol 2010;202(289):e1–9.
31. Blauer M, Rovio PH, Ylikomi T, Heinonen PK. Vitamin D inhibits myometrial and leiomyoma cell proliferation in vitro. Fertil Steril 2009;91:1919–25.
32. Donnez J, Tatarchuk TF, Bouchard P, Puscasiu L, Zakharenko NF, Ivanova T, Ugocsai G, Mara M, Jilla MP, Bestel E, Terrill P, Osterloh I, Loumaye E; PEARL I Study Group. Ulipristal acetate versus placebo for fibroid treatment prior to surgery. N Eng J Med 2012;366:409-20.
33. Donnez J, Tomaszewski J, Vázquez F, Bouchard P, Lemieszczuk B, Baró F, Nouri K, Selvaggi L, Sodowski K, Bestel E, Terrill P, Osterloh I, Loumaye E; PEARL II Study Group. Ulipristal acetate versus leuprolide acetate for uterine fibroids. N Eng J Med 2012;366:421-32.
34. Talaulikar VS and Manyonda IT. Ulipristal acetate: a novel option for the medical management of symptomatic uterine fibroids. Adv Ther 2012;29(8):655-63.
35. Cook H, Ezzati M, Segars JH, McCarthy K. The impact of uterine leiomyomas on reproductive outcomes. Minerva Ginecol 2010 Jun;62(3):225-36.
36. Klatsky PC, Tran ND, Caughey AB, Fujimoto VY. Fibroids and reproductive outcomes: a systematic literature review from conception to delivery. Am J Obstet Gynecol 2008 Apr;198(4):357-66.
37. Rackow BW, Arici A. Fibroids and in-vitro fertilization: which comes first? Curr Opin Obstet Gynecol 2005 Jun;17(3):225-31.
38. Hart R, Khalaf Y, Yeong CT, Seed P, Taylor A, Braude P. A prospective controlled study of the effect on intramural uterine fibroids on the outcome of assisted conception. Hum Reprod 2001:16(11):2411-7.
39. Surrey ES, Minjarez DA, Stevens JM, Schoolcraft WB. Effect of myomectomy on the outcome of assisted reproductive technologies. Fertil Steril 2005;83(5):1473-9.
40. Sunkara SK, Khairy M, El-Toukhy T, Khalaf Y, Coomarasamy A. The effect of intramural fibroids without uterine cavity involvement on the outcome of IVF treatment: a systematic review and meta-analysis. Hum Reprod 2010;25:418-29.
41. Lee DY, Norowitz ER, Shaw J. Contemporary management of fibroids in pregnancy. Rev Obstet Gynecol 2010;3(1):20-7.
42. Aharoni A, Reiter A, Golan D, Paltiely Y, Sharf M. Patterns of growth of uterine leiomyomas during pregnancy. A prospective longitudinal study. Br J Obstet Gynaecol 1988;95:510-3.
43. Rosati P, Exacoustos C, Mancuso S. Longitudinal evaluation of uterine myoma growth during pregnancy. A sonographic study. Ultrasound Med 1992;11:511-5.

44. Laughlin SK, Herring AH, Savitz DA, Olshan AF, Fielding JR, Hartmann KE, Baird DD. Pregnancy-related fibroid reduction. Fertil Steril 2010;94:2421–3.
45. Baird DD, Dunson DB. Why is parity protective for uterine fibroids? Epidemiology 2003;14:247–50.
46. Wise LA, Palmer JR, Harlow BL, Spiegelman D, Stewart EA, Adams-Campbell LL, Rosenberg L. Reproductive factors, hormonal contraception, and risk of uterine leiomyomata in African-American women: a prospective study. Am J Epidemiol 2004;159:113–23.
47. Marshall LM, Spiegelman D, Goldman MB, Manson JE, Colditz GA, Barbieri RL, Stampfer MJ, Hunter DJ. A prospective study of reproductive factors and oral contraceptive use in relation to the risk of uterine leiomyomata. Fertil Steril 1998;70:432–9.

Treatment options in the management of uterine fibroids

Michal Mara

Charles University in Prague, Prague, Czech Republic

Introduction

In the last 20 years, the treatment of uterine fibroids has become a very dynamic topic. This is due to multiple reasons. First, these benign tumors belong to the most common gynecological disorders. Second, even though the etiology remains unclear, the new data about decisive factors of genesis and the growth of myomas continuously accrue from the basic research studies (1). Third, due to socioeconomic factors the need to treat fibroids is relevant to ever increasing numbers of women wishing to preserve fertility. Finally, the number of therapeutic options has dramatically increased (2, 3). On the other hand, there are still lots of questions not only about the complex pathophysiology of fibroids but also very basic ones (i.e., questions about indication criteria, timing, and type of treatment).

The therapy of uterine fibroids could be classified based on the different parameters; however, the most logical way is to distinguish the patients with and without reproductive plans. For the purposes of this paper the preference will be given to women wishing to conceive.

Medical treatment

According to the fact that the fibroids may resemble a systematic disease with typical multiplicity and recurrence of tumors, there have always been the attempts to find an ideal pharmacological treatment. But, unfortunately, there has been no such medical therapy until now (4). The efforts to reach significant and persisting shrinkage of leiomyomas with different medical agents have especially failed repeatedly.

Except for hemostatic drugs, the analgesics, and the iron, various hormonal agents are often used in this indication. Both progestins as well as combined oral contraceptives seem to work effectively to decrease fibroid-related menorrhagia. If the uterine cavity is non-deformed by fibroids, the intrauterine system containing levonorgestrel (LNG-IUS) could also be applied (5). But some patients, and typically those with submucous location of myoma, are resistant to any of these therapies and require a surgical treatment.

The other drugs have higher ambitions than just to treat symptoms. Most of them affect ovarian steroids and their proliferative influence on leiomyomas. The injections with gonadotropin-releasing hormone analogues (GnRHa) belong to the most widespread medicaments in this area, but due to their side effects and low tolerability their use is limited to 3 months´ pretreatment before the surgery, which should be planned soon after the treatment because of well-known rebound phenomenon (6). GnRHa have been criticized for non-standard effect on shrinkage, higher risk of fibroid recurrence, and also for making myomectomy technically more difficult with higher risk of laparo-conversion (7).

The other medicaments from various drug groups like danazol, GnRH antagonists, selective estrogen receptor modulators, antiprogestins, or aromatase inhibitors have been tested to decrease the symptoms and size of uterine myomas with more or less similar outcomes. The results indicate mild to moderate effect on symptoms, many side effects, and limited impact on tumor´s shrinkage (2, 8, 9). None of these drugs have reached the standard clinical usage.

Recently, the promising results of two large multicenter randomized controlled trials, PEARL I and II, have been published (10, 11). The results have shown the reliable effect of oral ulipristal acetate (UPA), from the group of selective progesterone receptor modulators (SPRMs), on bleeding and pressure symptoms with a quick start of action and without significant side effects. The volume of myomas decreased by 12%–42% after 3 months of daily use of 5 mg or 10 mg of UPA. The shrinkage persisted 6 months after cessation of the treatment, but this parameter was analyzed only in selected group of patients that refused surgery. Unfortunately, the data describing the effect of UPA on fibroid volume could be criticized for inaccurate methodology. Not only *in vitro* but also *in vivo* studies have recently proved the induction of apoptosis in the cells of leiomyomas after the use of SPRM as one of their possible mechanisms of action (12).

Myomectomy

In the past, myomectomy was the only uterus-sparing modality of treatment. Nevertheless, it was seldom used because of the invasiveness of laparotomy, popularity of expectation strategy, rare use of precise diagnostic tools, lower interest in reproductive medicine (absence of assisted reproductive technologies), and often over-estimated risk of hysterectomy. With the development of gynecologic endoscopy as well as of in vitro fertilization (IVF) program, myomectomy has become one of the most common procedures in reproductive surgery.

Even today, in the co-existence of many new mini-invasive methods, myomectomy remains the treatment of choice in women with current reproductive plans and symptomatic uterine fibroids. It especially should be considered in cases with solitary mid-size (up to 7 cm) intramural or subserous fibroids accessible for laparoscopic resection (LM) or with submucous fibroids (up to 5 cm) eligible for transcervical resection (TCRM) (13, 14). This recommendation can be supported by good clinical and reproductive results of myomectomy and a very low incidence of serious complications like perioperative hysterectomy or uterine rupture during subsequent pregnancy (15).

There exist various recommendations for the crucial part of LM, which is the reconstruction of uterine anatomy using endoscopic suture. From my point of view, the particular technique of suturing is not so important. What is essential is to exactly close the cavity (in cases of intrauterine penetration), to enclose the whole defect of the uterine wall with at least 2-layers suture, and to avoid extensive coagulation. The patients are usually counseled to avoid conception from 4 to 6 months after myomectomy. The management of postmyomectomy labor could be analogous to patients after cesarean section (16).

A decision between open myomectomy (OM) and LM depends a lot on surgical endoscopic skills and experience. Certainly there are limits for safe LM determined by size, location, and number of myomas (15, 17). But in general, LM is now established as adequate procedure as OM for majority of pregnancy planning patients with fibroids due to lower invasiveness and comparable clinical and reproductive results (18). In some patients and especially in cases with fibroid multiplicity, the definitive decision about the approach and the extent of the procedure should be made intraoperatively and a surgeon should be prepared for all alternatives (LM, OM, TCRM) including eventual combination with occlusion of uterine arteries (19). Depending on fibroid size and location some authors advocate a combination of laparoscopy with minilaparotomy (laparoscopy-assisted myomectomy) or with vaginal approach (20, 21).

The dilemma between myomectomy and no intervention is uneasy and still incompletely covered by clinical data, mainly in patients without previous abortions or infertility treatment. Literature recommendations usually suggest treating women with voluminous fibroids that significantly alter normal pelvic anatomy, with myomas deforming the cavity, and with otherwise unexplained infertility, and especially with previous failure of IVF (2, 17, 22). Surprisingly, in the literature there is no randomized controlled study comparing fertility after myomectomy versus no treatment. The majority of data emphasize the importance of relation of the fibroid and the cavity indicating negative role of submucous and intramural fibroids that deform the endometrial cavity (23). On the other hand, recent meta-analysis covering 19 randomized trials and 6,047 IVF cycles amazingly showed that even women with intramural myomas without any cavity involvement had both live-birth rate and clinical pregnancy rate significantly lower than women without myomas (24).

Other surgical methods

As the reaction to the treatment performed by radiologists, several gynecologic surgeons started to treat myomas with laparoscopic uterine artery occlusion (LUAO) using bipolar electrosurgery, ultrasonically activated shears, or ligation or clips. They presented quite optimistic results in terms of decrease in volume and myoma-related symptoms (19, 25). Our own experience with more than 150 procedures showed that LUAO has a very low invasiveness and frequency of complications (including low incidence of pregnancy complications) but it often fails in causing complete infarction and sufficient shrinkage of the fibroids (26). It probably should not be recommended as the separate treatment of large fibroids but only as a support to myomectomy in cases with fibroid multiplicity where smaller fibroids remain in situ.

Some authors suggest vaginal approach to occlude the uterine arteries under the control of Doppler ultrasound (27). Focused laparoscopic destruction of the fibroid tissue called myolysis using electrosurgery, radiofrequency ablation, freezing (cryomyolysis), or laser has also been tested to treat the myomas but has never been widely recommended in women wishing gravidity, mainly due to a limited volume efficiency and significant risk of uterine rupture (28).

Non-surgical mini-invasive treatment

Thanks to the great popularity among the patients wishing to avoid hysterectomy, very good symptomatic results, and promising case reports about uneventful pregnancies, uterine artery embolization (UAE) seemed to be a useful alternative treatment of uterine fibroids even in women with fertility plans (29). However, later research indicated that women with fibroids treated by UAE are at risk of decreased ovarian reserve, or even ovarian failure, and impaired uterine cavity (30, 31). More than one third of women after UAE had major intrauterine abnormalities, mostly presence of necrotic fibroid tissue. Although post-UAE myomectomy could remove necrosis from uterine muscularity and cavity, these patients are still at increased risk of severe postoperative intrauterine adhesions. The only randomized trial comparing reproductive results of UAE and myomectomy showed superiority of the surgical treatment (32).

Other methods performed by radiologists have a similar mode of action like surgical myolysis (and completely different than selective catheterizing strategy of UAE) but with the use of the imaging methods instead of laparoscopy (33). Despite the presence of the case reports and small series of pregnancies, it hardly can be proposed as treatment of choice in young patients. The magnetic resonance-guided focused ultrasound (MRgFUS) seems to be the most developing method from this category (34).

Histopathological remarks

Not all tumors of the uterine corpus must be conventional leiomyomata. In our cohort of 968 patients planned for myomectomy to preserve fertility the histology finally showed atypical findings in 137 women (14%) including not only adenomyomas; benign mesotheliomas; and cellular, atypical, epithelioid, dissecting, and mitotically active leiomyomas, but also 2 cases of leiomyosarcoma, 2 endometrial stromal sarcomas, and 12 cases of smooth muscle tumor of uncertain malignant potential (STUMP). Preoperatively, only a minority of these patients had unusual clinical or imaging markers. Not even MRI has enough sensitivity to exclude uterine sarcoma, and especially STUMP (35). Experienced sonographers should recognize adenomyosis with typical higher echogenicity, diffuse vascularization, and wider junctional zone (36). From our experience, many of these abnormal tumors are technically harder to evacuate because of their atypical structure. In cases with suspicion of sarcoma, the frozen section and perioperative histology is indicated and laparoscopic morcellation of the tumor should be avoided.

Conclusion

Uterine fibroids are one of the most frequent diseases in women of reproductive age that could be associated with heavy menstrual bleeding, infertility, abortions, and other pregnancy complications. In women without current reproductive plans, medical treatment or LNG-IUS could be proposed to decrease menstrual symptoms. If pregnancy is desired, myomectomy should be considered, especially in patients with larger fibroids that involve the uterine cavity or in those with otherwise unexplained infertility.

Myomectomy should be performed hysteroscopically or laparoscopically in all suitable cases with the emphasis on preservation of compact uterine muscularity. LUAO could be added to myomectomy to reduce perioperative bleeding or in the presence of small residual fibroids. UAE should be avoided in all women with pregnancy plans and fibroids suitable for myomectomy due to its reproductive risks. Some of the new therapeutic possibilities like SPRM or MRgFUS are promising but their use in young patients with fibroids should be further studied.

References

1. Stewart EA, Morton CC. The genetics of uterine leiomyomata: what clinicians need to know. Obstet Gynecol 2006;107:917-21.
2. Olive DL, Lindheim SR, Pritts EA. Non-surgical management of leiomyoma: impact on fertility. Curr Opin Obstet Gynecol 2004;16:239-43.
3. Parker WH. Uterine myomas: management. Fertil Steril 2007;88:255-71.
4. Sankaran S, Manyonda IT. Medical management of fibroids. Best Pract Res Clin Obstet Gynaecol 2008;22:655-76.
5. Grigorieva V, Chen-Mok M, Tarasova M, Mikhailov A. Use of a levonorgestrel–releasing intrauterine system to treat bleeding related to uterine leiomyomas. Fertil Steril 2003;79:1194-8.
6. Lethaby A, Vollenhoven B, Sowter M. Efficacy of pre-operative gonadotrophin hormone releasing analogues for women with uterine fibroids undergoing hysterectomy or myomectomy: a systematic review. Br J Obstet Gynecol 2002;109:1097-108.
7. Campo S, Garcea N. Laparoscopic myomectomy in premenopausal women with and without preoperative treatment using gonadotrophin-releasing hormone analogues. Hum. Reprod 1999;14:44-8.
8. Eisinger SH, Meldrum S, Fiscella K, Le Roux HD, Guzick DS. Low-dose mifepristone for uterine leiomyomata. Obstet Gynecol 2003;101:243-50.
9. Shozu M, Murakami K, Segawa T, Kasai T, Inoue M. Successful treatment of symptomatic uterine leiomyoma in a perimenopausal woman with a nonsteroidal aromatase inhibitor. Fertil Steril 2003;79:628-31.
10. Donnez J, Tatarchuk TF, Bouchard P, et al. PEARL I Study Group. Ulipristal acetate versus placebo for fibroid treatment prior to surgery. N Engl J Med 2012;366:409-20.
11. Donnez J, Tomaszewski J, Vázquez F, et al. PEARL II Study Group. Ulipristal acetate versus leuprolide acetate for uterine fibroids. N Engl J Med 2012;366:421-32.
12. Horak P, Mara M, Dundr P, et al. Effect of a selective progesterone receptor modulator on induction of apoptosis in uterine fibroids in vivo. Int J Endocrinol 2012;2012:436174.

13. Darai E, Deval B, Darles C, Benifla JL, Guglielmina JN, Madelenat P. Myomectomy: laparoscopy or laparotomy. Contracept Fertil Sex 1996;24:751-6.
14. Di Spiezio Sardo A, Mazzon I, Bramante S, et al. Hysteroscopic myomectomy: a comprehensive review of surgical techniques. Hum Reprod Update 2008;14:101-19.
15. Dubuisson JB, Fauconnier A, Chapron C, Kreiker G, Norgaard C. Reproductive outcome after laparoscopic myomectomy in infertile women. J Reprod Med 2000;45:23-30.
16. Kumakiri J, Takeuchi H, Kitade M, et al. Pregnancy and delivery after laparoscopic myomectomy. J Minim Invasive Gynecol 2005;12:241-6.
17. Bajekal N, Li TC. Fibroids, infertility and pregnancy wastage. Hum Reprod Update 2000; 6:614-20.
18. Seracchioli R, Rossi S, Govoni F, et al. Fertility and obstetric outcome after laparoscopic myomectomy of large myomata: a randomized comparison with abdominal myomectomy. Hum Reprod 2000;15:2663-8.
19. Holub Z, Jabor A, Luká , J, et al. The effect of lateral uterine artery dissection on clinical outcomes in laparoscopic myomectomy: a prospective randomized study. Gynec Surg 2004;1:253-8.
20. Nezhat C, Nezhat F, Bess O, Nezhat CH, Mashiach R. Laparoscopically assisted myomectomy: a report of a new technique in 57 cases. Int J Fertil Menopausal Stud 1994;39:39-44.
21. Wang CJ, Zen CF, Lee CL, Soong YK. Laparoscopic-assisted vaginal myomectomy. J Am Assoc Gynecol Laparosc 2000;7:510-4.
22. Rackow BW, Arici A. Fibroids and in-vitro fertilization: which comes first? Curr Opin Obstet Gynecol. 2005;17:225-31.
23. Pritts EA, Parker WH, Olive DL. Fibroids and infertility: an updated systematic review of the evidence. Fertil Steril 2009;91:1215-23.
24. Sunkara SK, Khairy M, El-Toukhy T, Khalaf Y, Coomarasamy A. The effect of intramural fibroids without uterine cavity involvement on the outcome of IVF treatment: a systematic review and meta-analysis. Hum Reprod 2010;25:418-29.
25. Liu WM. Laparoscopic bipolar coagulation of uterine vessels to treat symptomatic leiomyomas. J Am Assoc Gynec Laparosc 2000;7:1251-9.
26. Mara M, Maskova J, Kubinova K, Horak P, Novotna M, Kuzel D. Uterine Artery Embolization versus Laparoscopic Uterine Artery Occlusion: the outcomes of prospective, nonrandomized clinical trial. Cardiovasc Intervent Radiol 2012;35:1041-52.
27. Vilos GA, Vilos EC, Romano W, Abu-Rafea B. Temporary uterine artery occlusion for treatment of menorrhagia and uterine fibroids using an incisionless Doppler-guided transvaginal clamp: case report. Hum Reprod 2006;21:269-71.
28. Nisolle M, Smets M, Malvaux V, Anaf V, Donnez J. Laparoscopic myolysis with the Nd:YAG laser. J Gynecol Surg 1993;9:95-9.
29. Carpenter TT, Walker WJ. Pregnancy following uterine artery embolisation for symptomatic fibroids: a series of 26 completed pregnancies. Br J Obstet Gynaecol 2005; 112:321-5.
30. Tulandi T, Sammour A, Valenti D, Child TJ, Seti L, Tan SL. Ovarian reserve after uterine artery embolization for leiomyomata. Fertil Steril 2002;78:197-8.
31. Mara M, Horak P, Kubinova K, Dundr P, Belsan T, Kuzel D. Hysteroscopy after uterine fibroid embolization: evaluation of intrauterine findings in 127 patients. J Obstet Gynaecol Res 2012;38:823-31.
32. Mara M, Maskova J, Fucikova Z, Kuzel D, Belsan T, Sosna O. Midterm clinical and first reproductive results of a randomized controlled trial comparing uterine fibroid embolization and myomectomy. Cardiovasc Intervent Radiol 2008;31:73-85.

33. Hindley JT, Law PA, Jockey M, et al. Clinical outcomes following percutaneous magnetic resonance image guided laser ablation of symptomatic uterine fibroids. Hum Reprod 2002;17: 2737-41.
34. Stewart EA, Rabinovici J, Tempany CM, et al. Clinical outcomes of focused ultrasound surgery for the treatment of uterine fibroids. Fertil Steril 2006;85:22-9.
35. Guntupali SR, Ramirez PT, Anderson ML, Milam MR, Bodurka DC, Malpica A. Uterine smooth muscle tumor of uncertain malignant potential: A retrospective analysis. Gynecol Oncol 2009;113:324-6.
36. Reinhold C, Tafazoli F, Wang L. Imaging features of adenomyosis. Hum Reprod Update 1998;4:337-49.

Trilogy 10. Preimplantation genetic diagnosis

Meiotic errors and polar body diagnosis

Anver Kuliev

Reproductive Genetics Institute, Chicago, United States

Introduction

It is well known that chromosomal abnormalities originate predominantly from female meiosis. As demonstrated by DNA polymorphism studies performed in families with aneuploid spontaneous abortions or live-born babies with trisomy syndromes, these abnormalities derive predominantly, or even exclusively, from meiosis I. It was suggested that the age-related increase of common trisomies is probably determined by the age-related reduction of meiotic recombination, resulting in premature separation of bivalents and chromosomal nondisjunction. Meiosis II errors were also postulated to derive from meiosis I, as a result of the increased meiotic recombination rate, which may lead to separation failure of bivalents.

The polar body (PB) sampling was introduced 20 years ago for direct testing of the outcome of the first and second meiotic divisions. PB1 is extruded following maturation of oocytes and represents a by-product of meiosis I, while PBII is a by-product of meiosis II and is extruded following the exposure of oocytes to sperm or intracytoplasmic sperm injection (ICSI). In contrast to previous traditional meiotic studies, direct testing of meiotic outcome using PB1 and PB2 analysis showed a higher prevalence of meiotic errors and also significant contribution of chromatid, rather than chromosomal, errors. This was demonstrated in the study of simultaneous testing of metaphase II (MII) oocytes with their corresponding PBI, which showed that a normal chromosome pattern is represented by paired fluorescent signals for each chromosome, while the lack or addition of one or both signals in either oocyte or PB1 reflects an exact opposite pattern in the corresponding MII oocytes or PB1, suggesting a high accuracy of PB testing for the oocyte genotype prediction.

Based on this data, PB testing was applied clinically for the preselection of aneuploidy-free oocytes, which demonstrated the practical relevance of PB1 testing for in vitro fertilization (IVF) patients of advanced reproductive age. The data also demonstrated that the genotype of the resulting zygotes could not be accurately predicted without information about the outcome of the second meiotic division, which may be inferred from PB2 testing. The present experience includes fluorescence in situ hybridization (FISH) and microarray-based analysis on over 20,000 oocytes, demonstrating the accuracy of the oocyte genotype evaluation by PB1 and PB2 testing and providing an attractive approach for the study of the origin of human aneuploidies. The PB aneuploidy testing provides the least noninvasive method for preselection of oocytes and embryos with the highest developmental potential, which is of obvious interest for improving the assisted reproductive technology (ART) efficiency.

Aneuploidy in human oocytes

According to our data, based on the study of 20,986 oocytes obtained from 3,953 preimplantation genetic diagnosis (PGD) cycles performed for 2,830 (IVF) patients of an average age of 38.8 years, 46.81% of oocytes are with aneuploidies, of which 29.8% had errors in both PB1 and PB2, 30.4% in only PB1 and 39.8% in only PB2. As expected, the aneuploidy rates rose with increasing maternal age, from 20% in patients 35 years of age, to over 40% in patients of 40 years of age.

Comparable proportions of detectable aneuploidies were observed in PB1 (31.1%) and PB2 (33.7%), suggesting that the observed aneuploidies originate equally from both meiosis I and II, which is in contrast to the well-established concept of predominant meiosis I origin of chromosomal abnormalities in spontaneous abortions and live-born infants. Almost one third of the chromosomally abnormal oocytes were outcomes of sequential meiosis I and meiosis II errors; so, significant proportion of meiosis II errors are in fact associated with the preceding errors in meiosis I. However, half of meiosis II errors are still observed independent from meiosis I errors, emphasizing their clinical significance, as the genotype of the resulting zygote cannot be predicted without testing the outcomes of both meiotic divisions, inferred from PB1 and PB2. The biological significance of both meiotic errors may also be obvious from the age dependence of isolated errors of meiosis I and meiosis II, as well as sequential meiosis I and meiosis II errors. At least two times higher frequency for PB1s with nullisomy, compared to those with disomy, was observed, in contrast to a comparable distribution of missing and extra signals in PB2. Over 10 times higher frequency of chromatid errors, compared to chromosomal ones, was also evident. The results are of clinical relevance, as the genotype of the resulting zygote cannot be predicted without testing of the outcomes of both meiotic divisions, inferred from PB1 and PB2. However, even testing of meiosis I errors alone reduces aneuploidy rate in the resulting embryos at least by two thirds. Despite the fact that over one third of these oocytes will still be aneuploid following the second meiotic division, PB1 testing still could sufficiently improve the implantation and pregnancy rates in poor prognosis IVF, or ICSI patients, by applying ICSI selectively to the oocytes with aneuploidy-free PB1. On the other hand, only close to half of the abnormalities deriving from the second meiotic division may be detected by PB1 analysis as complex errors; therefore, to avoid the transfer of all the embryos resulting from aneuploid oocytes, testing of both PB1 and PB2 is required. As PB1 and PB2 are extruded in a normal process of oocyte maturation and fertilization, having no biological significance in pre- and post-implantation development, their removal and testing is potentially a useful tool in ART practices to identify the oocytes without nuclear abnormalities, which should help in the preselection of oocytes with the highest potential for establishing a viable pregnancy, improving significantly the IVF efficiency.

Impact of PB testing on detection and avoidance of aneuploid embryos from transfer

The above data may indicate the practical relevance of PGD for poor prognosis patients, as more than half of the tested oocytes or embryos are with aneuploidies, which may clearly affect the developmental competence and the embryo potential to implant, if not removed from transfer. In contrast to the data obtained in traditional meiotic studies, the above data on the direct testing of the meiotic outcomes in patients of advanced reproductive age show that chromosomal abnormalities originate comparably from meiosis I and meiosis II and are predominantly of chromatid origin.

Of special practical relevance is the analysis of the chromosome-specific origin of errors, which for some individual chromosomes are predominantly of meiosis II origin, such as for chromosomes 22 and 16. These data are opposite to that observed in spontaneous abortions and live-born children and may indicate a poor viability of embryos resulting from the oocytes with the chromosome 16 and 22 errors of the second meiotic division, which are probably incompatible with implantation and post-implantation development. This is obvious from the fact that despite similar overall prevalence of meiosis I and meiosis II errors, the observed aneuploidies in spontaneous abortions and live-born children are predominantly or even exclusively of meiosis I origin. This may provide a strong evidence for differential viability of embryos depending on the meiotic origin, with meiosis II errors being incompatible with implantation. Therefore, avoiding transfer of the embryos originating from meiosis II errors may be expected to improve implantation rate. Although there is no clear explanation of the biological differences of aneuploidies depending on the meiotic origin, a possible explanation may be a loss of heterozygosity or higher homozygosity of the embryos originating from meiosis II errors for the genes located in the chromosomes involved, through the imprinting of paternal or maternal genes in these chromosomes.

It is also of note that, in addition to the isolated errors in meiosis I and meiosis II, significant proportion of oocytes with meiosis I errors also had sequential meiosis II errors, resulting in apparently balanced zygotes in over one third of cases, similar to the well-known phenomenon of aneuploidy rescue. However, our follow-up study of the resulting balanced embryos showed that they were predominantly aneuploid, suggesting the inherent predisposition of these zygotes to the postzygotic chromosomal errors, following sequential errors in meiosis I, and meiosis II. Comparison of the types of chromosomal aneuploidies, and the prevalence of each chromosome-specific error in oocytes and embryos, detected by FISH and DNA fingerprinting, suggests that the majority of chromosomal aneuploidies in embryos originating from female meiosis predisposes to further sequential postzygotic errors, which may explain the high rate of mosaicism in preimplantation embryos. The introduction of both PB and blastomere testing and the technique of DNA fingerprinting also demonstrated the occurrence of uniparental disomies, the possible impact of which is still to be documented. This may also indicate the requirements for both the oocyte and embryos testing in PGD for aneuploidies to exclude the transfer of embryos with aneuploidies originating from meiosis and mitotic errors.

Therefore, the PB1 and PB2 testing in conjunction with embryo biopsy should help in the preselection of oocytes with the highest potential for establishing a viable ongoing pregnancy, significantly improving IVF efficiency. Significant improvement in the implantation rate was reported even by PB1 preselection of oocytes in infertile patients. The further improvement could have been achieved by detection of the remaining meiosis II errors, representing at least one third of the overall number of abnormal oocytes. This is in agreement with the available clinical outcome data, which demonstrated the utility of PB1 and PB2 testing in detecting and avoiding the transfer of aneuploid embryos. The overall impact was particularly obvious from the reduction in spontaneous abortion rate, which was much lower than observed in patients of comparable reproductive age without aneuploidy testing.

Summary

The presented results of aneuploidy testing of the world's largest series of oocytes provide the evidence of the usefulness of PB-based aneuploidy testing as part of accurate preselection of aneuploidy-free embryos for transfer, which is performed by removal and analysis of both PB1 and PB2. The data also provide the evidence for a strong relationship between embryo viability and meiotic origin of chromosomal errors, affecting their impact on preimplantation and post-implantation development. The data demonstrate a high accuracy of PB-based diagnosis for chromosomal disorders and its practical value in detection and avoidance from transfer of embryos with chromosomal anomalies.

Recommended references

ESHRE Preimplantation Genetic Diagnosis (PGD) Consortium. Best practice guidelines for preimplantation genetic diagnosis/screening (PGD/PGS). Hum Reprod 2011; 26: 14-46

Fragouli E, E Escalona, Guttieres Mateo C et al. Comparative genomic hybridization of oocytes and first polar bodies from young donors. Reproductive BioMedicine Online; 2009; 19:228-237

Gabriel AS, Thornhill AR, Ottolini CS et al. Array comparative genomic hybridization on first polar bodies suggests that non-disjunction is not the predominant mechanism leading to aneuploidy in humans. J Med Genet 2011; 48:433-437

Geraedts J, Montag M, Magli C et al. Polar Body array CGH for prediction of the status of the corresponding oocyte. Part I: clinical results. Hum Reprod 2011; 26:3172-3180

Hassold T, Merril M, Adkins K, Freemen S, Sherman S Recombination and maternal age-dependent nondisjunction: molecular studies of trisomy 16. Am J Hum Genet 1995; 57, 867-874

Kuliev A. Practical Preimplantation Genetic Diagnosis. Second Edition. Springer,London, New York, 2012 pp. 304

Kuliev A, Cieslak J, Verlinsky Y. Frequency and distribution of chromosomal abnormalities in human oocytes. Cytogenet Genome Res 2005; 111:193-198

Kuliev A, Zlatopolsky Z, Kirillova I, Spivakova J, Cieslak-Janzen G. Meiosis errors in over 20,000 oocytes studied in the practice of preimplantation aneuploidy testing. Reproductive BioMedicine Online 2011; 22: 2-8

Lamb NE, Freeman S, Savage-Austin A, et al. Susceptible chiasmate configurations of chromosome 21 predispose to nondisjunction in both maternal meiosis I, and meiosis II. Nat Genet 1996; 14, 400-405

Magli C, Montag M, Koster M et al. Polar Body array CGH for prediction of the status of the corresponding oocyte. Part II: technical aspects. Hum Reprod 2011; doi:10.1093/humrep/der295

Preimplantation Genetic Diagnosis International Society (PGDIS). Guidelines for good practice in PGD: program requirements and laboratory quality assurance. Reprod BioMed Online 2008;16:134-147.

Sherman SL, Peterson MB, Freeman S.B. et al. Nondisjunction of chromosome 21 in maternal meiosis I: evidence for a maternal age-dependent mechanism involving reduced recombination. Hum Mol Genet 1994; 3,1529-1535.

Microarray-comparative genomic hybridization

Dagan Wells

University of Oxford, Oxford, United Kingdom

This year sees the 20th anniversary of the first attempts to improve in vitro fertilization (IVF) success rates by assessing embryos for chromosome abnormalities (aneuploidy), a strategy sometimes referred to as preimplantation genetic screening (PGS). The underlying theory of PGS is based upon three simple facts: 1) human oocytes and embryos are frequently chromosomally abnormal; 2) aneuploidy is almost always lethal; 3) chromosome abnormalities have little if any effect on embryo morphology. This means that in a typical IVF cycle many of the embryos produced will carry chromosome abnormalities and yet these embryos will often be chosen for transfer because they look just as 'good' as their chromosomally normal siblings. Inevitably, the transfer of nonviable embryos, at the expense of healthy embryos from the same cohort, will harm pregnancy rates.

The theory underlying PGS seems extremely attractive and yet the clinical utilization of PGS has been controversial. For the most part, the controversy stems from data produced during a series of randomized controlled trials (RCTs) that aimed to quantify the improvements to IVF outcomes (if any) delivered by PGS. None of the trials were able to demonstrate any benefits attributable to PGS (See Fragouli and Wells, 2012 for review). This was followed by a highly polarized and sometimes acrimonious debate within the field of preimplantation genetic diagnosis and has led many clinics to abandon the use of PGS. There followed a collapse in the number of cases referred for PGS. In the United States the utilization of PGS fell from about 5% of all IVF cycles to just 1%-2%, while in several European countries PGS ceased altogether.

So where are we now? The entire concept of PGS has been revitalized in the last few years by the introduction of new technologies for chromosome analysis. Data now beginning to emerge have indicated that the failure of the earlier randomized clinical trials was primarily a consequence of deficiencies in the embryological and/or genetic techniques used. In particular, the strategy of using fluorescence in situ hybridization (FISH) to assess a relatively small number of chromosomes in cleavage-stage embryos seems to have been problematic. Information from studies using the new generation of genetic technologies, which permit a comprehensive chromosomal analysis, strongly supports the concept of PGS.

There is now excellent data confirming that, even at the blastocyst stage, many embryos are aneuploid and that this problem rapidly worsens with advancing female age (Fragouli et al., 2012). For women aged 30-35 years, ~40% of blastocysts are chromosomally abnormal, while for those aged 40-42 aneuploidy affects ~70%. Additionally, it has recently been proven that transfer of chromosomally abnormal embryos leads to implantation failure of miscarriage in at least 95% of cases (Scott et al., 2012). Furthermore, data from thousands of embryos clearly demonstrate that the impact of aneuploidy on morphology is too subtle for this problem to be avoided by assessing the morphological appearance of embryos (Alfarawati et al., 2011). These facts all suggest that PGS should work, but what evidence is there that it can really make a difference in the clinic? After the disappointments of the first generation of PGS technologies, doctors and embryologists in many centers are understandably cautious about the utilization of the new chromosome screening methods.

Evidence that PGS does indeed improve outcomes is now accumulating at a rapid rate. By the end of 2012 three randomized controlled trials had reported significantly elevated implantation and/or pregnancy rates per cycle and dramatically reduced rates of miscarriage (Scott et al., 2010; Schoolcraft et al., 2012; Yang et al., 2012). Two of the trials involved elective single embryo transfer for 'good-prognosis' patients and reported that on-going (third trimester) pregnancy rates were ~50% higher in the PGS group. The third trial was focused on women of advanced reproductive age (average age ~40 years) and similarly showed a large improvement in the ability of chromosomally normal embryos to implant and create a sustained, healthy pregnancy. Several additional trials, still ongoing, have reported interim data that also strongly support the use of PGS. As a result of this evidence the uptake of PGS in the United States has rebounded to levels exceeding the previous high water mark. In the United States the number of cases referred continues to grow rapidly.

Arguments that PGS does not improve IVF outcomes appear to be fading and even some of the most fervent critics of chromosome testing have reassessed their position and begun to offer PGS to their patients. However, publication of further randomized trials in peer-review journals will be needed before the case for PGS can be considered irrefutable. At present, several important questions concerning the use of PGS still need to be answered: There are several methods available for chromosome analysis, does it matter which is used? There is data to support the use of PGS in good prognosis patients and poor prognosis patients, so should it be offered to all couples or are their specific patient groups that benefit more than others? Most of the randomized trials supporting the use of PGS employed biopsy at the blastocyst stage. Does PGS also work when applied to polar bodies or blastomeres biopsied at the cleavage stage?

There are now at least five genetic methods capable of providing a comprehensive analysis of chromosome copy number in samples from embryos. The most widely used is microarray comparative genomic hybridization, also referred to as array-CGH or aCGH. The method has been validated in multiple laboratories, using a wide variety of strategies and has been consistently shown to yield accuracy rates of ~95% in polar bodies and higher still in embryos (e.g., Geraedts et al., 2011; Christopikou et al., 2013; Fragouli et al., 2011; Gutierrez-Mateo et al., 2011). Other methods allowing analysis of all 24 types of chromosome are single nucleotide polymorphisms (SNP) microarrays, real-time quantitative polymerase chain reaction (PCR), metaphase CGH, and next generation sequencing. Which is the best method to use for embryo analysis? Some scientists and clinicians never waste an opportunity to promote their favorite method, criticizing all other technologies and implying that their chosen strategy is the only one acceptable for PGS. However, the truth of the matter is that none of the techniques is perfect. Each has benefits and deficiencies. The key requirement for PGS is that the genetic method used accurately assesses the copy number of all 24 chromosomes, and it is likely that all of the techniques mentioned above are capable of providing such an assessment.

Several large clinics in the United States, Europe, and Australia are now routinely using PGS in ~20% of all IVF cycles and at least one center is applying it to over half of all cycles and reporting a substantial upsurge in pregnancy rates. The patients who have traditionally received PGS can be divided into four groups: couples who have experienced several unsuccessful IVF treatments; patients with a history of recurrent miscarriage; couples who have had a previous aneuploid pregnancy; couples where the woman is of advanced reproductive age. Clinical data from cycles employing comprehensive chromosome analysis suggest that all these patients may benefit from PGS. However, some patients falling within these categories produce such a high proportion of aneuploid embryos that PGS may not be able to improve the pregnancy rate. For example, a woman of advanced reproductive age will typically produce fewer embryos than a younger woman and each of her embryos will have an elevated risk of aneuploidy (due to her age). The combination of high probability of abnormality and few embryos to choose from creates a significant risk that no viable embryos will be identified. In such an event, no transfer is carried out and PGS could be said to have failed to provide the patient with an improved pregnancy rate, although it may have helped to avoid a miscarriage or birth of a child affected by serious abnormalities.

It should never be forgotten that PGS is a selection technique. It does not improve the viability of the embryos tested, it simply helps to guide physicians and embryologists to those that are chromosomally normal and therefore have a better chance of yielding a sustained pregnancy. For this reason, PGS might actually yield the most dramatic benefits for patients outside the traditional PGS categories: patients of better prognosis who typically produce more embryos and have lower aneuploidy rates. Such patients almost always produce at least one euploid embryo and therefore achieve an embryo transfer (and a pregnancy) in the vast majority of cases.

At the time of writing, the embryonic stage at which biopsy should ideally be carried out is unclear. There is very little information concerning pregnancy rates or other outcome measures after PGS with comprehensive chromosome analysis carried out on polar bodies or blastomeres. Randomized clinical trials of PGS at both of these stages are underway, but it may still be some time before a definitive conclusion can be reached. What can be said right now is that there is strong data supporting the use of trophectoderm biopsy on days-5/-6. As described above, clinical trials have shown improved implantation and pregnancy and miscarriage rates for certain patient groups for fresh cycles (day-6 transfer) and vitrified cycles. Biopsy at the blastocyst stage seems to be associated with little if any risk to the embryo, although more data are needed before this can be accurately quantified.

While genetic analysis at the blastocyst stage may prove to be ideal, there could still be a place for PGS at other stages. Patients who produce few oocytes or have a history of poor embryo development might not be considered appropriate for extended in vitro culture and consequently testing may need to be carried out at an earlier stage. Although PGS performed on polar bodies only reveals the maternal contribution to aneuploidy, this is likely to account for ~90% of all chromosome abnormalities detected at later stages. The polar bodies are essentially waste products of meiosis and their removal should not therefore interfere with subsequent embryo development. Additionally, polar body analysis has the advantage that it is not affected by chromosomal mosaicism (cells of the same embryo having different chromosomal make ups, potentially leading to diagnostic error).

Unlike removal of polar bodies, concerns have been raised about the impact of cleavage-stage biopsy. Another problem is that this stage is associated with the highest levels of mosaicism, posing a problem for accurate diagnosis. Despite these issues, analysis of single blastomeres could still prove valuable for some groups of patients (e.g., those unable to form several blastocysts, especially in cases where there is also a significant male-derived contribution to aneuploidy). Diagnosis of aneuploidy in single blastomeres has been shown to accurately reveal abnormal embryos that have a high probability of implantation failure or miscarriage (Scott et al., 2012).

While many questions remain to be answered, it appears that PGS is finally beginning to deliver the advantages long anticipated. With improved embryo selection, pregnancy rates can potentially be improved while the number of embryos transferred is reduced, finally eliminating the problem of multiple gestations.

References

Alfarawati S, Fragouli E, Colls P, Stevens J, Gutiérrez-Mateo C, Schoolcraft WB, Katz-Jaffe MG, Wells D. Fertil Steril. 2011 Feb;95(2):520-4.

Christopikou D, Tsorva E, Economou K, Shelley P, Davies S, Mastrominas M, Handyside AH. Hum Reprod. 2013 Mar 10.

Fragouli E, Alfarawati S, Daphnis DD, Goodall NN, Mania A, Griffiths T, Gordon A, Wells D. Hum Reprod. 2011 Feb;26(2):480-90.

Fragouli E, Alfarawati S, Spath K, Jaroudi S, Sarasa J, Enciso M, Wells D. Human Genetics. 2013 In press.

Fragouli E, Wells D. Semin Reprod Med. 2012 Aug;30(4):289-301.

Geraedts J, Montag M, Magli MC, Repping S, Handyside A, Staessen C, Harper J, Schmutzler A, Collins J, Goossens V, van der Ven H, Vesela K, Gianaroli L. Hum Reprod. 2011 Nov;26(11):3173-80.

Gutiérrez-Mateo C, Colls P, Sánchez-García J, Escudero T, Prates R, Ketterson K, Wells D, Munné S. Fertil Steril. 2011 Mar 1;95(3):953-8.

Schoolcraft WB, Surrey E, Minjarez D, Gustofson RL, Scott RT, Katz-Jaffe MG. Fertil Steril. 2012 98, Issue 3, Supplement, Page S1

Scott R, Tao X, Taylor D, Ferry KM, Treff NR. Fertil Steril 2010;94:S2.

Scott RT Jr, Ferry K, Su J, Tao X, Scott K, Treff NR. Fertil Steril. 2012 Apr;97(4):870-5.

Yang Z, Liu J, Collins GS, Salem SA, Liu X, Lyle SS, Peck AC, Sills ES, Salem RD. Mol. Cytogenet. 2012 May 2;5(1):24.

Does preimplantation genetic diagnosis improve live birth rates?

Luca Gianaroli, M. Cristina Magli, Ilaria Stanghellini, Anna P. Ferraretti

Società Italiana Studi di Medicina della Riproduzione (S.I.S.Me.R.), Bologna, Italy

Introduction

During the last decade, the field of assisted reproduction confronted a substantial change in the policy of embryo transfer with the concept of single, healthy delivery becoming the first priority. This happens in a scenario where women tend to delay the time to first pregnancy resulting in an increased demand for fertility treatments along with growing awareness and acceptance of available treatment options.

As a general concept, assisted reproductive technology (ART) can be viewed as part of preventive medicine due to its capacity of restoring parenthood to couples that otherwise would remain childless. Its preventive label is reinforced by the implementation of those techniques related to preimplantation genetic diagnosis (PGD) and screening (PGS) by which specific genetic diseases and chromosomal abnormalities can be identified in the corresponding oocytes or embryos.

Social, economic, and political considerations

Assisted reproduction is a relatively recent discipline and includes some innovative techniques like PGD. Now, differently from the past, decisions about new technologies are based not only on data on clinical efficacy, safety, and effectiveness, but also on economic aspects, and particularly on cost-effectiveness ratios. In many European countries, health economic analysis is now required before introducing new health care technologies into national programs. The large differences existing in health care systems, budgets, screening programs, and vaccination policies make the results from economic evaluations from one country not easily transferable to other countries.

Despite the increasing demand for ART cycles, health authorities often view infertility as a low health priority. Consequently, access to treatments is frequently restricted by rationing and limiting funds. This situation is exacerbated by financial constraints, which make not only national health providers but also private insurers restrain access. As a result, most couples must pay out-of-pocket for these services, while many of those unable to afford the cost of an ART cycle withdraw from treatment. In the current economic crisis, the ratio between affordability and utilization of services suggests that an increasing number of couples are unable to undergo treatment. As a result, fewer children are born every year leading to the consequent negative impacts related to this phenomenon. In addition, the exclusion of PGD precludes the earliest form of genetic or chromosomal disease prevention.

ART: A health investment for the state

Assisted reproductive technologies are unique among all medical interventions in the sense that their success leads to a birth. This new life would not have existed had the technology not been available and accessible to the infertile couple. Therefore, it is possible to estimate lost tax revenue to the state resulting from children who have not been born due to the limited public access to ART that is currently observed in many countries.

According to several studies considering different aspects, such as future earnings, health care consumption, and life expectancy, to calculate the cost-effectiveness of an ART cycle an *in vitro* conceived child represents a net positive return to the government. It was estimated that the lifetime net taxes paid from an average employed individual born in 2005 from in vitro fertilization (IVF), relative to the initial IVF investment, represent a 700% net return to the government. The projected net lifetime tax contribution is US $606,200; taking into consideration the costs of an ART cycle and all direct financial interactions, the net present value is US $155,870.

A similar model was developed in the United Kingdom to evaluate whether state-funded IVF programs represent sound fiscal policies. These calculations took into account the average investment cost to conceive an IVF child and the net taxes derived from gross taxes paid minus direct government transfers received (e.g., education, health, pension) over the lifetime of the child. The results showed that an investment to achieve an IVF child is worth 8.5-times the amount to the United Kingdom Treasury in discounted future tax revenue. More specifically, the lifetime discounted value of net taxes from an IVF-conceived child with mother aged 35 is pound 109,939 compared with pound 122,127 for a naturally conceived child. Therefore, an investment of pound 12,931 to achieve an IVF singleton is actually worth 8.5-times this amount to the United Kingdom Treasury in discounted future tax revenue.

In other words, besides the many humanistic reasons for offering IVF treatment to infertile couples, the above reported figures suggest that removing barriers to IVF would have positive tax benefits for the government, notwithstanding its beneficial effect on overall economic growth. Nevertheless, the birth of a child affected by a genetic or chromosomal disease would heavily modify the above calculations.

Embryo transfer policy: single vs. double embryo transfer

Adopting the right policy for embryo transfer optimizes the cost-effectiveness of ART procedures by maximizing the chances of term pregnancy while reducing the risk of multiple implantations. A Swedish study shows that single embryo transfer (SET) represents a better economic investment in women aged <36 years resulting in lower costs per delivery. In this category of patients, transfer of more than one embryo exposes the patient to a high multiple birth rate with the consequent increased morbidity and high costs for neonatal care. Conversely, a SET strategy, possibly including one fresh SET followed by one additional frozen SET, leads to the same live birth rate as a double embryo transfer (DET), but with a markedly reduced incidence of multiple births.

When the costs for maternal health care, productivity losses, and pediatric care for SET and DET are compared in relation to the corresponding maternal and pediatric outcomes, the SET strategy has a lower average total cost calculated from treatment until 6 months after delivery. In the DET group, the incremental cost per extra delivery is significantly higher (71,940) as well as is the rates of prematurely born and low birth weight children. Twin pregnancies and complications during pregnancy and delivery (including preterm labor, preterm premature rupture of the membranes, severe hemorrhage, and rates of caesarean section) were significantly more common in the DET group. On the contrary, fewer maternal and pediatric complications have been observed in the SET group. To make the above calculations, multiple parameters were evaluated, like costs of IVF treatment in relation to the used drugs, the adopted technique, possible complications related to the ART treatment, and the costs of early abortions. Additional costs comprise the cost for prenatal care.

The evaluation of working status was also considered as well as the number of days of absence from work (including sick, maternity, and parental insurance leave). Also in this case, women in the SET group had on average significantly fewer days of sick leave during pregnancy as compared with the DET group, resulting in a significantly lower total mean cost for absence from work. In the Swedish study, the mean health cost per randomized woman was

9,309 in the SET group and 12,318 in the DET group. With a given budget of 4 million and an extensive list of couples waiting for an ART cycle, more women could have been treated if a SET strategy was chosen (437 vs. 331 with DET strategy).

As already mentioned, a cost-effective strategy implies the adoption of the correct transfer policy to be established in relation to the patient's category and reproductive history. It is actually clear that not all women benefit from SET. This is the case of poor responders that generally have overall lower live birth rates compared with normal responders even after DET with a modest increase in multiple birth rates. There is no doubt that crucial factors in determining the success of a SET program are the selection of the patient and the selection of the embryo. At this respect, a customized approach is recommended that also needs to take into consideration the relevance of time-to-pregnancy. With the recent technological advances, the analysis of the chromosomal status in the *in vitro*-generated embryos could represent an important extra tool.

Preimplantation genetic screening

PGS was proposed in the early 1990s based on the rationale of improving IVF results by selecting for transfer those embryos having a euploid setting. This approach was designed specifically for women of advanced reproductive age, who are known to be exposed to a higher incidence of aneuploid concepti, and to represent a category of patients for which the likelihood to obtain a pregnancy is lower. The incidence of chromosomal aneuploidy that increases proportionally with age could be responsible for the diminished oocyte viability. In order to select euploid embryos for transfer and to prevent early abortions and aneuploid births, PGS began to be offered to these women.

Some initial reports showed promising results, including the reduction in the spontaneous miscarriage rate, particularly evident in women older than 40 years and in patients with idiopathic recurrent pregnancy losses. A decreased risk of trisomic offspring was also documented. Nevertheless, other papers showed that PGS was both expensive and ineffective and even detrimental, suggesting that avoidance of PGS may save millions of euros and prevent the loss of hundreds of pregnancies. Based on these data, PGS was not considered entitled to receive a reimbursement. A cost-effectiveness analysis performed in 2008 comparing conventional treatment with prenatal diagnosis versus PGS showed that conventional IVF was the least costly strategy per healthy infant ($118,713 in PGS vs. $68,026 in conventional IVF) in women aged 38-40 years. In women aged >40, conventional IVF and PGS were shown to be essentially equal in terms of cost-effectiveness ($122,000 vs. $118,713), suggesting that some selected category of patients may benefit from PGS.

These results were quite disappointing and also surprising since the scientific foundation supporting the methodology was certainly correct. A study published in 2005 demonstrated that from 1,247 embryos generated by 208 pregnant patients, 687 carried chromosomal abnormalities. Of these abnormal embryos, 160 were aneuploid for one of those chromosomes compatible with implantation, suggesting that PGS avoided exposing receptive uteri to the risk of an aneuploid implantation.

However, the majority of the studies published so far, including those derived from randomized controlled trials (RCTs), present some objective limitations, such as the frequent biopsy of two cells from day 3 embryos, which has been proven to negatively affect the following development. In addition, the use of the fluorescence in situ hybridization (FISH) technology, which only tests a limited number of chromosomes, may result in the transfer of embryos with abnormalities in the untested chromosomes.

More recently, new strategies have been introduced in PGS. These include the development of techniques such as comparative genomic hybridization (CGH) that evaluates all chromosomes and the biopsy of trophectoderm cells at the blastocyst stage that bypasses the risk of mosaicism typical of day 3 embryos. The corresponding results on the effectiveness of PGS are extremely encouraging, yielding double implantation rates in comparison with the controls. Further data are needed to confirm these findings and RCTs on polar bodies and on trophectoderm cells are currently ongoing. If the theoretically predictable advantage of PGS is confirmed, a significant decrease of costs compared with conventional treatments is expected due to both an increased rate of healthy births and a reduced incidence of spontaneous or therapeutic abortions. Once these data are available, the calculation of the cost-benefit of PGS must also take into consideration the range of immediate and long-term economic costs derived from the birth of a child with disabilities consequent to the transfer of an aneuploid embryo, an event much more likely to occur after conventional IVF than after PGS. The consequent implications, although difficult to quantify and variable among different situations, also include indirect costs for the families involving, for example, decisions about employment. Having a child with disabilities increases the likelihood that the parents, mostly the mother, need to shorten hours of work or stop working completely. In the longer term, disabilities can severely compromise a child›s schooling and the capacity to get employment as an adult. It is useless to say that an efficient PGS program, particularly indicated in specific cases, helping to prevent and reduce childhood disability would be justified by a cost-benefit calculation.

Preimplantation genetic diagnosis

PGD can be applied in cases of couples carrying a specific genetic disorder. Its large-scale implementation at the national level to prevent the birth of individuals affected with a debilitating genetic disease is a form of preventive medicine. For example, cystic fibrosis (CF) is the most common life-shortening inherited disease in Caucasians, with a prevalence of around 1 in 2,500 live births. Each year in the United States, more than 1,000 babies affected with CF are born. It was estimated that as of the year 2000 more than $1.3 billion represented the total direct medical costs spent each year to treat CF patients. This estimate is destined to increase given that the advances in the treatment and management of respiratory and pancreatic disorders have significantly increased the life expectancy of patients with CF.

Since PGD is a realistic alternative to raising a sick child or to aborting an affected fetus, a cost–benefit analysis would be important to evaluate a PGD program as a strategy to prevent CF. Therefore, a calculation was made to compare the cost to deliver healthy children for CF carrier-couples by PGD with the average annual and lifetime direct medical costs per CF patient avoided. The study performed in the United States reported that treating annually about 4,000 CF carrier-couples with PGD would result in 3,715 deliveries of non-affected children at a cost of $57,467 per child. Considering an average annual direct medical cost per CF patient of $63,127 with a life expectancy of 37 years, savings would be $2.3 million per patient and $2.2 billion for all new CF patients annually in lifetime treatment costs. Cumulated net saving of a PGD program for all carrier-couples for 37 years would be $33.3 billion. In this way, most births of individuals affected with a debilitating genetic disease and thousands of abortions would be prevented. There is no doubt that a national PGD program for CF would be a highly cost-effective novel modality of preventive medicine.

When analyzing these data in more detail in relation to maternal age, when used for women younger than 35 years of age the net benefit of PGD over natural conception (NC) followed by prenatal testing and termination of affected pregnancies was $182,000. For women aged 35-40 years, the net benefit of PGD over NC was $114,000, while for women older than 40 years, the net benefit of PGD over NC was -$148,000. Since success rates are considerably lower in advanced reproductive age, in older women more than one cycle is usually necessary to achieve a live birth.

Similar calculation could be performed for other genetic pathologies.

In Europe, access to PGD is regulated differently in each state with great diversity in health care arrangements or therapeutic cultures. This diversity makes PGD fundamentally different in the single realities, where access and exclusion are dependent on the different health care provision practices rather than regulation alone. As a result, individual couples end up with different rights, opportunities, and financial compensation schemes. While these differences have enormous consequences for the access of individual patients to PGD throughout Europe, in some way they also contribute to the process of turning PGD into regular health care, supporting the value of diversity for innovation in health care provision practices.

References

Aarden E, Van Hoyweghen I, Vos R, Horstman K Providing preimplantation genetic diagnosis in the United Kingdom, The Netherlands and Germany: a comparative in-depth analysis of health-care access. Hum Reprod. 2009;24:1542-7.

Chang LJ, Chen SU, Tsai YY, Hung CC, Fang MY, Su YN, Yang YS. An update of preimplantation genetic diagnosis in gene diseases, chromosomal translocation, and aneuploidy screening. Clin Exp Reprod Med 2011;38:126-34.

Connolly M, Gallo F, Hoorens S, Ledger W. Assessing long-run economic benefits attributed to an IVF-conceived singleton based on projected lifetime net tax contributions in the UK. Hum Reprod 2009;24:626-32.

Davis LB, Champion SJ, Fair SO, Baker VL, Garber AM. A cost-benefit analysis of preimplantation genetic diagnosis for carrier couples of cystic fibrosis. Fertil Steril 2010;93:1793-804.

Gianaroli L, Magli MC, Ferraretti AP, Tabanelli C, Trengia V, Farfalli V, Cavallini G. The beneficial effects of preimplantation genetic diagnosis for aneuploidy support extensive clinical application. Reprod Biomed Online 2005;10:633-40.

Gianaroli L, Magli MC, Gambardella L, Giusti A, Grugnetti C, Corani G. Objective way to support embryo transfer: a probabilistic decision. Hum Reprod 2013 doi:10.1093/humrep/det030.

Gianaroli L, Racowsky C, Geraedts J, Cedars M, Makrigiannakis A, Lobo R. Best practices of ASRM and ESHRE: a journey through reproductive medicine. Hum Reprod 2012;27:3365-79 / Fertil Steril 2012;98:1380-94.

Kjellberg AT, Carlsson P, Bergh C. Randomized single versus double embryo transfer: obstetric and paediatric outcome and a cost-effectiveness analysis. Hum Reprod 2006;21:210–6.

Mersereau JE, Plunkett BA, Cedars MI. Preimplantation genetic screening in older women: a cost-effectiveness analysis. Fertil Steril 2008;90:592-8.

Munné S, Fischer J, Warner A, Chen S, Zouves C, Cohen J; Referring Centers PGD Group. Preimplantation genetic diagnosis significantly reduces pregnancy loss in infertile couples: a multicenter study. Fertil Steril 2006;85:326-32.

Stabile M, Allin S. The economic costs of childhood disability. Future Child 2012;22:65-96.

Trilogy 11. Multiple pregnancy (evidence-based practice)

Embryo selection

Arne Sunde

St. Olav's University Hospital, Trondheim, Norway

This summary is based in part on a manuscript submitted to Fertility and Sterility as an invited contribution to Views and Reviews (Fertility and Sterility, Volume 100, Issue 2, August 2013).

Introduction

The clinical results of assisted reproductive technology (ART), judged by the annual European IVF-monitoring (EIM) reports published by the European Society of Human Reproduction and Embryology (ESHRE), have improved annually since the end of the 1990s. Delivery rates per embryo transfer have improved and, perhaps more importantly, the multiple delivery rates have gone down (1, 2). In individual countries, and even more pronounced at individual clinics, the variation in clinical results are, however, surprisingly large. Recent data from a prospective randomized multi-center study suggest that the US clinics participating in the study, in general, have better results than the European clinics (3). Visiting different ART laboratories can be quite revealing. There is a large variation concerning the physical organization of the laboratory, the equipment used, and consumables such as culture dishes and pipettes as well as culture media and culture protocols. The algorithms used to select embryos for replacement or cryopreservation also show considerable variation among clinics. Quality control and quality assurance vary from rigorous and validated by certifying bodies to being almost absent.

The clinical part of ART has seen a strong development towards evidence-based clinical practice. New drugs and new treatment protocols are tested in properly powered prospective controlled trials before being introduced in general clinical practice. Concerning the ART laboratory, most of our understanding is still based on research in animal models (4). Although this research may be of high quality in itself, the issue is always to what extent the animal data are relevant for the human gametes and embryos (5).

It is still an exception that changes in protocols and consumables used in the ART laboratory are based on the results of sufficiently large prospective randomized clinical trials. Large clinical trials are laborious and expensive, and it is difficult to find the necessary funds to run sufficiently large clinical trials on consumables and treatment protocols in the ART laboratory. One way forward is that ART units collaborate to organize large multi-center trials and share the cost among them. The ART units in the The Netherlands are exemplary in this respect. They have set up a large multi-center double-blind randomized controlled trial of two culture media for human ART (6).

Success criteria

The purpose of selecting embryos in ART is presumably to increase the success of the treatment. A complicating factor is that there is no uniform agreement on the most relevant success criteria in ART (7) (Table 1). It is more complicated than just recording number of pregnancies per embryo replacement since it is well established that the likelihood of obtaining a viable pregnancy after ART is dependent on many variables. Factors like the infertility diagnosis, female age, obesity, hormonal status, ovarian stimulation protocols, the quality of the ART laboratory, and number of embryos replaced all play a role (8).

Success criteria also may be different in different regulatory and financial environments. In cases where the patients have to bear all costs of the ART treatment, it is understandable that they will focus on the likelihood of obtaining a delivery after the first attempt and will accept multiple embryo transfer even with the increased risk of high-order multiple birth (9, 10). ART clinics will, therefore, tend to use pregnancy rate per fresh embryo transfer as their success criterion and marketing parameter. In environments where the cost of ART treatment is covered by the government or health insurance, the health provider will focus on the total cost and can introduce economic incentives or regulations to increase the use of elective single-embryo transfer (11-13). In countries like Sweden, Belgium, and Turkey, elective single-embryo transfer must be done in cases where prognostic factors such as female age, first treatment cycle, and previous fertility history indicate a good prognosis. In these circumstances, the cumulative delivery rate per oocyte recovery is perhaps the most relevant success criterion both for the clinic and for the couple treated (14, 15). A disadvantage of this criterion is that it may take a long time before all frozen embryos are used and it requires a system for keeping track of all patients treated. In the Nordic countries this is done through official health registries using the unique personal identification number allocated at birth to all individuals (16).

For the ART laboratory, one of the most relevant parameters for continuous monitoring of the quality of the laboratory is on-going implantation rate per number of embryos replaced.

The health of the child should be an obvious success criterion. ART is associated with a less favorable outcome for the offspring. Multiple pregnancy is likely a major contributor to this (17), but even in singleton pregnancies, children born after ART have an increased chance of being small for gestational age and born prematurely (18). Studies of families where two singletons are born, one after ART and the other spontaneously conceived, have indicated that infertility may contribute to the reduced gestational length and birth weight (19, 20), but there is also evidence that ART as such may have an influence on perinatal complication or the health of the child (21-23). Linking specific events in the ART procedure to obstetric or neonatal problems or the phenotype of the offspring demands huge databases and long-term follow-up. This is not the case currently. The large Nordic collaborative database may form the basis for such studies in the future (16).

Embryo selection

Selection rationale

A reasonable assumption is that in a given cohort of embryos there are embryos of different developmental potential. An optimal selection algorithm should be able to rank these embryos according to their potential. An algorithm that only identifies the top-quality embryos is of limited value since it is of no use in all the cases where there are no top-quality embryos present.

Cryopreservation of human embryos has become very successful, and in stimulated cycles the endometrium may be suboptimal (24). This has led to a suggestion of a strategy where all embryos are cryopreserved and then replaced later in cycles where the endometrium is more optimal. A prospective randomized study showed that this is an attractive option (25). It can then be argued that the only variable embryo selection can influence is time to pregnancy (26).

Elective single-embryo transfer is only done because one wishes to avoid multiple pregnancies. With embryos of equal quality, two embryos transferred at a time gives higher pregnancy rate from the first transfer of fresh embryos than just transferring one fresh embryo. Cumulative delivery rate with one fresh plus one frozen embryo is, however, comparable with delivery rate following transfer of two fresh embryos (27). The multiple delivery rate is, of course, different (28). Again, it can be argued that embryo selection in conjunction with elective single-embryo transfer is primarily influencing time-to-pregnancy and not cumulative delivery rate. If the single most important success criterion is the pregnancy rate in the fresh cycle, then selecting the embryo in the cohort with the highest implantation potential becomes important.

Subjective embryo scoring, keep it simple?

Traditionally, embryo selection has been done subjectively based on morphology and growth kinetics as seen in the microscope. A very large number of variables may be observed and recorded, each one of them with some predictive power to select embryos with implantation potential (29). Organizations such as ESHRE and Alpha have jointly tried to standardize scoring of both fresh and frozen embryos and have issued published consensus papers on the topic (29, 30).

A critical issue is, however, an assessment of the relative predictive power of each variable recorded (Table 2). It is a waste of time to assess and record a number of variables that do not give independent selection power. Holte et al. (31) did a statistical analysis of the selection variables they used for selection of embryos for day 2 transfer. In a univariate analysis, degree of fragmentation, relative size of blastomeres, number of blastomeres, and symmetry and absence of multinucleated blastomeres all had predictive power. Testing these variables against each other in a multivariate regression analysis showed that only blastomere number, relative blastomere size, and absence of multinucleated cells had independent predictive power (31). Since multinucleated cells tend to be bigger than mononucleated cells, one could argue that for selection for day 2 transfer, most of the selection power would be available just by counting number of blastomeres and their relative size. If one chooses to assess and record more variables one should also judge whether the marginal increase in selection power justifies the increase in time and exposure of the embryos to potentially adverse conditions that could reduce their developmental potential. To observe and record a lot of redundant information is not only a waste of time, but can potentially be harmful to oocytes, zygotes, and embryos and reduce their developmental potential.

Many clinics have excellent clinical results with replacement of embryos at the blastocyst stage. Blastocyst selection is usually done based on a variant of the scoring system suggested by Gardener et al. (32, 33). The embryos are scored based on variables such as blastocoel expansion, zona thinning, inner cell mass morphology, and size and number and morphology of the trophectoderm cells. Randomized studies have been done comparing different scoring systems for blastocysts (34). Recently, Ahlström et al. published data from a study where they have been trying to assess the predictive power of the classical variables used for selection of blastocyst. Their conclusion was that, of these variables, the morphology of the trophectoderm was the only statistically independent predictor of pregnancy (35).

Objective embryo scoring

Scoring of embryo morphology and growth kinetics has traditionally been done subjectively. The advantage is that skilled and experienced embryologists have acquired a sense of how good embryos should look and behave. The disadvantage is that a lot of this intuition of embryo quality is difficult to translate into objective quantifiable terms and it takes a long time to train new embryologists to be excellent in scoring embryos. It is therefore potentially a major step forward that objective methods for evaluation of embryos are being developed. Evaluation of zona pellucida structure can be done automatically and user-independent (36). By using multi-level images of embryos, Paternot et al. have shown that an objective measurement of morphology and morphometrics will improve embryo selection (37, 38).

Another approach is using time-lapse-based systems. This gives a dynamic evaluation of morphology, cleavage patterns, and growth kinetics. Initially, time-lapse was used as a tool for negative selection; some embryos that would pass the normal selection criteria had aberrant cleavage pattern and subsequently low developmental potential (39, 40). It is possible to devise a system for ranking embryos according to developmental potential based on growth kinetics (39, 41, 42). Data from time-lapse recordings also suggested that the time-points one traditionally used for looking at embryos are not optimal (42). A potentially very important observation is that the pattern and kinetics of embryo development may be predictive for the ploidy of the embryo and may thus be an alternative to more laborious genetic methods for identifying embryos with normal chromosomal complement (43).

A major potential advantage with objective embryo scoring is that one can compare different ART laboratories and, by using very large datasets, identify and quantify a range of factors (embryological and others) that have an influence on the developmental potential of human embryos. This may lead to a major step forward in the understanding of critical parameters in the human ART laboratory.

Biomarkers as tool for embryo selection

Identification of a biomarker that could be useful as a tool for objective embryo selection has been the focus for a lot of research since the end of the 1980s. To be clinically useful, selection variables based on the metabolism, the secretome, the epigenome, or the genome must give information that is statistically independent from selection variables obtained by morphology and growth kinetics (i.e., they should provide additional information that would increase the selection ability) (44).

Analysis of carbohydrate metabolism and amino acid turnover may correlate to the viability of the embryos (45-48, 49). It is, however, still unknown whether this type of information will enable selection of embryos with a higher implantation potential than more traditional selection methods based on embryo morphology and growth kinetics. Potential advantages of selection methods based on embryo metabolism are that they give objective information and they may be integrated in new culture platforms that enable inline automatic analysis of embryo quality (50, 51).

Analysis of spent culture media by near–infrared spectroscopy, although initially promising (52, 53), failed in prospective randomized trials and it currently does not look like this approach is a promising, viable option (54, 55).

With the advent of preimplantation genetic diagnosis (PGD) (56), it was obvious that one had a technique available that had the potential to select chromosomally normal embryos for transfer in routine in vitro fertilization (IVF), and the concept of preimplantation genetic screening (PGS) was introduced (57). PGS based on fluorescence in situ hybridization (FISH) analysis of selected chromosomes was rapidly introduced in routine clinical practice in clinics all over the world. This technique was not tested in sufficiently large randomized controlled trials until more than 10 years after being introduced in clinical routine. Unexpectedly, it was shown that PGS did not improve embryo selection; on the contrary, it could even reduce the likelihood of pregnancy (58-61). The reasons for this failure may be due to several factors such as the detection technique used (62), the procedure or timing of embryo biopsy (63), or the fact that human embryos frequently are mosaic and show chromosomal instability (64, 65). A lesson to be learned from the controversy around PGS is that new techniques or interventions should not be introduced in routine clinical use before they have been properly tested in sufficiently large prospective randomized trials.

Summary

The ART laboratory must gradually move towards evidence-based practice for equipment, consumables, and procedures tested and validated for ART in humans.

Selection of human embryos in routine IVF should be evidence-based using variables and methods that have been shown to have statistically independent selection power.

New methods and strategies for the culture and selection of human embryos must be tested in prospective trials before being widely introduced in clinical routine.

Parameter	Denominator to calculate rate	Pro and Con
hCG rise **Viable fetus delivery**	**Started cycle (start of medication)** **Completed cycle (embryo replacement)**	**Pro: An indication of success rate of ART**
		Con: Dependent on number of embryos replaced
Number of viable fetuses	**Number of embryos replaced**	**Pro: Marker of embryo quality**
		Con: Dependent on endometrial receptivity
Multiple delivery	**Delivery**	**Dependent on number of embryos replaced** **Linked to health of the child** **Of interest for the heath provider**
Cumulative delivery rate (deliveries from fresh and frozen embryos in the same cohort)	**Oocyte recovery**	**Pro: Marker of quality of the cohort of embryos** **Very relevant for the patients**
		Con: Can take several years from oocytes recovery until last delivery from frozen embryos
Time to pregnancy **(Time from first ART treatment until first viable pregnancy)**	**None, not a rate**	**Pro: Relevant for the patients**
		Con: Can be complicated to track the patients if they are treated at different clinics
Healthy child	**Children**	**Pro: Important endpoint for all involved parties** **Paramount for the standing of ART in the society**
		Con: Can take many years from ART treatment until the health of the child can be assessed

Table 1. Success criteria for assisted reproduction.

Type of assessment	Stage	Parameters recorded	Reference
Subjective assessment	**Cleavage stages**	**Blastomere number** **Relative blastomere size** **Mononucleated cells**	**Holte et al. (31)**
Subjective assessment	**Blastocyst stage**	**Trophectoderm cell morphology**	**Ahlström et al. (35)**
Computer-assisted assessment	**Cleavage stages**	**Embryo and blastomere volumes**	**Paternot et al. (38)**
Time-lapse-based assessment	**Cleavage stages**	**Time intervals between developmental stages**	**Meseguer et al. (39)** **Chen et al. (41)** **Dal Canto et al. (42)**

Table 2. Morphology and growth kinetics parameters shown to be independent markers for developmental potential.

References

1. Ferraretti AP, Goossens V, de Mouzon J, Bhattacharya S, Castilla JA, Korsak V et al. Assisted reproductive technology in Europe, 2008: results generated from European registers by ESHRE. Human reproduction 2012;27:2571-84.
2. Nygren KG, Nyboe Andersen A. Assited reproductive technology in Europe, 1997. Results genrated from European registries by ESHRE. Human Reprod 2001;16:384-91.
3. Boostanfar R, Mannaerts B, Pang S, Fernandez-Sanchez M, Witjes H, Devroey P et al. A comparison of live birth rates and cumulative ongoing pregnancy rates between Europe and North America after ovarian stimulation with corifollitropin alfa or recombinant follicle-stimulating hormone. Fertility and sterility 2012;97:1351-8.
4. Cohen J, Rieger D. Historical background of gamete and embryo culture. Methods in molecular biology 2012;912:1-18.
5. Menezo Y, Lichtblau I, Elder K. New insights into human pre-implantation metabolism in

vivo and in vitro. Journal of assisted reproduction and genetics 2013.
6. A multi-center double-blind randomized controlled trial of two media for the in vitro culture of human preimplantation embryos. Nederlands Trial Register no. NTR1979. (http://www.trialregister.nl/trialreg/admin/rctview.asp?TC=1979. In.
7. Alper MA, Brinsden PR, Fisher R, Wikland M. Is your IVF programme good? Human Reprod 2002;17:8-10.
8. Group. ECW. Failures (with some successes) of assisted reproduction and gamete donation programs. Human reproduction update 2013.
9. Stillman RJ, Richter KS, Banks NK, Graham JR. Elective single embryo transfer: a 6-year progressive implementation of 784 single blastocyst transfers and the influence of payment method on patient choice. Fertility and sterility 2009;92:1895-906.
10. Connolly MP, Hoorens S, Chambers GM, Reproduction E, Society Task F. The costs and consequences of assisted reproductive technology: an economic perspective. Human reproduction update 2010;16:603-13.
11. Gerris J, De Sutter P, De Neubourg D, Van Royen E, Vander Elst J, Mangelschots K et al. A real-life prospective health economic study of elective single embryo transfer versus two-embryo transfer in first IVF/ICSI cycles. Human Reprod 2004;19:917-23.
12. Kallen B, Finnstrom O, Lindam A, Nilsson E, Nygren KG, Otterblad Olausson P. Trends in delivery and neonatal outcome after in vitro fertilization in Sweden: data for 25 years. Human reproduction 2010;25:1026-34.
13. Maheshwari A, Griffiths S, Bhattacharya S. Global variations in the uptake of single embryo transfer. Human reproduction update 2011;17:107-20.
14. Sundstrom P, Saldeen P. Cumulative delivery rate in an in vitro fertilization program with a single embryo transfer policy. Acta obstetricia et gynecologica Scandinavica 2009;88:700-6.
15. Garrido N, Bellver J, Remohi J, Simon C, Pellicer A. Cumulative live-birth rates per total number of embryos needed to reach newborn in consecutive in vitro fertilization (IVF) cycles: a new approach to measuring the likelihood of IVF success. Fertility and sterility 2011;96:40-6.
16. Henningsen AK, Romundstad LB, Gissler M, Nygren KG, Lidegaard O, Skjaerven R et al. Infant and maternal health monitoring using a combined Nordic database on ART and safety. Acta obstetricia et gynecologica Scandinavica 2011;90:683-91.
17. Zollner U, Dietl J. Perinatal risks after IVF and ICSI. Journal of perinatal medicine 2012.
18. Pinborg A, Wennerholm UB, Romundstad LB, Loft A, Aittomaki K, Soderstrom-Anttila V et al. Why do singletons conceived after assisted reproduction technology have adverse perinatal outcome? Systematic review and meta-analysis. Human reproduction update 2013;19:87-104.
19. Romundstad LB, Romundstad PR, Sunde A, von During V, Skjaerven R, Gunnel D et al. Effects of technology or maternal factors on perinatal outcome of assisted reproduction: a population-based cochort study. The Lancet 2008;372:737-43.
20. Henningsen AK, Pinborg A, Lidegaard O, Vestergaard C, Forman JL, Andersen AN. Perinatal outcome of singleton siblings born after assisted reproductive technology and spontaneous conception: Danish national sibling-cohort study. Fertility and sterility 2011;95:959-63.
21. Romundstad LB, Romundstad PR, Sunde A, von During V, Skjaerven R, Vatten LJ. Increased risk of placenta previa in pregnancies following IVF/ICSI; a comparison of ART and non-ART pregnancies in the same mother. Human reproduction 2006;21:2353-8.
22. Dumoulin JC, Land JA, Van Montfoort AP, Nelissen EC, Coonen E, Derhaag JG et al. Effect of in vitro culture of human embryos on birthweight of newborns. Human reproduc-

tion 2010;25:605-12.
23. Scherrer U, Rimoldi SF, Rexhaj E, Stuber T, Duplain H, Garcin S et al. Systemic and pulmonary vascular dysfunction in children conceived by assisted reproductive technologies. Circulation 2012;125:1890-6.
24. Balaban B, Urman B, Ata B, Isiklar A, Larman MG, Hamilton R et al. A randomized controlled study of human Day 3 embryo cryopreservation by slow freezing or vitrification: vitrification is associated with higher survival, metabolism and blastocyst formation. Human reproduction 2008;23:1976-82.
25. Aflatoonian A, Oskouian H, Ahmadi S, Oskouian L. Can fresh embryo transfers be replaced by cryopreserved-thawed embryo transfers in assisted reproductive cycles? A randomized controlled trial. Journal of assisted reproduction and genetics 2010;27:357-63.
26. Mastenbroek S, van der Veen F, Aflatoonian A, Shapiro B, Bossuyt P, Repping S. Embryo selection in IVF. Human reproduction 2011;26:964-6.
27. Thurin AT, Hausken J, Hillensjö T, Jablonowska B, Pinborg A, Strandell A et al. Elective Single-Embryo Transfer versus Double-Embryo Transfer in in Vitro Fertilization. N Engl J Med 2004;351:2392-402.
28. McLernon DJ, Harrild K, Bergh C, Davies MJ, de Neubourg D, Dumoulin JCM et al. Clinical effectiveness of elective single versus double embryo transfer: meta-analysis of individual patient data from randomised trials. Bmj 2010;341:c6945-c.
29. Alpha Scientists in Reproductive M, Embryology ESIGo. The Istanbul consensus workshop on embryo assessment: proceedings of an expert meeting. Human reproduction 2011;26:1270-83.
30. Alpha Scientists In Reproductive M. The Alpha consensus meeting on cryopreservation key performance indicators and benchmarks: proceedings of an expert meeting. Reproductive biomedicine online 2012;25:146-67.
31. Holte J, Berglund L, Milton K, Garello C, Gennarelli G, Revelli A et al. Construction of an evidence-based integrated morphology cleavage embryo score for implantation potential of embryos scored and transferred on day 2 after oocyte retrieval. Human reproduction 2007;22:548-57.
32. Gardner DK, Phil D, Lane M, Stevens J, Schlenker T, Schoolcraft WB. Blastocyst score affects implantation and pregnancy outcome: towards a single blastocyst transfer. Fertility and sterility 2000;76:1155-8.
33. Hardarson T, Van Landuyt L, Jones G. The blastocyst. Human reproduction 2012;27 Suppl 1:i72-91.
34. Balaban B, Yakin K, Urman B. Randomized comparison of two different blastocyst grading systems. Fertility and sterility 2006;85:559-63.
35. Ahlstrom A, Westin C, Reismer E, Wikland M, Hardarson T. Trophectoderm morphology: an important parameter for predicting live birth after single blastocyst transfer. Human reproduction 2011;26:3289-96.
36. Ebner T, Balaban B, Moser M, Shebl O, Urman B, Ata B et al. Automatic user-independent zona pellucida imaging at the oocyte stage allows for the prediction of preimplantation development. Fertility and sterility 2010;94:913-20.
37. Paternot G, Debrock S, D'Hooghe T, Spiessens C. Computer-assisted embryo selection: a benefit in the evaluation of embryo quality? Reproductive biomedicine online 2011;23:347-54.
38. Paternot G, Debrock S, De Neubourg D, D'Hooghe TM, Spiessens C. Semi-automated morphometric analysis of human embryos can reveal correlations between total embryo volume and clinical pregnancy. Human reproduction 2013;28:627-33.
39. Meseguer M, Herrero J, Tejera A, Hilligsoe KM, Ramsing NB, Remohi J. The use of mor-

phokinetics as a predictor of embryo implantation. Human reproduction 2011;26:2658-71.
40. Kirkegaard K, Agerholm IE, Ingerslev HJ. Time-lapse monitoring as a tool for clinical embryo assessment. Human reproduction 2012;27:1277-85.
41. Chen AA, Tan L, Suraj V, Reijo Pera R, Shen S. Biomarkers identified with time-lapse imaging: discovery, validation, and practical application. Fertility and sterility 2013;99:1035-43.
42. Dal Canto M, Coticchio G, Mignini Renzini M, De Ponti E, Novara PV, Brambillasca F et al. Cleavage kinetics analysis of human embryos predicts development to blastocyst and implantation. Reproductive biomedicine online 2012;25:474-80.
43. Chavez SL, Loewke KE, Han J, Moussavi F, Colls P, Munne S et al. Dynamic blastomere behaviour reflects human embryo ploidy by the four-cell stage. Nature communications 2012;3:1251.
44. Palmer SS, Barnhart KT. Biomarkers in reproductive medicine: the promise, and can it be fulfilled? Fertility and sterility 2013;99:954-62.
45. Leese HJ, Hooper MAK, Edwards RG, Ashwood-Smith MJ. Uptake of pyruvate by early human embryos determined by a non- invasive technique. Human reproduction 1986;1:181-2.
46. Gott AL, Hardy K, Winston RML, Leese HJ. Non-invasive measurement of pyruvate and glucose uptake and lactate production by single human preimplantation embryos. Human reproduction 1990;5:104-8.
47. Gardner DK, Wale PL, Collins R, Lane M. Glucose consumption of single post-compaction human embryos is predictive of embryo sex and live birth outcome. Human reproduction 2011;26:1981-6.
48. Picton HM, Elder K, Houghton FD, Hawkhead JA, Rutherford AJ, Hogg JE et al. Association between amino acid turnover and chromosome aneuploidy during human preimplantation embryo development in vitro. Molecular human reproduction 2010;16:557-69.
49. Brison DR, Houghton FD, Falconer D, Roberts SA, Hawkhead J, Humpherson PG et al. Identification of viable embryos in IVF by non-invasive measurement of amino acid turnover. Human reproduction 2004;19:2319-24.
50. Smith GD, Takayama S, Swain JE. Rethinking in vitro embryo culture: new developments in culture platforms and potential to improve assisted reproductive technologies. Biology of reproduction 2012;86:62.
51. Heo YS, Cabrera LM, Bormann CL, Shah CT, Takayama S, Smith GD. Dynamic microfunnel culture enhances mouse embryo development and pregnancy rates. Human reproduction 2010;25:613-22.
52. Seli E, Sakkas D, Scott R, Kwok SC, Rosendahl SM, Burns DH. Noninvasive metabolomic profiling of embryo culture media using Raman and near-infrared spectroscopy correlates with reproductive potential of embryos in women undergoing in vitro fertilization. Fertility and sterility 2007;88:1350-7.
53. Scott R, Seli E, Miller K, Sakkas D, Scott K, Burns DH. Noninvasive metabolomic profiling of human embryo culture media using Raman spectroscopy predicts embryonic reproductive potential: a prospective blinded pilot study. Fertility and sterility 2008;90:77-83.
54. Hardarson T, Ahlstrom A, Rogberg L, Botros L, Hillensjo T, Westlander G et al. Noninvasive metabolomic profiling of Day 2 and 5 embryo culture medium: a prospective randomized trial. Human reproduction 2012;27:89-96.
55. Vergouw CG, Kieslinger DC, Kostelijk EH, Botros LL, Schats R, Hompes PG et al. Day 3 embryo selection by metabolomic profiling of culture medium with near-infrared spectroscopy as an adjunct to morphology: a randomized controlled trial. Human reproduction

2012;27:2304-11.
56. Handyside AH, Pattison JK, Penketh RJA, Delhanty JDA, Winston RML, Tuddenham WG. Biopsy of human preimplantation embryos and sexing by DNA amplification. The Lancet 1989;8634:347-9.
57. Munné S, Lee A, Rosenwaks Z, Grifi J, Cohen J. Diagnosis of major chromosome aneuploidies in human preimplantation embryos. Human Reprod 1993;8:2185-99.
58. Mastenbroek S, Twisk M, van Ecten-Arends J, Sikkema-Raddatz B, Korevaar JC, Verhoeve HR et al. In Vitro Fertilization with Preimplantation Genetic Screening. N Engl J Med 2007;357:9-17.
59. Twisk M, Mastenbroek S, Hoek A, Heineman MJ, van der Veen F, Bossuyt PM et al. No beneficial effect of preimplantation genetic screening in women of advanced maternal age with a high risk for embryonic aneuploidy. Human reproduction 2008;23:2813-7.
60. Hardarson T, Hanson C, Lundin K, Hillensjo T, Nilsson L, Stevic J et al. Preimplantation genetic screening in women of advanced maternal age caused a decrease in clinical pregnancy rate: a randomized controlled trial. Human reproduction 2008;23:2806-12.
61. Twisk TM, Mastenbroek S, van Wely M, van der Veen F, Repping S. Preimplantation genetic screening for abnormal number of chromosomes (aneuploidies) in in vitro fertilisation or intracytoplasmic sperm injection (Review). Cochrane Database of Systematic Reviews 2006 2010;1:Art. No. CD005291.
62. Rubio C, Rodrigo L, Mir P, Mateu E, Peinado V, Milan M et al. Use of array comparative genomic hybridization (array-CGH) for embryo assessment: clinical results. Fertility and sterility 2013;99:1044-8.
63. Capalbo A, Bono S, Spizzichino L, Biricik A, Baldi M, Colamaria S et al. Sequential comprehensive chromosome analysis on polar bodies, blastomeres and trophoblast: insights into female meiotic errors and chromosomal segregation in the preimplantation window of embryo development. Human reproduction 2013;28:509-18.
64. Vanneste E, Voet T, Le Caignec C, Ampe M, Konings P, Melotte C et al. Chromosome instability is common in human cleavage-stage embryos. Nature medicine 2009;15:577-83.
65. Mertzanidou A, Wilton L, Cheng J, Spits C, Vanneste E, Moreau Y et al. Microarray analysis reveals abnormal chromosomal complements in over 70% of 14 normally developing human embryos. Human reproduction 2013;28:256-64.

Single-blastocyst transfer

Osamu Ishihara

Saitama Medical University, Saitama, Japan

Introduction

Safety and quality are the key target issues of every aspect of medical practice, and assisted reproductive technology (ART) is not an exception. The recent progress and worldwide growth of ART have attracted the attention of infertile couples as well as the general public and media. They are especially interested in the effectiveness of treatment as reflected by pregnancy rates of different techniques in each clinic. However, most of the clinicians in this field are now aware that safety and quality issues are the highest priority of every kind of clinical assessment. This attention has now extended especially to issues regarding perinatal and fetal-maternal safety after ART treatment. Among indicators of safety and quality, multiple pregnancy rates can be one of the best tools to assess ART.

Single-embryo transfer and frozen-thawed embryos

The International Committee Monitoring Assisted Reproductive Technologies (ICMART) world report for 2004 (1), the most recent and the most comprehensive ART worldwide data, indicated that multiple birth rates due to ART had decreased considerably in response to reduced number of transferred embryos that occurred in various developed countries. At the same time, the number of frozen embryo replacement/transfer (FER/T) cycles increased to 31% of the total initiated cycles in 2004; it had only been 23.8% in the previous year. More recent national data from the US national summary reported that 20.7% of the total non-donor cycles were FET in 2010 (2). In contrast, the national registry of Japan recorded 34.6% of the cycles being FET in the same year (3). This wide gap mainly seems due to the difference in the proportion of single embryo transfer (SET) and the spread of vitrification method in these two countries. Although data regarding methods of freezing and the stage of embryos are not available, the better obstetric and perinatal outcomes being suggested by recent studies of FET are reassuring with respect to safety and are likely to encourage the wider application of embryo freezing (4). Furthermore, recent improvements of cryopreservation techniques involving vitrification have resulted in highly successful outcomes (5). And it is important to remember that FET is indispensable for the transition to SET.

Assurance of clinical outcome and additional strategies

The transition to SET is indeed a milestone in the development of ART. However, the possibility of lower pregnancy rates due to the reduction of the number of embryos transferred has been the major concern for both patients and clinicians. But it was elegantly demonstrated that the cumulative live birth rate of fresh embryo transfer followed by the transfer of frozen embryo resulted in equivalent effectiveness to fresh double embryo transfer protocols (6). However, there remained concerns about the wider application of SET, in particular SET in cases of recurrent implantation failure and for older patients. An additional strategy to improve pregnancy rates with SET included blastocyst transfer because of its higher implantation rate. Improved laboratory standards and refined culture media made longer embryo culture feasible and even favorable in terms of live birth rate after blastocyst transfer (7). Therefore, we can easily imagine the dominance of single embryo transfer with fresh/frozen-thawed blastocyst transfer in the future.

Safety and quality of ART revisited

Vitrification methods and blastocyst culture are relatively new techniques in our field. Therefore, it will take some time before we know the long-term effect of these methods on growth of and health implications to newborn babies and children. However, we may be able to describe some short-term effects based on recently published data.

A population-based study using the Swedish national registry (8) suggested higher malformation rates and possible higher rates of preterm birth after blastocyst transfer. There was also a report that suggested higher incidence of placenta previa and preeclampsia after blastocyst transfer, although the finding was not statistically significant (9). However, a recent systematic review suggested that general perinatal outcomes of blastocyst transfer were similar to those of cleaved-stage transfer (10). Moreover, frozen-thawed blastocyst transfer presented no adverse neonatal outcomes and had heavier birth weights (11). The significance of a higher neonatal weight was reconfirmed as the general tendency of FET in a large-scale registry-based study from Japan (12). The data suggested that fresh embryo transfer would not be the optimal timing for further embryonic and fetal growth in the uterus since overall birth weight after fresh embryo transfer was significantly less than that in spontaneously conceived neonates. The superiority of FET to fresh transfer is also suggested by recent meta-analysis in terms of better ongoing pregnancy rate (13).

Adverse events during pregnancy and the perinatal period are also the main issues for discussion related to the safety and quality of the vitrification method and blastocyst transfer. However, a vast number of well-controlled cases are required to verify a hypothesis if the studied events happen relatively rarely. For example, a significant reduction of ectopic pregnancy was reported after frozen-thawed blastocyst transfer in Japan after analyzing 10,312 pregnant cycles after SET (14). Recent meta-analysis also reported better outcome of FET in postpartum hemorrhage, preterm birth, small for gestational age, low birth weight, and perinatal mortality (4).

Limitations and future scope

It seems almost impossible to plan a large-scale prospective randomized comparative study with enough power to distinguish differences in relatively rare adverse events during pregnancy and the perinatal period after ART. Therefore, meta-analysis is the best possible way at the moment to address safety and quality issues and has actually been repeated at certain intervals by the same authors to produce important results (15). Apart from multiple limitations of meta-analysis, however, the obvious problem is the wide variety of times and places of the studies that were included in the meta-analysis. The rapid progress of technologies and techniques in ART has resulted globally in very heterogeneous settings, protocols, and practices. For example, there are wide regional differences in the proportion of intracytoplasmic sperm injection (ICSI) cycles to the total number of ART cycles (16). In addition, the recent introduction of so-called “freeze-all policy” in some practices and countries should affect outcomes and safety in the future (17).

Therefore, alternative methods for ensuring the safety and quality of ART could be affected in the near term by analysis of data in carefully managed observational registries. We need to remain steady and focused on continuously monitoring ART outcomes in the world to create valuable information regarding safety and quality issues.

References

1. Sullivan EA, Zegers-Hochschild F, Mansour R, Ishihara O, de Mouzon J, Nygren KG, Adamson GD. International Committee for Monitoring Assisted Reproductive Technologies (ICMART) world report: assisted reproductive technology 2004. Hum. Reprod. Advance Access published February 26, 2013. doi:10.1093/humrep/det036
2. http://apps.nccd.cdc.gov/art/Apps/NationalSummaryReport.aspx
3. http://plaza.umin.ac.jp/~jsog-art/report2010.pdf (in Japanese)
4. Maheshwari A, Pandey S, Shetty A, Hamilton M, Bhattacharya S. Obstetric and perinatal outcomes in singleton pregnancies resulting from the transfer of frozen thawed versus fresh embryos generated through in vitro fertilization treatment: a systematic review and meta-analysis. Fertil Steril 2012;98:368-77.
5. Cobo A, de los Santos MJ, Castello D, Gamiz P, Campos P, Remohi J. Outcomes of vitrified early cleavage-stage and blastocyst-stage embryos in a cryopreservation program: evaluation of 3,150 warming cycles. Fertil Steril 2012;98:1138-46.
6. Thurin-Kjellberg A, Olivius C, Bergh C. Cumulative live-birth rates in a trial of single-embryo or double-embryo transfer. N Engl J Med 2009;361:1812-3.
7. Blake DA, Farquhar CM, Johnson N, Proctor M. Cleavage stage versus blastocyst stage embryo transfer in assisted conception. Cochrane Database Syst Rev 2007;4:CD002118.
8. Kallen B, Finnstrom O, Lindam A, Nilsson E, Nygren KG, Olausson PO. Blastocyst versus cleavage stage transfer in in vitro fertilization: differences in neonatal outcome? Fertil Steril 2010;94:1680-3.
9. Fernando D, Halliday JL, Breheny S, Healy DL. Outcomes of singleton births after blastocyst versus non-blastocyst transfer in assisted reproductive technology. Fertil Steril 2012;97:579-584.
10. Pinborg A, Wennerholm UB, Romundstad LB, Loft A, Aittomaki K, Soderstrom-Anttila V, Nygren KG, Hazekamp J, Bergh C. Why do singletons conceived after assisted reproduction technology have adverse perinatal outcome? Systematic review and meta-analysis. Hum Reprod Update 2013;19:87-104.
11. Wikland M, Hardarson T, Hillensjo T, Westin C, Westlander G, Wood M, Wennerholm UB. Obstetric outcomes after transfer of vitrified blastocysts. Hum Reprod 2010;25:1699-1707.
12. Nakashima A, Araki R, Tani H, Ishihara O, Kuwahara A, Irahara M, Yoshimura Y, Kuramoto T, Saito H, Nakaza A, Sakumto T. Implications of assisted reproductive technologies on term singleton birth weight: an analysis of 25,777 children in the national assisted reproduction registry of Japan. Fertil Steril 2013;99(2):450-5.
13. Roque M, Lattes K, Serra S, Sola I, Geber S, Carreras R, Checa MA. Fresh embryo transfer versus frozen embryo transfer in in vitro fertilization cycles: a systematic review and meta-analysis. Fertil Steril 2013;99:15662.
14. Ishihara O, Kuwahara A, Saito H. Frozen-thawed blastocyst transfer reduces ectopic pregnancy risk: an analysis of single embryo transfer cycles in Japan. Fertil Steril 2011;95:1966-9.
15. Hansen M, Kurinczuk JJ, Milne E, de Klerk N, Bower C. Assisted reproductive technology and birth defects: a systematic review and meta-analysis. Hum Reprod Update Advance access published February 28 2013 doi:10.1093/humupd/dmt006
16. Zegers-Hochschild F, Nygren KG, Ishihara O. The impact of legislation and socioeconomic factors in the access to and global practice of assisted reproduction. In Gardner et al "Textbook of Assisted Reproductive Medicine Vol 2, Informa 2012"
17. Maheshwari A, Bhattacharya S. Elective frozen replacement cycles for all: ready for prime time? Hum Reprod 2013;28:6-9.

Economics in the development of embryo transfer policies

G. David Adamson

Fertility Physicians of Northern California, Palo Alto, United States

Introduction

While it has long been recognized that costs associated with assisted reproductive technology (ART) affect delivery of care and embryo transfer policies, the complexities of the many relationships are just being realized. Economic theory tells us that the cost willing to be paid is equivalent to the perceived benefit gained, but traditional tools used in health economic evaluations do not lend themselves well to valuing a medical intervention that performs such a fundamental human function as reproduction. Striking economic differences in ART services are due to global socioeconomic disparities, health care systems, and public and third-party subsidization. Relative cost differences affect not only who can afford to access ART treatment but how ART is practiced in terms of embryo transfer practices, which in turn significantly impacts the health outcomes and costs of caring for ART-conceived children. Costs can be categorized and analyzed in different ways, which can affect conclusions regarding embryo transfer policies. A societal viewpoint of costs considers all direct and indirect costs regardless of who incurs them, while consumer (patient) costs generally refer to either the direct or the indirect net market charges. Aspects of economics in the development of embryo transfer policies will be reviewed.

Costs of performing embryo transfers

The first is Direct Costs, which include medical consultations, medications, laboratory and embryology services, medical procedures, hospital charges, nursing and counseling services, and administrative and overhead charges. The average cost of a single fresh in vitro fertilization (IVF) cycle in 33 high- and middle-income countries is USD $4,950, ranging from $1,800 to $12,500 per cycle, and in some low-income countries approximately $500 (1). From a societal perspective, the direct costs of treatment relate not only to the per cycle costs but also to the volume of treatments undertaken and what proportion of the total health care dollar this consumes. In Australia and the Nordic countries, ART consumes around 0.25% of the total health care expenditure, compared with 0.06% in the United States. Therefore, direct costs of ART treatment may be expensive from a patient's perspective in the United States but not from a societal perspective. While empirical evidence indicates that ART treatment is 'good value for money' from a societal and patient perspective, there remains a challenge to communicate this to policymakers, primarily because fertility treatments are not easily accommodated by traditional health economic methods.

Cost-effectiveness Analysis, which measures the outcomes of alternate medical interventions in natural units (e.g., pregnancy rates, live birth rates) can easily accommodate competing fertility treatments and embryo transfer strategies. The cost of a live birth in the United States has been calculated at $41,132 compared to Japan at $24,329 and an average of 33 countries of $32,727 (1). Other analyses have shown that ART is cost-effective compared to gonadotropins and intrauterine insemination (2). Additional studies have shown that IVF is cost-effective for certain types of infertility problems (3).

Cost-utility Analysis is the primary method used by governments to guide decisions about the allocation of public health care resources because it allows for economic comparison between disparate interventions that result in different health outcomes (e.g., immunization, cancer treatment). This is usually measured in Quality of Life Years (QALYs). Under most clinically appropriate circumstances, access to ART treatment and single-embryo transfer (SET) represents good value for money from a societal perspective (4, 5).

Affordability of treatment to patients is another way to analyze costs (6). Affordability is based on societal economic status, disposable income, insurance, and other coverage. Because of the considerable variation in funding arrangements of ART worldwide among and even within countries, the actual net cost to the consumer can be much reduced after subsidies. Public financing of ART ranges from very little subsidization in the United States and many developing countries to complete funding of a limited number of cycles for eligible patients in most European countries to unrestricted subsidization with co-payments in Australia (7). The latest estimates from the International Federation of Fertility Societies (IFFS) Surveillance indicate that in 2010 64% of reporting countries offered some form of ART financing through national health services or third-party insurers. This compares to 46% in 2004 (8). The economic burden that ART treatment represents to a consumer (that is, how affordable it is) is a function of the underlying cost of treatment, the level of public or third-party insurance to subsidize this cost, and the available income of consumers. A review of the affordability of ART treatment among countries shows even more variation in net consumer costs than in unsubsidized (gross) costs in terms of the economic burden of paying for treatment. The cost of a single fresh IVF cycle represented 52% of average annual disposable income in US states without mandates compared to 13% of average annual disposable income in the 5 US states with mandates in 2007/08. One of the most notable disparities exists between the United States and Nordic countries. The Nordic countries perform 2½ times more ART cycles per woman of reproductive age than the United States and do single-embryo transfer (SET) in 56% of fresh embryo treatment cycles compared with 13% in the United States. ART treatment is generally more affordable in European countries than in the United States. There is a strong correlation between consumer affordability and uptake of ART treatment. Price elasticity suggests that in the mid-range of prices for developed countries ($3,956 to $2,775) a 10% reduction in price would theoretically be associated with a 17.8% increase in demand (1). The behavior of consumers to lower consumer costs is not uniform. Certain ethnic groups and lower socioeconomic groups are less likely to access ART treatment even when access is improved through lower consumer costs. Studies using US data found that patients who seek treatment in response to lower cost in mandated states may include those with both better and poorer prognoses from ART treatment than those in non-mandated states.

While theoretically the correct cost of any resource is its opportunity cost (that is, the value of foregone benefits because money is spent on other societal opportunities), this is rarely quantifiable in imperfect markets such as health care. Opportunity cost in ART would be the value of babies not born because ART (and therefore embryo transfers) is not performed. The opportunity cost, discussed below, is much greater than the other costs noted and, therefore, suggests that it is worth paying for embryo transfers.

Contingent evaluation techniques to elicit society's willingness-to-pay (WTP) for ART treatments also fall into the category of Cost-benefit Analysis. While there is a lack of empirical evidence to validate whether these methods are applicable to fertility treatments, one pilot study did attempt to quantify ART treatment from an ex-post (user-based) perspective and ex-ante (insurance-based) perspective finding that the implied willingness-to-pay for a baby was $177,730 for potential child bearers in the event that they were infertile and $1.8 million for society to pay for insurance to allow couples access to ART (9). This willingness-to-pay amount greatly exceeds the cost of obtaining a baby through ART. Additionally, when employers have been willing to cover infertility costs, they have generally found the cost acceptable (10).

Indirect costs include the costs of infertility patient complications secondary to ART and maternal pregnancy complications that are increased because of ART. Generally, these complications are increased because of the population being treated, a few possibly as a consequence of the ART procedure, and the majority because of multiple pregnancy. Indirect costs include the cost of treatment complications (e.g., ovarian hyperstimulation syndrome or OHSS), patient travel costs, lost productivity, and, most significantly, the downstream costs associated with the caring for multiple birth infants.

Baby and child care and complications for singleton, twin, and higher-order births (indirect costs) are greater for ART patients than the general population. Many countries persist in having very high iatrogenic multiple birth rates. The ART multiple birth rate is 34% for the United States and 24% in the United Kingdom. These compare to rates of less than 10% in Australia, Sweden, Belgium, and Japan. The medical complications associated with multiple births and the resultant financial costs incurred in caring for infants and mothers are substantial. The maternal and infant costs of a twin pregnancy during the perinatal period are approximately three times that of singletons. In addition, the costs of caring for multiple birth infants has been shown to extend beyond the perinatal period. For example, compared to normal birth weight children, low birth weight children use more health care and educational resources to at least the age of 8-9 years. A recent cost analysis of preterm infants born in the United States as a result of ART multiple births estimated that the total health care cost was approximately USD $1 billion annually, which approximates the total direct cost of ART treatment in the United States (11). Analyses of United Kingdom and Australia data have shown that the savings in caring for multiple birth infants has theoretically cross-subsidized much of the increase in ART utilization in those countries (12).

Many treatment factors related to embryo transfer influence these costs. Controlled ovarian stimulation (COS) protocols vary from very minimal stimulation in some countries to much higher gonadotropin dosing in others. The economic assessment of different approaches to ovarian stimulation warrants more investigation because there is limited literature in this area. A non-inferiority effectiveness trial of mild ovarian stimulation with single-embryo transfer versus standard stimulation with two embryos transferred reported similar cumulative live birth rates over a 1-year period and lower costs per live birth, primarily due to lower indirect costs associated with caring for multiple birth infants and cases of OHSS in the standard ART group (13).

The day of embryo transfer affects the economics of ART. The day 2/3 cleaved live birth rate of 31% on the initial transfer after retrieval is less than the 38.8% on day 5/6 blastocyst transfer that has been calculated through meta-analysis. However, cumulative pregnancy rates are 56.8% on day 2/3 compared with 46.3% on day 5/6, which significantly favors early cleavage transfer because of better embryo freezing rates and lower rate of failure to transfer (14). Furthermore, concerns over epigenetic changes, a possible increase in twinning, and other issues with growth to blastocyst exist. Some data suggest that there is a 1.53 times increased risk of adverse neonatal outcomes with blastocyst transfer and only 1.11 with day 3 transfer compared with the general population (15, 16).

Diagnostic tests performed on the embryos (e.g., preimplantation genetic diagnosis/screening) also affect the economics of embryo transfer. While live birth rate may be higher on the first transfer of selected embryos, there are no high-quality studies showing higher or even equivalent live birth rates from an equivalent cohort of eggs at the initial retrieval. Furthermore, embryo biopsy is increasingly performed at the blastocyst stage and, while quite possibly, is superior to day 3 biopsy, has also clinically been associated with increasing twin rates because of the transfer of 2 screened blastocysts, in many cases exceeding ASRM/SART guidelines. Oocyte cryopreservation by vitrification is associated with markedly improved pregnancy rates compared with slow freezing, and newer treatment paradigms such as "freeze-all" cycles further complicate analysis of the economics of embryo transfer. As new ART techniques and treatment options enter the market they should do so based on both their clinical and cost effectiveness. However, very few economic evaluations have been undertaken before such technologies enter the market. Newer techniques are almost universally not covered by either public or third-party insurance plans. Newer technologies enabling selection of higher potential embryos through genetic testing, optical methods, proteomics, metabolomics, or other biomarkers will increase the probability of pregnancy through ART and likely encourage more use of ART for elective reproduction through the use of technology, further confounding economic analysis and subsequent policies surrounding embryo transfer. Nevertheless, careful assessment through well-designed trials is necessary before these technologies become standard of care.

One of the most common findings from studies is that the number of embryos/blastocysts transferred is related to treatment affordability. States and countries with comprehensive insurance mandates transfer lower average numbers of embryos than those with limited or no insurance mandates. These differences cannot be fully explained by differences in patient population characteristics. In a bid to reduce ART multiple birth rates, a number of jurisdictions, including Belgium, Turkey, New Zealand, and Quebec, have made public funding contingent on clinical practice guidelines that dictate the number of embryos to be transferred. Such arrangements have dramatically reduced ART multiple birth rates but have also removed clinician and patient autonomy. In contrast, Australia is a prime example of a jurisdiction in which embryo transfer practices have not been directly tied to public funding yet has achieved an equivalently low ART multiple live birth delivery rate of 8%, presumably with the assistance of a policy of supportive public funding that minimizes the incentive to achieve pregnancy at the expense of safe embryo-transfer practices (6). Also, the publication of clinic-specific pregnancy rates, especially in markets with low affordability, results in clinical practices that focus on highest possible initial transfer live birth rates, often at the cost of higher multiple rates, other pregnancy and baby safety issues, and lower cumulative live birth rates. A 10 percentage-point decrease in affordability (for example, an increase in cost of an IVF cycle from 16.7% to 26.7% of annual disposable income) would predict an average increase of 0.14 embryos transferred in fresh cycles and conversely a decrease in the percentage of SET cycles of about 5.1%, not to mention a decrease in utilization of 32%. The market incentive to attract patients over-rides the incentive to conservative embryo practices (17).

Value added by performing embryo transfers

The costs noted above have to be balanced against the benefits, including the economic value, of singleton, twin, and higher order births for both healthy and unhealthy babies (18). Despite a literature replete with the additional costs associated with ART babies, especially twins, regardless of the approach taken to valuing ART treatment the implied or explicit monetary value of providing ART treatment far exceeds the cost per child conceived. This suggests that ART treatment is indeed good value for money - particularly if ART children are born as singletons. It remains, however, necessary to meet the challenge of demonstrating the value and cost-effectiveness of ART compared to other medical interventions in order to make ART more attractive for public funding.

One of the economic values of any individual to society is his/her tax contributions. A number of studies have used investment evaluation techniques to quantify the return on government investment in ART treatment in terms of future net tax revenues over an ART child's lifetime. Using data from the United Kingdom, the discounted net tax revenue of an ART singleton child born in 2005 was found to be roughly USD $208,400, representing an eight-fold return on investment for the government (19). Of course, it only represents a good investment for couples who would not have reasonably been expected to achieve a pregnancy without ART treatment. While it is doubtful that an unconceived life is valued in the same way as a life already being lived, it is informative to look to other sectors that value human life in economic terms such as the insurance industry and transportation safety agencies. Although health care is found to elicit lower valuations of human life than other sectors, the value of a statistical life is often quoted in the vicinity of $1–$6 million. The US 9/11 government fund compensation estimates for victims are about $3.1 million (range $0.25 to $7.1 million), with an average across studies of approximately $2-$3 million per life (20). Given these numbers, even when ART results in twins the overall net benefit to society is very positive economically.

There are also many non-economic benefits of ART babies, such as "happiness," "a meaningful life," and the role that parenthood plays in life goals. The empirical research of whether parenting indeed increases levels of happiness is conflicting. However, the vast majority of people consider parenthood as a vital mode of fulfillment and there is near consensus that parenting provides for a satisfying and meaningful life. This generally remains true even when the outcome is a less-than-healthy baby.

Other factors affecting the economics of embryo transfer policy

The incidence of infertility in resource-poor countries displays wide geographic variation but is estimated to be similar to those in developed countries, at around 9% of couples. The etiology of infertility in these countries differs to those in developed countries with higher rates of secondary infertility and tubal factor infertility associated with high rates of sexually transmitted infections (STI) and postpartum infections. Patients in less-developed countries tend to be younger. So, the economics of embryo transfer will be different based on these population differences. The benefits of embryo transfer need to be considered relative to societally heterogeneous perspectives on families, children, infertility, ART treatment, and the more innovative ART technologies, as well as the regulatory environment (21). Fertility treatments are intrinsically different to other types of medical care because they are judged on their ability to create new life rather than to extend or improve the quality of existing life. Therefore, they do not lend themselves to usual health economic methods. Demographic considerations, fertility rates, and the value placed in increasing a nation's population will partially determine the desirability of investing in ART treatment, even though ART by itself cannot solve any nation's population problems. Given the strong sociocultural norms associated with ART, and the increasing use of ARTs to create nontraditional families, it is likely that other considerations such as equity of access and the perceived role of ART in population growth will play just as an important role in funding decisions as do traditional health economic methods. Education of patients, the public, and physicians about the evidence-based outcomes and economics of ART is an important factor affecting how societies will deal with embryo transfer policies. Policies that provide financial support programs, including lending and refund guarantee programs, as well as psychological support programs that reduce patient dropout rates will also affect embryo transfer policies. Appropriate and effective treatment sooner will result in shorter duration of infertility, reduced patient anxiety, and more conservative decision-making regarding embryo transfer.

ART is primarily treatment used in advanced economies such as North America, the Euro Zone, Japan, and Australia/New Zealand. Especially in these countries, ART is increasingly being used to treat people who don't have infertility in the classical sense. Emerging market economies such as China and India have grown and strengthened impressively over the last decade. It is predicted that ART demand will correspondingly increase. In resource-poor developing countries infertility is not widely recognized as a priority because the countries are overpopulated and have health care systems struggling to provide basic health care needs. Nevertheless, a growing middle and upper-middle class in these countries will also want more access to ART. Overall, ART utilization should continue to increase.

Health care systems need to ensure that any funding is directed to those patients who will gain the most benefit from them. All societies need to be educated about the role that ART plays in maximizing reproductive desires. ART treatment is not cost-effective or necessary in couples who are likely to conceive naturally in a reasonable period of time. Over-utilization of ART treatment serves neither patients nor society.

The increasing demand for donor gametes and embryos is likely to continue. The degree of legislation and commercialization governing donor treatment is greatly influenced by sociocultural and religious norms. The increasing growth of cross-border reproductive care for such services will alter the economics of embryo transfer policies.

Conclusion

With global demand for ART treatment likely to increase, it is important that future funding decisions are informed by what has been learned about how costs and economic incentives influence equity of access, effectiveness, safety, and the health outcomes of ART children. The reasons for global disparities are multifactorial and include the diversity of regulatory and funding environments, demographic differences, and the influence of sociocultural norms. The cost of treatment provides an important explanation for differences in utilization rates and embryo transfer practices. Such differences have important ethical implications in terms of equity of access, safe clinical practice, and ultimately the health outcomes and future health care resource consumption by ART mothers and babies.

The empirical evidence that does exist indicates that ART is indeed 'good value for money' from a societal and patient perspective. The total expenditure on ART remains low in most societies, and especially low in the United States, given the importance of children to most people. Economic incentives not only affect who and how many can afford to access ART treatment but how ART is practiced, especially with respect to number and day of embryo transfer and cryopreservation. Both factors have significant implications for health of mothers and even more so for short and long-term health outcomes of ART children. Increased affordability results in safer embryo transfer policies for mothers and babies. Reasonable data suggest that the money currently spent on complications arising from multiple pregnancy is sufficient to fund most of the needed IVF cycles in many countries.

In summary, based on economics, the following embryo transfer policies should be developed: 1) make ART affordable for all who need treatment, 2) single-embryo transfer be performed in a majority of patients, 3) more research be performed to understand the role of blastocyst culture, and 4) preimplantation genetic screening and other new embryo assessment technologies in order to maximize the cumulative delivery rate with at least one live born baby and the total reproductive potential for all patients (22).

References

1. Chambers GM, Sullivan EA, Ishihara O, Chapman MG, Adamson GD. The economic impact of assisted reproductive technology: a review of selected developed countries. Fertil Steril 2009 Jun;91(6):2281-94.
2. Reindollar RH, Regan MM, Neumann PJ, Levine BS, Thornton KL, Alper MM, Goldman MB. A randomized clinical trial to evaluate optimal treatment for unexplained infertility: the fast track and standard treatment (FASTT) trial. Fertil Steril 2010 Aug;94(3):888-99.
3. Van Voorhis BJ, Stovall DW, Allen BD, Syrop CH. Cost-effective treatment of the infertile couple. Fertil Steril 1998 Dec;70(6):995-1005.
4. National Collaborating Centre for Women's and Children's Health. Fertility: assessment and management (update). Commissioned by the National Institute for Clinical Excellence (NICE). Available at: http://guidanceniceorguki/GC/WaveR/90 2012.
5. Scotland GS, McLernon D, Kurinczuk JJ, McNamee P, Harrild K, Lyall H, Rajkhowa M, Hamilton M, Bhattacharya S. Minimising twins in in vitro fertilisation: a modelling study assessing the costs, consequences and cost-utility of elective single versus double embryo transfer over a 20-year time horizon. BJOG 2011 Aug;118(9):1073-83.
6. Chambers GM, Adamson GD, Eijkemans MJC. Views and Reviews. Optimal IVF in 2020: the global perspective. Acceptable cost for the patient and society. Fertility and Sterility. Accepted for publication August 2013.
7. Stovall DW, Allen BD, Sparks AE, Syrop CH, Saunders RG, VanVoorhis BJ. The cost of infertility evaluation and therapy: findings of a self-insured university healthcare plan. Fertil Steril 1999 Nov;72(5):778-84.
8. Jones HW Jr, Cooke I, Kempers R, Brinsden P, Saunders D. International Federation of Fertility Societies Surveillance 2010: preface. Fertil Steril 2011 Feb;95(2):491.
9. Neumann PJ, Johannesson M. The willingness to pay for in vitro fertilization: a pilot study using contingent valuation. Med Care 1994;32:686-99.
10. Issacs JC. Infertility coverage is good business. Fertil Steril 2008 May;89(5):1049-52.
11. Bromer JG, Ata B, Seli M, Lockwood CJ, Seli E. Preterm deliveries that result from multiple pregnancies associated with assisted reproductive technologies in the USA: a cost analysis. Current Opinion in Obstetrics & Gynecology 2011;23:168-73.
12. Chambers GM, Illingworth PJ, Sullivan EA. Assisted reproductive technology: public funding and the voluntary shift to single embryo transfer in Australia. Medical Journal of Australia 2011;195:594-8.
13. Polinder S, Heijnen EMEW, Macklon NS, Habbema JDF, Fauser BJCM, Eijkemans MJC. Cost-effectiveness of a mild compared with a standard strategy for IVF: a randomized comparison using cumulative term live birth as the primary endpoint. Human Reproduction 2008;23:316-23.
14. Glujovsky D, Blake D, Farquhar C, Bardach A. Cleavage stage versus blastocyst stage embryo transfer in assisted conception Cochrane Database Syst Rev. 2012 Jul 1;7:CD002118.
15. Practice Committee of the Society for Assisted Reproductive Technology and Practice Committee of the American Society for Reproductive Medicine. Elective single embryo transfer. Fertil Steril 2012;97:835–42.
16. Practice Committee of the American Society for Reproductive Medicine. Multiple gestation associated with infertility therapy. Fertil Steril 2012;97:825–93.

17. Chambers GE, Hoang VP, Sullivan E, Chapman M, Ishihara O, Zegers Hochschild F, Nygren K-G, Adamson GD. The impact of consumer cost on access to assisted reproductive technologies and embryo transfer practices: an international analysis. Fertil Steril Accepted for publication. August, 2013.
18. Adamson GD. Financial aspects of ART throughout the world. The Best of ESHRE and ASRM. American Society for Reproductive Medicine. Bahamas. March 9, 2012.
19. Connolly M, Gallo F, Hoorens S, Ledger W. Assessing long-run economic benefits attributed to an IVF-conceived singleton based on lifetime net tax contributions in the UK. Human Reproduction 2009;24:626-32.
20. RAND Institute for Civil Justice. Research Brief: Compensating the Victims of 9/11. Available at: http://www.rand.org/pubs/research_briefs/RB9087/index1.html . Accessed May 17, 2013.
21. Zegers-Hochschild F, Nygren K, Ishihara O. The Impact of legislation and socioeconomic factors in the access to and global practice of assisted reproductive technology (ART). in: Gardner, Weissman, Howles & Shoham (eds) Textbook of Assisted Reproductive Techniques, (2012) Volume two, chapter 69,; 441-450: Clinical Perspective, 4th Edition, London, UK.
22. Zegers-Hochschild F, Adamson GD, de Mouzon J, Ishihara O, Mansour R, Nygren K, Sullivan E, Vanderpoel S for ICMART and WHO. International Committee for Monitoring Assisted Reproductive Technology (ICMART) and the World Health Organization (WHO) revised glossary of ART terminology, 2009*. Fertil Steril 2009;92:1520–4.

Trilogy 12. Safety in assisted reproductive technology

Towards an ovarian hyperstimulation syndrome-free clinic

Edgar V. Mocanu and Joan Kelly

HARI, Rotunda Hospital, Dublin, Ireland

Introduction

Ovarian hyperstimulation syndrome (OHSS) is a potentially life-threatening complication of assisted reproductive technology (ART) treatment using gonadotropin ovarian stimulation. The full manifestations of the syndrome occur only after oocyte retrieval (OR). They are almost invariably triggered by the pre-OR administration of human chorionic gonadotropin (hCG) (Schenker and Weinstein, 1978). Clinically, OHSS manifests as abdominal discomfort and distension, nausea and vomiting, oliguria, respiratory complaints, and rarely, thromboembolic events. Severe OHSS may include pleural and pericardial effusions, profound hypovolemia, multiple organ failure, and adult respiratory distress syndrome (ARDS). Deaths from OHSS have been reported on occasion in the literature (Cluroe & Synek, 1995; Semba et al., 2000; Fineschi et al., 2006).

The reported OHSS incidence is between 0.6% and 14% (Al Ramahi, 1999; Fluker et al., 2000). According to its severity, three types have been described: mild, moderate, and severe (Golan et al., 1989). Severe OHSS represents only 0.5%-2% of the total number of cases (Forman et al., 1990; Abramov et al., 1999; Al-Ramahi, 1999). Groups of patients with a greater potential of developing OHSS (Table 1) are the ones with polycystic ovary syndrome (PCOS) (Navot et al., 1988; MacDougall et al., 1992; Buyalos & Lee, 1996), age less than 35 years (Golan et al., 1988), and lean habitus (Navot et al., 1988; Delvigne et al., 1993). These patients can be identified before stimulation. This process is, however, not perfect and any patient has the potential to overreact unpredictably. In fact, no single identifiable risk factor can accurately predict the potential, the onset, and the severity of OHSS (Delvigne & Rozenberg, 2002). For this reason, prevention of OHSS should be a major priority among ART practitioners.

From a prevention perspective, understanding the clear separation between early and late OHSS and the separate etiology is paramount. Early OHSS presents within 9 days after the hCG trigger. It reflects either overstimulation of ovaries or excessive ovarian response. It can only be prevented by not administering the hCG trigger and cancelling the treatment cycle. In the case of cycle cancellation, an endogenous luteinizing hormone (LH) surge still could trigger OHSS; thus, prevention of such surge by antagonist or agonist use should be employed until a period ensues.

Late OHSS (occurring more than 9 days after oocyte retrieval), a condition initiated by the production of hCG by an establishing pregnancy, is more likely to be severe and last longer than early OHSS (Mathur et al., 2000). Avoiding embryo transfer and affecting a freeze-all protocol when all suitable embryos are cryostored can prevent late OHSS.

Increase in number of patients affected by OHSS

Published European Society of Human Reproduction and Embryology (ESHRE) data from 1999 to 2008 show a constant incidence of OHSS (0.7%-1.2%). Yet, the number of OHSS cases reported in 2008 was 2,947, an increase of nearly 500 cases compared to year 2007 (see

Figure 1). A phenomenal 300% increase (2,947 vs. 1,083) in the annual number of OHSS cases reported by ESHRE has occurred in the 9 years of published data (Figure 1). The true number of OHSS occurring at European or worldwide level is truly unknown as significant under-reporting occurs.

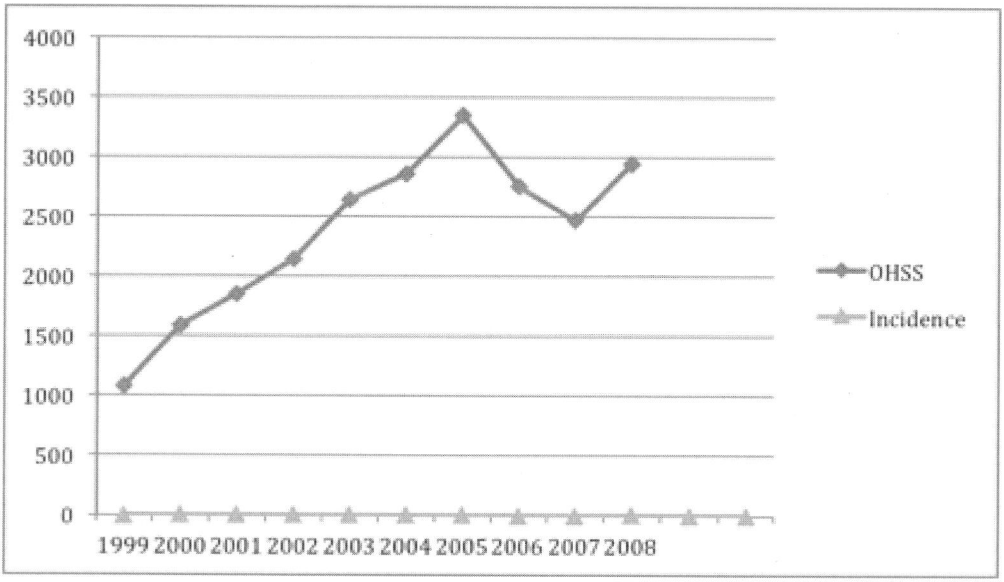

Figure 1. Continuous increase in the number of OHSS cases reported by ESHRE (1999-2008).

In the United Kingdom, the "Saving Mothers' Lives" 8th and latest publication (2006-2008) does not report any deaths due to OHSS but mentions that "*Gratifyingly, no maternal deaths appeared to have occurred as a direct result of pregnant women dying of ovarian hyperstimulation syndrome following assisted fertility therapy…, but one or two cases did occur in non-pregnant women, which are not currently classified as maternal deaths*." Of note, the 7th report drew attention to the importance of including OHSS among measured causes as 4 maternal deaths related to in vitro fertilization (IVF)-OHSS complications occurred between 2003 and 2005. Notably, 3 deaths occurred in cases of pregnant women (late OHSS).

Certain parts of the world have seen an enormous expansion in ART therapy and, as the same areas have a higher incidence of PCOS as a cause of infertility, the number of OHSS cases and subsequent severe complications is increasing. For obvious reasons, OHSS complications such as death are not routinely reported in the literature or by professional societies. While a number of professional bodies have produced OHSS treatment guidelines, there is a lack of guidelines for the prevention of OHSS at professional body level.

The OHSS prevention strategy

The main players in OHSS occurrence are the patient background risk, the medical intervention planned, and the establishment (or not) of a pregnancy (Figure 2).

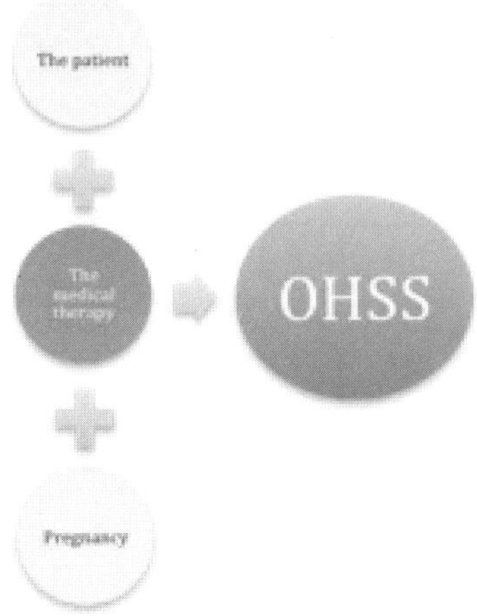

Figure 2. Main players in OHSS prevention strategy.

OHSS can only be prevented by not administering hCG for final follicular maturation, cancelling the cycle of treatment, and continuing down-regulation until a period ensues. All other methods cannot guarantee elimination of OHSS. Prevention can be optimized by initially recognizing the risk factors and individualizing ovulation induction regimens, using the minimum dose and duration of gonadotropin therapy necessary to achieve the therapeutic goal.

Yet, the assessment of OHSS risk is dynamic, a continuous feedback before, during treatment, and after oocyte collection. As the goal post changes so does the decision-making process. Every measure initiated early contributes to the reduction of OHSS occurrence.

Step I. Identification of "high-risk groups"

The first safety net is the initiative to identify patients at higher than average risk of developing OHSS. Table 1 details such well-established risk groups and suggested interventions to reduce the risk of OHSS.

The pre-treatment identification facilitates the choice of medical therapy that has been proven to reduce the risk of OHSS. Women receiving antagonists have been shown to have a lower incidence of OHSS. A recent update of a previous Cochrane Review (Al-Inany et al., 2011) analyzing 45 randomized controlled trials (RCTs) (n=7,511) comparing the antagonist to the long agonist protocols showed no statistically significant difference in rates of live births (9 RCTs; odds ratio (OR) 0.86, 95% confidence interval (CI) 0.69-1.08) but a statistically significant lower incidence of OHSS in the gonadotropin-releasing hormone (GnRH) antagonist group (29 RCTs; OR 0.43, 95% CI 0.33-0.57). Assuming comparable clinical outcomes for the antagonist and agonist protocols, these benefits could justify a change from the standard long agonist protocol to antagonist regimens.

Studies also have shown that a lower starting dose of follicle-stimulating hormone (FSH) resulted in a nearly 3-fold reduction (3.7% vs. 1.4%) in OHSS incidence compared to standard treatment FSH doses (Heijnen et al., 2007). As such, all women belonging to a high OHSS risk group should be advised to pursue antagonist and low-dose FSH stimulation, particularly women with PCOS. Furthermore, in PCOS patients the use of metformin has been shown (Tso et al., 2009) to reduce the risk of OHSS (pooled OR 0.27, 95% CI 0.16- 0.47). Although the medication has significant side effects, this intervention should be considered in patients with good tolerance once they pursue ART.

PRE-TREATMENT
PCOS
Thin habitus (low body mass index)
Elevated antimüllerian hormone (AMH) levels
Increased ovarian volume
Increased number of antral follicles
Previous OHSS
Younger than 30 years
- START ANTAGONIST protocol - Low dose FSH (150 IU or less) - If PCOS, can use metformin

Table 1. High-risk categories and proposed interventions.

Step II. Stimulation and trigger control (early OHSS prevention)

Early during the controlled ovarian stimulation treatment certain monitoring parameters can indicate that OHSS is likely to develop. A list of such clinical and biochemical parameters is presented in Table 2. Kahnberg et al., 2009, tried to identify independent factors that can predict the occurrence of OHSS. The authors showed that the only independent predictor of OHSS before hCG administration was the total number of medium/large-sized follicles. A corresponding receiver operating characteristic (ROC) found a sensitivity of 82.1% and specificity of 79.4%.

As a consequence, when a large number of follicles are evident at the time of first scan, particularly if estradiol levels are very high, reducing the dose of FSH is the first step in preventing OHSS. This will inhibit new follicular recruitment and temper both estradiol elevation and the increase in the number of follicles.

Our group (Mocanu et al., 2007) identified an estradiol level at hCG ($\geq$15,000 pmol/L) and number of oocytes ($\geq$20) above which the odds of being admitted with OHSS increases significantly. As such, our current practice dictates, apart from a lower hCG dose (5,000 IU), a delay in administering the hCG trigger until the estradiol (E2) level is <15,000 pmol/L. In our practice, it is also routine in these circumstances that a freeze-all policy is effected if more than 20 oocytes are collected.

A high E_2 result on the day of hCG is the last opportunity to modify therapy in order to eliminate or reduce the OHSS risk as shown below:

Risk elimination

1. Withholding the ovulatory trigger injection of human chorionic gonadotropin (hCG), if ovarian response is significantly high (number of follicles and estradiol level above threshold) in agonist cycles.
2. GnRH analogue trigger if an antagonist protocol was used.
3. A freeze-all protocol to prevent late OHSS.

Risk reduction

1. Reducing the dose of the hCG trigger to 5,000 IU instead of the standard 10,000 IU if the FSH dose has been reduced during the stimulation or more than 12 dominant follicles are present in agonist treatments.

DURING STIMULATION
Large number of follicles over 11 mm (>12)
High E2 levels at first scan and trigger time
Ascites
Patient discomfort, abdominal distention
- Reduce FSH dose - Establish a threshold for E_2 level at trigger - Allow E_2 levels to fall below your accepted limit prior to trigger - Cancel treatment if E_2 above threshold and not falling - In antagonist cycles, trigger with agonist - In agonist cycles, trigger with low dose hCG ONLY if safe. - If treatment cancelled continue antagonist until period starts.

Table 2. Clinical and biochemical indicators of high risk of OHSS and proposed interventions.

Step III. Luteal phase (Late OHSS prevention)
Once the hCG trigger has been administered, only late OHSS can be prevented by a freeze-all policy. In antagonist treatments, the lower pregnancy rate after transfer makes a freeze-all policy a better choice than luteal supplementation with hCG, not proven to prevent late OHSS. Measures to reduce the risk of late OHSS are detailed in Table 3.

No hCG for luteal support

Progesterone and only progesterone! A recent publication (van der Linden, et al., 2011) set to determine the relative effectiveness and safety of methods of luteal phase support in subfertile women undergoing assisted reproductive technology and showed that hCG, or hCG plus progesterone, was associated with a higher risk of OHSS. The authors suggested that the use of hCG should therefore be avoided. As the type of luteal support used does not influence the likelihood of pregnancy, the elimination of hCG use for luteal support could be the first step in reducing the occurrence of OHSS globally.

Cabergoline

Tang et al., 2012, reviewed the use of cabergoline 0.5 mg daily as means of preventing OHSS. The data showed a statistically significant reduction in OHSS in the cabergoline treated group (OR 0.40, 95% CI 0.20-0.77; 2 RCTs, 230 women). The indication for cabergoline use is women with a large number of oocytes collected and when a freeze-all policy was pursued, particularly in long protocol agonist treatments.

POST OOCYTE COLLECTION
Large number of follicles aspirated
Large number of oocytes (>15)
Ascites
Severe abdominal discomfort
- Establish a threshold in number of oocytes collected above which a freeze-all policy is effected. - Freeze-all if above threshold irrespective of protocol used* - Use progesterone only for luteal support - Use cabergoline 0.5 mg daily

Table 3. Clinical indicators of high risk of OHSS and proposed interventions.
*Where the risk of OHSS has been established to be high and a GnRH analogue has been used for trigger, an embryo transfer is contraindicated as pregnancy rates are lower and supplementation with hCG has not been proven to prevent late OHSS.

As regards to the differences between long and antagonist protocols, while customization of interventions is possible in both, differences exist and underline the enhanced risk of OHSS in long protocols (Table 4).

Intervention/ Protocol	Long protocol	Antagonist
Initial assessment	√	√
FSH dose reduction/Coasting	√	√
GnRH antagonist trigger	-	√
Reduced hCG dose (5,000 IU)	√	√
Dopamine agonist course	√	√
Freeze all	√	√
OHSS risk	**1%-6%**	**0%**

Table 4. OHSS prevention methods and type of treatment protocol.

Discussion

OHSS is a condition that can be prevented. The modern practitioners cannot, for professional and legal reasons, ignore the dangers of OHSS and pursue therapy "at any costs" any longer. The armamentarium available is extensive, from initial assessment, wise protocol choice, monitoring of follicular recruitment, and FSH dose adjustment to trigger with GnRH analogue or a reduced dose of hCG in long protocol cycles and culminating with a freeze-all approach to eliminate late OHSS. In the circumstances of ever-increasing numbers of patients receiving

ART and the explosion of IVF/intracytoplasmic sperm injection (ICSI) as first rather than last resort therapy, the number of patients diagnosed with OHSS is on the increase particularly as many young females embark on therapy, many with donor eggs.
All evidence to date suggests that in cases of "identified" OHSS high-risk patient, antagonist treatment is the ONLY CHOICE of therapy. For the same reasons, it has become unethical not to use an antagonist protocol with agonist trigger in donor and oncofertility treatments where OHSS must be avoided.
The recommendations below summarize best practice towards the elimination of OHSS in ART.

All stimulated oncology cryopreservation cycles should employ antagonist protocol and trigger with GnRH agonist.
All donor egg cycles should be stimulated with an antagonist protocol and GnRH should be used for trigger.
All PCOS patients should receive antagonist protocol. When high E2 levels or more than 12 dominant follicles are present, a GnRH analogue trigger is recommended and "elective freeze" could be considered depending on the number of oocytes collected.
Luteal support should be provided only with progesterone.
Patients where over-response was evident during previous treatments should receive a lower FSH starting dose in subsequent treatments.
Dopamine agonists should be used in patients where the risk of OHSS is present.
Final trigger should not be used unless E_2 levels are below clinic's measured threshold.
Elective embryo cryopreservation is the only method to prevent late OHSS and should be used where the oocyte number is above threshold.
All ART services should develop patient risk profiles including risk of OHSS at different E2 levels and number of oocytes collected.
Where the risk of OHSS is very significant, hCG administration should be cancelled.
While this condition cannot be eliminated, the use of correct protocols and careful monitoring with appropriate adjustment of therapy in patients identified at high risk should ensure a very rare occurrence.

Conclusions

While natural cycle IVF, in vitro maturation of oocytes, and cycle cancellation (withholding the hCG administration) are the only methods to eliminate OHSS, despite clinical and pharmacological tools existing to globally reduce the number of patients affected by OHSS, their application in clinical practice is lagging behind the evidence. Every effort should be made by professional bodies to establish and support implementation of OHSS prevention measures to safeguard patient health.

References

Abramov Y, Elchalal U, Schenker JG. (1999) Severe OHSS: An 'epidemic' of severe OHSS: a price we have to pay? Human Reproduction, 14, 2181-2185.

Al-Inany HG, Youssef MAFM, Aboulghar M, Broekmans FJ, Sterrenburg MD, Smit JG, Abou-Setta AM. Gonadotrophin-releasing hormone antagonists for assisted reproductive technology. Cochrane Database of Systematic Reviews 2011, Issue 5. Art. No.: CD001750. DOI: 10.1002/14651858.CD001750.pub3.

Al-Ramahi M. (1999) Severe OHSS: Decreasing the risk of severe ovarian hyperstimulation syndrome. Human Reproduction, 14, 2421-2422.

Buyalos RP, Lee CT. (1996) Polycystic ovarian syndrome: pathophysiology and outcome with in vitro fertilization. Fertility and Sterility, 65, 1-10.

Centre for Maternal and Child Enquiries (CMACE). Saving Mothers' Lives: reviewing maternal deaths to make motherhood safer: 2006–08. The Eighth Report on Confidential Enquiries into Maternal Deaths in the United Kingdom. BJOG 2011;118 (Suppl. 1):1–203.

Cluroe AD, Synek BJ. (1995) A fatal case of ovarian hyperstimulation syndrome with cerebral infarction. Pathology, 27, 334-346.

Delvigne A, Demoulin A, Smitz J, Donnez J, Koninckx P, Dhont M, Englert Y, Delbeke L, Darcis L, Gordts S, Puttemans P, Gerris J, Schoysman R, Leroy F. (1993) The ovarian hyperstimulation syndrome in in-vitro fertilization: a Belgian multicentric study. I. Clinical and biological features. Human Reproduction, 8, 1353-1360.

Delvigne A, Rozenberg S. (2002) Epidemiology and prevention of ovarian hyperstimulation syndrome (OHSS): a review. Human Reproduction Update, 8, 559-577.

Fineschi V, Neri M, Di Donato S, Pomara C, Riezzo I, Turillazzi E. (2006) An immunohistochemical study in a fatality due to ovarian hyperstimulation syndrome.
Int J Legal Med. Sep;120(5):293-9.

Fluker MR, Copeland JE, Yuzpe AA. (2000) An ounce of prevention: outpatient management of the ovarian hyperstimulation syndrome. Fertility and Sterility, 73, 38-45.

Forman RG, Frydman R, Egan D. (1990) Severe ovarian hyperstimulation syndrome using agonists of gonadotropin releasing hormone for in vitro fertilization: a European series and a proposal for prevention. Fertility and Sterility, 53, 502-509.

Golan A, Ron-El R, Herman A, Soffer Y, Weinraub Z, Caspi E. (1989) Ovarian hyperstimulation syndrome: an update review. Obstetrical and Gynaecological Survey, 44, 430-440.

Golan A, Ron-El R, Herman A, Weinraub Z, Soffer Y, Caspi E. (1988) Ovarian hyperstimulation syndrome following D-Trp-6 luteinising hormone releasing hormone microcapsules and menotrophin for in vitro fertilization. Fertility and Sterility, 50, 912-916.

Heijnen EM, Eijkemans MJ, De Klerk C, Polinder S, Beckers NG, Klinkert ER, Broekmans FJ, Passchier J, Te Velde ER, Macklon NS, Fauser BC. (2007) A mild treatment strategy for in-vitro fertilisation: a randomised non-inferiority trial. Lancet. Mar 3;369(9563):743-9.

Kahnberg A, Enskog A, Brännström M, Lundin K, Bergh C. (2009) Prediction of ovarian hyperstimulation syndrome in women undergoing in vitro fertilization. Acta Obstet Gynecol Scand. 88(12):1373-81.

Lewis, G (ed) 2007. The Confidential Enquiry into Maternal and Child Health (CEMACH). Saving Mothers' Lives: reviewing maternal deaths to make motherhood safer - 2003-2005. The Seventh Report on Confidential Enquiries into Maternal Deaths in the United Kingdom. London: CEMACH.

MacDougall MJ, Tan SL, Jacobs HS. (1992) In-vitro fertilization and the ovarian hyperstimulation syndrome. Human Reproduction, 7, 597-600.

Mathur RS, Akande AV, Keay SD, Hunt LP, Jenkins JM. (2000) Distinction between early and late ovarian hyperstimulation syndrome. Fertil Steril. May;73(5):901-7.
Mocanu E, Redmond ML, Hennelly B, Collins C, Harrison R. (2007) Odds of ovarian hyperstimulation syndrome (OHSS) - time for reassessment. Hum Fertil (Camb). Sep;10(3):175-81.
Navot D, Bergh PA, Laufer N. (1992) Ovarian hyperstimulation syndrome in novel reproductive technologies: prevention and treatment. Fertility and Sterility, 58, 249-261.
Navot D, Relou A, Birkenfeld A, Rabinowitz R, Brzezinski A, Margalioth EJ. (1988) Risk factors and prognostic variables in the ovarian hyperstimulation syndrome. American Journal of Obstetrics and Gynecology, 159, 210-215.
Schenker JG, Weinstein D. (1978) Ovarian hyperstimulation syndrome: a current survey. Fertility and Sterility, 30, 255-268.
Semba S, Moriya T, Youssef EM, Sasano H. (2000) An autopsy case of ovarian hyperstimulation syndrome with massive pulmonary edema and pleural effusion. Pathology International, 50, 549-552.
Tang H, Hunter T, Hu Y, Zhai SD, Sheng X, Hart RJ. Cabergoline for preventing ovarian hyperstimulation syndrome. Cochrane Database of Systematic Reviews 2012, Issue 2. Art. No.: CD008605. DOI: 10.1002/14651858.CD008605.pub2.
Tso LO, Costello MF, Andriolo RB, Freitas V. Metformin treatment before and during IVF or ICSI in women with polycystic ovary syndrome. Cochrane Database of Systematic Reviews 2009, Issue 2. Art. No.: CD006105. DOI: 10.1002/14651858. CD006105.pub2
van der Linden M, Buckingham K, Farquhar C, Kremer JAM, Metwally M. Luteal phase support for assisted reproduction cycles. Cochrane Database of Systematic Reviews 2011, Issue 10. Art. No.: CD009154. DOI:10.1002/14651858.CD009154.pub2

Safety analysis of assisted reproductive technology laboratory procedures

Kersti Lundin

Sahlgrenska University Hospital, Göteborg, Sweden

Safety "culture"

During the last decade safety issues and safety management of assisted reproduction has become an increasing part of our work. As in every aspect of health care – and of life – there are a huge number of things that potentially can go wrong. It is important to be open-minded, to try to look forward to see and prevent what might happen, and to be able to learn from mistakes and correct if and when they happen. There are a number of ways to implement a safety culture, such as;

- Having a quality management system in place (as is a demand in, for example, the European Union [EU] tissue directives)
- Continuous self-assessment analyses of the clinic and laboratory/clinic/work, including process mapping of all procedures; making sure that stated procedures are being followed
- Performing risk analyses of critical processes/tasks
- Setting up a risk assessment strategy, where potential risks can be identified, and the routines for risk analyses are documented
- Performing event analyses (root cause analyses) when things have gone wrong
- Monitoring and analyzing own results, as well as comparing to other clinics (benchmarking)

It is important in this work not to see the laboratory as a separate entity, but as part of the whole reproductive clinic. It is equally important that we do not see a mistake as the error of a separate human being, but that we look at the whole process (*why* was it possible to make this mistake). The discovery of a mistake should be seen as a chance to improve our work. Mistakes will be made and errors will occur, but we should do all we can to prevent or minimize them and, in particular, not to repeat them.

A prerequisite for being able to learn from our mistakes is that staff members are encouraged to tell when things have gone wrong. And the prerequisite for this is the lack of a blame culture and the existence of a safety culture, where safety aspects are always present in everything we do. The climate in the clinic, all the way from the top of the management, has to be allowing enough so that someone who has made or discovered a mistake can feel confident to tell what has happened.

Quality system

The official definition of a quality system from ISO (the International Organization for Standardization) is "the management system used to direct and control an organization with regard to quality." A quality system is set up by establishing a quality manual defining the organizational structure, including staff and management, responsibilities, procedures and processes, resources, and documentation.

The main goals of setting up a quality system are to prevent and correct errors, to detect deviations as early as possible, to improve efficiency, and thereby reduce costs. We want to have a "robust process that consistently produces an output with minimal variation that adheres to quality criteria." This can be rather difficult in the assisted reproductive technology (ART) business, where we have a large built-in biological variation (i.e., our patients). However, learning the variation of our processes means that we can also define the control limits and in that way limit the risk for uncontrolled variation.

Process mapping

Process mapping can be defined as a structured analysis of a process flow (such as an order-to-delivery cycle), by distinguishing how work should be done from how it is actually done, and what functions a system should perform from how the system is built to perform those functions. The strength of having your processes mapped is that you see the entirety of what you are doing, understand each other's work, may reach a common ground for future work, and may thereby improve efficiency. In this technique, main activities, information flows, and interconnections are depicted, usually in a flowchart. It is something that we do in order to understand and improve what we are doing and how we are doing it. Thus, a process map must not be drawn as "wishful thinking" of how we think the process *should* be carried out; it is important that it shows how a process is *being* carried out.

Standard operational procedures (SOPs)

SOPs are the detailed manuals for each procedure, the "cook-book." They have to be updated and easily accessible at all times. It is up to the quality management to decide the level of detail of the SOPs. Too little detail may make the procedure difficult to follow; too much detail will make the SOP difficult to read. It should be at a sufficient level to allow an experienced ART laboratory person to go in to the laboratory and perform the procedure, but not at the detailed level that someone who is not trained within in vitro fertilization (IVF) should be able to do the same.

Risk analysis and risk assessment (safety analysis): A risk = a threat

In order to identify and prevent/minimize threats and vulnerabilities of the organization and of the processes, risk analyses should be carried out for critical and "sensitive" processes. A risk analysis can be performed for a laboratory procedure as well as for an instrument or for an information technology (IT) system.

A job safety analysis (JSA) is a form of risk assessment, which details step by step how the task is to be carried out safely. Methodology is based on the idea that safety is an integral part of every job and not a separate entity. It does not have to be a huge task; it may be more valuable and effective to perform several smaller analyses within one area than one large.

A risk or job safety analysis is proactive, with the aim to prevent errors *before* they happen. Risk analyses should be part of an overall risk management strategy, where risks are continuously being identified, analyzed, and eliminated or minimized. Risk management strategies should be proactive at all levels, and can also be coupled to, for instance, an education plan.

Working with risk or safety analyses, the main process to be analyzed is broken down into a sequence of steps, the potential for risk is identified and listed for each step, and the preventive measures to overcome – or minimize - the identified risks are determined. Care must be taken not to make the steps too general. On the other hand, if the steps are too detailed, the process may become too complex to perform a proper analysis.

Questions to be answered/monitored in a risk analysis are, for instance:

- What is the likelihood of an error?
- What is the error frequency?
- How severe may the consequences be?
- What may be the cause behind the error?
- What is the efficiency of recommended measures (eliminating, minimizing, or accepting a risk)?

Event analysis

Event analysis, or root cause analysis, is the reactive measurement *after* a mistake has occurred. It is in many ways similar to a risk analysis, and it should answer the questions:

- What happened?
- Why did it happen?
- How can we prevent it from happening again?

Like in a risk analysis, the event analysis should identify the causes and compose measures for prevention and methods for follow-up.

Adverse events in the IVF laboratory

How can these procedures be translated into the ART laboratory/clinic? Performing risk and safety analyses and setting up risk management are time- and energy-consuming exercises. The ART clinic is often a very busy place, having a high workload with many things being carried out in parallel. The sad truth also is that many IVF laboratories are understaffed. These are some reasons why in general we do not do as much preventive work as we should be doing. Another reason is probably ignorance, or the inherent human way of thinking "it won't happen to me." Thus, in many organizations we do too little of proactive risk analysis and too much reactive event analysis. It is important to realize that putting more energy into preventing errors from occurring instead of analyzing and correcting afterwards usually saves time and money. So the question to put to ourselves is "Can we afford *not* to work proactively"?
Looking specifically at ART laboratory issues, we can identify a number of different types of things that can go wrong, the most common being:

- Identification errors – mix-up during handling of gametes and embryos, or during patient identification
- Technical errors – e.g., an incubator, heating block, or cryopreservation machine that is either handled incorrectly or that breaks down
- Storing problems – in incubators, cryopreservation tanks, e.g., insufficient labelling

So, why do errors occur?

Going through event analyses, the most common explanations for *why* errors occur are:

- Communication failure between staff members
- Handling errors – staff not properly trained, inattention
- Working environment factors (e.g., disturbances by other personnel, by cell phones, by internet surfing, by noise)
- Equipment failure

It is a responsibility of the management to make sure that the laboratory and the staff have proper resources and working conditions, but it also is a responsibility of everyone working in the laboratory and the clinic to follow procedures and regulations. The aim is that it should be less complicated to do right than to do wrong, and, in this, having standardized ways of working is necessary.

Mix-ups

The gravest error that can be made in the ART laboratory is mix-up of samples between patients. Working in the laboratory, often with many patients per day, demands a very high level of focus during long periods. Only a short moment of defocusing or a quick disturbance can cause a mix-up error.

In some countries (like the United Kingdom) the regulation demands that a double witnessing system, whereby a second person witnesses and signs all critical procedures, is in place. However, this system has also been criticized on the grounds that in doing this, you will continuously be asking someone else to break off from their own work in order to witness yours. In addition, the fact that two people are responsible might even be a negative factor, in that if you "hand over" the responsibility to someone else, who is actually responsible? In the long run, there might be a risk for over-confidence and attention slack.

A sort of double-witnessing can also be performed by an automatic system, using barcode labelling and alarm systems that react when barcodes that don't match are put into the same workstation. This system still requires that some procedures are manually double-witnessed by two actual persons (e.g., delivery and labelling of the sperm sample, ovum pick-up (OPU), and oocyte identification), since barcodes may still be put onto the wrong dish/tube. Thus, with a system like this it is equally important to determine which steps should be witnessed by another person.

Overall issues of prevention

To be able to prevent errors, we should have highly standardized systems. It is easier to perform correctly if you have strict guidelines and correct and updated SOPs that have been communicated to all relevant staff. And if everything is in the right place, with well-functioning equipment and being handled correctly by the right person, life will be easier as well as safer.
It is important to remember that quality pays. It will show as less waste (of time, money, and resources), more efficiency, and in the end, improved quality with lower cost.
However, quality cannot be expected to translate directly into "better" results such as higher pregnancy rates. Also, the concept of "quality" is not necessarily conceived equally in all places. Things to consider are, for example:

- Do we have enough staff? Is the workload too high or too low?
- Do we have enough of and accurate equipment? And are they validated, updated, user-friendly?
- Do we have the correct number of SOPs and is the level of detail optimal? Not enough detail or too complex? Does our staff follow the SOPs?
- Do we have conformity in procedures and handling? Are they being continuously updated and communicated?
- Are we able to track everything we do and the material we use?

In the aim to go forward and improve, there is a need and a demand for upgrading both methods and equipment. This is always a potential risk, and it is crucial for laboratories to perform a strict validation before changing any critical processes. According to the Food and Drug Administration (FDA), the goal of validation is to "establish documented evidence, which provides a high degree of assurance that a specific process will consistently produce a product meeting its predetermined specifications and quality attributes."

Processes, in addition to individual equipment, must be continuously validated. Thereby it is possible to discover divergences in performance, to create action plans, and to improve. The goal is to create a robust process that consistently produces an output with minimal variation and that adheres to quality criteria. In the end, continuous process validation should ensure a robust process that is highly reproducible over time.

In addition, "validation" (= education and evaluating performance) of staff is extremely important. It is essential that everybody working in the laboratory - or anywhere in the clinic - understands *why* and *why not*. It is important not only to know *that* you should not have the dish outside the incubator too long but also *why* (temperature, spindle disassembling, aneuploidy, pH, stress, etc.), or *why* the frozen/vitrified samples must be transferred from container to cryo tank extremely fast (recrystallization, membrane instability, etc.). To know and understand the biology and background of what you are doing is the best way to ensure that you will follow the established procedures. In the EU tissue directives (Commission Directive 2006/86/EC Annex I. B .Personnel) it is stated that a) staff should be available in sufficient numbers, b) a training program should be available, and c) that work descriptions must be clearly documented.

How do we know where we are? Benchmarking

There are also events that may not be quite as grave, for instance, that result not in the wrong sperm, oocytes, or embryos being mixed, inseminated, or transferred, but in shorter or longer periods of lower success rates. Examples of things that were not noticed and that may cause a reduction in results can be:

- Suboptimal handling of gametes and embryos (too slow handling, loss of gametes or embryos)
- Suboptimal environment (culture conditions, contamination, poor cryopreservation methods)
- Supplier changed composition (culture media, hormones)
- Machinery that performs badly over time (e.g., temperature)

In order to know how we are doing success-wise, and to see that we do not have an unidentified problem that needs trouble-shooting, key performance indicators should be monitored. For the ART laboratory, they can be:

- Percentage of mature oocytes at OPU
- 2PN (pronuclei) fertilization (and also 1 and 3 PNs)
- Intracytoplasmic sperm injection (ICSI) vs. IVF (fertilization, development, implantation)
- Cleavage rates
- Number of good-quality embryos
- Blastocyst rates
- Cryosurvival rates
- Rates of implantation, miscarriage, birth
- Adverse events
- Technical equipment errors

The question, especially for smaller units, is how often should we calculate results, how much material do we need to draw conclusions, how long a period should each measurement cover? We all know that the results may vary quite a lot for different periods, depending also on the patient population.

Summary

IVF today is a routine treatment and must be subjected to strict quality and safety routines. A majority of safety breaches in the IVF laboratory are due to problems that could and *should* be easily corrected, like risk analyses not being performed, staff not following standard operation procedures, communication problems within the unit, disturbances (breakdown of focus/attention), and breakdown of technical equipment. However, we are only human beings, and we need routines and technical/IT solutions to help us to focus, to remember, and to perform in the correct way. And most of all, the clinic's management must be driving and supporting all through the process.

References

Adams S and Carthey J. IVF witnessing and electronic systems- Final report. HFEA 2006

Bielanski A., and Vajta G. Risk of contamination of germplasm during cryopreservation and cryobanking in IVF units. Hum Reprod 2009;24: 2457-2467.

Brison D et al. Reducing the risk in the IVF laboratory: implementation of a double-witnessing system. Clinical Risk 2004;10:176-180.

European Union. Directive 2004/23/EC of the European Parliament and of the Council of 31 March 2004 'On setting standards of quality and safety for the donation, procurement, testing, processing, preservation, storage, and distribution of human tissue cells. Official Journal of the European Union 2004. L102/48.

European Union. Commission Directive 2006/17/EC of 8 February 2006 implementing Directive 2004/23/EC of the European Parliament and of the Council as regards certain technical requirements for the donation, procurement and testing of human tissues and cells. Official Journal of the European Union 2006. L38/40.

European Union. Commission Directive 2006/86/EC of 24 October 2006 implementing Directive 2004/23/EC of the European Parliament and of the Council as regards traceability requirements, notification of serious adverse reactions and events and certain technical requirements for the coding, processing, preservation, storage and distribution of human tissues and cells. Official Journal of the European Union 2006. L294/32.

http:/www.ccohs.ca/oshanswers/hsprograms/job-haz.html#_1_1

Magli C, Van den Abbeel E, Lundin K, Royere D, Van der Elst J and Gianaroli L. Revised guidelines for good practice in IVF laboratories. Hum Reprod 2008; 23:1253-1262

Mayer JF, Jones EL, Dowling-Lacey D, Nehchiri F, Muasher SJ, Gibbons WE, Oehninger SC. Total quality improvement in the IVF laboratory: choosing indicators of quality. Reprod Biomed Online. 2003;7:695-9.

Mortimer D and Mortimer ST. Quality and risk management. Cambridge University Press, 2005.

Socialstyrelsen. Riskanalys & Händelseanalys (Swedish Board of Health and Welfare. Risk analysis and event analysis). 2009.

Toft B. Independent review of the circumstances surrounding four adverse events that occurred in the Reproductive Medicine Units at The Leeds Teaching Hospitals NHS Trust, West Yorkshire, Department of Health, June 2004.

Birth defect risk following assisted reproductive technology (ART)

Richard Kennedy

University of Warwick, Coventry, United Kingdom

Introduction

Assisted reproductive technology (ART) accounts for a significant proportion of births in developed economies, and it is estimated that more than 5 million children have been conceived by this technology worldwide. An increased incidence of birth defects in ART-conceived children has been repeatedly reported, but this observation is confounded by underlying characteristics of the infertile population and the effect of infertility itself (1). This paper reviews the evidence for risk of birth defect following ART, examines the reported associations with specific abnormalities, and considers some of the possible factors implicated.

Does ART increase the likelihood of an abnormal baby?

Bergh et al. (2) reported from a national cohort of 5,856 children conceived following in-vitro-fertilization (IVF) that malformations occurred in 5.4% of all babies in the IVF group (odds ratio [OR] 1.39; 95% confidence interval [CI], 1.25-1.54). Ericson and Kallen (3), investigating the Swedish Medical Birth Registry, found an excess of birth defects in children conceived following ART (OR 1.47) that disappeared when confounders were taken into consideration (OR 0.89). Hansen et al. (4) reported infants conceived with use of intracytoplasmic sperm injection (ICSI) or IVF to have twice the risk of major birth defect as naturally conceived children. Anthony et al. (5) reported a small increase in birth defects observed in IVF children but concluded that this was attributable to differences in maternal characteristics and not to any aspect of the IVF procedure. Hansen et al. (6), in their meta-analyses of 7 reviewer-selected studies, found an OR of 1.40 (95% CI, 1.28-1.53) associated with infants conceived following IVF and ICSI. The National Birth Defects Prevention Study in the United States, investigating a population-wide case group of 30 major defects, found significant associations between cardiac and gastrointestinal defects and ART compared to natural conception (7), whereas Yan et al. (8) reported similar birth defect rates in 15,405 offspring conceived through IVF/ICSI at 7 centers in China compared to a naturally conceived comparative group. Rimm et al. (9) analyzed data from 18 studies and found an overall OR of 1.14 (95% CI, 0.94-1.4) and, after adjustment for the effect of infertility, an OR of 1.01 (95% CI, 0.82-1.23). Wen et al. (10), in their meta-analysis, found the combined effect of IVF with ICSI compared to natural conception showed a significant risk, OR 1.37 (95% CI, 1.26-1.48). Davies et al. (11) reported the prevalence of birth defects from an Australian population-wide study an unadjusted OR of 1.43 (95% CI, 1.26-1.62) compared with births following natural conception in fertile women. After multivariate analysis the OR fell to 1.24 (95% CI, 1.09-1.41).

Though the reported risk of birth defects following ART is consistently raised, caution is required in its interpretation as a number of methodological problems exist including lack of proper controls, failure to take into account potential confounding variables, anomaly surveillance subject to reporting bias, definition of birth defect, inclusion or exclusion of minor anomalies, those evident only on ultrasound, or those resulting in late miscarriage or subject to termination (12).

What are the possible causes of this effect?

Effect of infertility

The observed increase in birth defect incidence is in part explained by the underlying causes of infertility. This view is supported in several publications. Zhu et al. (13), using a Danish national birth cohort, found, compared to fertile couples, those whose time to spontaneous conception was greater than 12 months had a significantly increased chance of a birth defect (OR 1.20; 95% CI, 1.07-1.35), which was further increased in those conceiving after ART (OR 1.39; 95% CI, 1.23-1.57).

Davies et al. (11) reports births from spontaneous conception in women who had had a previous birth with assisted conception were associated with an increased overall risk of any birth defect (OR 1.25; 95% CI, 1.01-1.56).

ART process

The increasing complexity of ART exposes the developing gametes and embryos to many potential hazards. This adds to the difficulty in disentangling the impact of any given intervention on birth defect risk, and it is beyond the scope of this review to cover all the possible permutations.

a) Ovarian stimulation

Ovarian stimulation is ubiquitous with ART, and its possible adverse impact on both placentation and birth defects has been reported; however, others have found no differences in birth defects following natural conception compared to low dose and superovulation in ART. Possible mechanisms for ovarian stimulation include altered endocrine milieu affecting meiotic competence and disrupting acquisition of imprints in developing oocytes (14).

b) Culture media

Little has been published about the impact of embryo culture media on the likelihood of a birth defect, although one recent study compared two commercial culture systems and reported no significant difference in the incidence of birth defect (15).

c) IVF vs. ICSI

Intuitively, the use of ICSI should be associated with a greater risk of birth defect and there have been many studies comparing outcomes with IVF with varying conclusions as to their differential effects. A recent study from South Australia reported an OR for birth defects associated with IVF of 1.07 (95% CI, 0.90-1.26) and ICSI 1.57 (95% CI, 1.30-1.90). In the side to side comparison with ICSI, IVF was associated with a reduced risk of any birth defect (OR 0.68; 95% CI, 0.53-0.87) (11). Wen et al. (10) concluded from their meta-analysis (excluding the Davies study) no difference (OR 1.05; 95% CI, 0.91-1.20), although the combined effect of IVF with ICSI compared to natural conception showed a significant risk (OR 1.37; 95% CI, 1.26-1.48).

d) Source of sperm

In their systematic review Woldringh et al. (16) found no differences in the karyotype or incidence of birth defects. Fedder et al. (17) conducted a population-based cohort study including all births following ART in Denmark from 1995 to 2009 and concluded the rate of hypospadias, cardiac malformations in singleton boys, and undescended testicles for singleton as well as twin boys were each significantly increased from natural conception to IVF and ICSI ($P < 0.001$).

e) Extended embryo and in vitro gamete culture

Prolonged culture increases embryonic exposure to potentially harmful influences such as altered epigenetic influences, and a recent Swedish study supports the concern in outcomes. An additional risk relates to a reported increased rate of monozygotic twinning in blastocyst conceptions. What little data are available for in vitro maturation of oocytes are reassuring.

f) Cryopreservation

There has been no evidence to date that cryopreservation confers any additional risk of birth defect to the underlying ART process (11,18).

g) Blastomere biopsy/preimplantation genetic diagnosis/screening (PGD/S)

From limited data there is no evidence of an additional adverse effect on birth defect incidence when PGD/S is applied to the ART process. A single center prospective cohort study conducted by Desmyttere et al. included 995 consecutive live-born children following PGD/PGS and reported an OR of 0.868 (95% CI, 0.492-1.496) compared to outcomes from a standard ART cohort (19). Further assurance has come from Beukers et al. in a recent randomized controlled trial comparing PGS + ICSI vs. IVF/ICSI without PGS in which no significant differences were found (20).

What are the possible associations between ART and specific congenital abnormalities?

Imprinting disorders

Genomic imprinting is a normal mechanism of transcriptional regulation occurring during the preimplantation period. Disorder at any stage of this process may result in phenotypic expression as an imprinting disorder, the most well-recognized of which are Angelman syndrome and Beckwith-Weidemann syndrome (BWS). Altered DNA methylation related to the ART process is thought to disrupt normal imprinting.

Halliday et al. reported a prevalence nine times greater in children conceived through ART than in the general population whilst others have been unable to confirm this association (21). Currently, given the rarity of these disorders, it is unlikely that the risk associated with ART will ever be defined.

Cancer

Many studies have been conducted to examine the association between infertility, infertility treatment, and childhood cancer. Kallen et al. reported from a Swedish national cohort study a risk estimate of 1.42 (95% CI, 1.09-1.87) (22). Most other studies have shown no increased risk but have been based on small numbers of cancers and are also confounded by the known association of some childhood cancers and very low birth weight.

Specific childhood cancer association has been investigated with no definitive positive associations with infertility treatment including infant leukemia, hepatoblastoma, and retinoblastoma.

Cardiac

Several cohort studies have shown an association between ART and congenital heart disease in the offspring. In a recent case-controlled study in Paris by Tararbit et al., exposure to ART was significantly higher for tetralogy of Fallot, than controls (6.6% vs. 3.5%, $P = 0.002$) although this was not the case with other diagnoses (23).

Autism

Two recent large national studies from Scandinavia have shown no increase in the incidence of children with autism spectrum disorder following conception with ART.

Urogenital

Several studies have reported an association between hypospadias in children conceived following ICSI, although Silver et al. reported a 5-fold increased risk of hypospadias after IVF (24). However, van der Zenden et al., in a systematic review, reports inconsistent results and concludes that other factors, both genetic and environmental, may impact on the incidence of hypospadias (25).

Asthma

Carson et al. reported from the UK Millennium Study that asthma, wheezing, and the use of anti-asthmatic medications are higher among children born to subfertile couples than those who conceived in less than 12 months and that children born after ART have a much higher risk (26).

Longer-term outcomes

Several studies have shown that children resulting from ART conception are more likely to use health care resources. This likely stems from complications of prematurity related to multiple pregnancy and the observed increase in birth defects. Hediger et al. has recently reviewed neurodevelopmental disorder outcomes in ART-conceived children and concludes that these children do not have a uniformly higher risk (27). Longer-term data are limited, but there is no concern to date that ART adolescents do less well than their naturally conceived peers.

Conclusions

The observed data indicate a small but significant increase in birth defects in children conceived following ART. There is no clear evidence to link this risk with a specific treatment process nor is there unequivocal evidence to link ART with a specific birth defect. Given the rarity of certain disorders this latter point may never be proven. Undoubtedly, any effect is multifactorial and not least related to the underlying causes of infertility, but as ART processes increase in complexity and particularly as new techniques develop, it is essential that outcomes are recorded and linkages enabled among ART, birth, and child health data nationally and internationally.

References

1. Pinborg A, Henningsen AKA, Malchau SS, Loft A. Congenital anomalies after assisted reproductive technology. Fertil Steril. 2013; 99: 327-332.
2. Bergh T, Ericson A, Hillensjö T, Nygren KG, Wennerholm UB Deliveries and children born after in-vitro fertilisation in Sweden 1982-95: a retrospective cohort study. Lancet. 1999;354(9190):1579-85.
3. Ericson A, Källén B. Congenital malformations in infants born after IVF: a population-based study.Hum Reprod. 2001;16:504–509.
4. Hansen M, Kurinczuk JJ, Bower C, Webb S. The risk of major birth defects after intracytoplasmic sperm injection and in vitro fertilization. N Engl J Med. 2002; 346:725-30.
5. Anthony S, Buitendijk SE, Dorrepaal CA, Lindner K, Braat DD, den Ouden AL.Congenital malformations in 4224 children conceived after IVF. Hum Reprod 2002;17:2089-2095.
6. Hansen Mle, Bower C,Milne E,de Klerk N, Kurinczuk JJ. Assisted reproductive technologies and the risk of birth defects—a systematic review Human Reproduction 2005; 20: 328–338.
7. Reefhuis J, Honein MA, Schieve LA, Correa A, Hobbs CA, Rasmussen SA. Assisted reproductive technology and major structural birth defects in the United States. The National Birth Defects Preventive Study. Hum Reprod. 2009;24:360–366.
8. Yan J, Huang G, Sun Y, Zhao X, Chen S, Zou S, Hao C, Quan S, Chen ZJ. Birth defects after assisted reproductive technologies in China: analysis of 15,405 offspring in seven centers (2004 to 2008). Fertil Steril. 2011;95: 458-60.
9. Rimm AA, Katayama AC, Katayama KP. A meta-analysis of the impact of IVF and ICSI on major malformations after adjusting for the impact of subfertility. J Assist Reprod Genet 2011; 28: 699-705.
10. Wen J, Jiang J, Ding C, Dai J, Liu JD, Xia Y, Liu J, Hu Z. Birth defects in children conceived by in vitro fertilization and intracytoplasmic sperm injection: a meta-analysis. Fertility and Sterility 2012; 97: 1331-1337.
11. Davies MJ, Moore VM, Willson KJ, Van Essen P, Priest K., Scott H, Haan EA. Chan A. Reproductive technologies and the risk of birth defects. N Engl J Med 2012; 366: 1803-1813.
12. Simpson JL, Liebaers I. Assessing congenital anomalies after preimplantation genetic diagnosis. J Assist Reprod Genet. 1996;13:170-6.
13. Zhu JL, Basso O, Obel C, Bille C, Olsen J. Infertility, infertility treatment, and congenital malformations: Danish national birth cohort. BMJ 2006;333: 679.
14. Santos AM, Kuijk EW, Macklon NS. The impact of ovarian stimulation for IVF on the developing embryo Reproduction January 1, 2010; 13923-34.
15. Nelissen EC, Van Montfoort AP, Coonen E, Derhaag JC, Geraedts JP, Smits LJ, JA, Evers JL, Dumoulin JC. Further evidence that culture media affect perinatal outcome: findings after transfer of fresh and cryopreserved embryos Hum. Reprod. 2012; 27:1966-1976.
16. Woldringh GH, Besselink DE, Tillema AHJ, Hendriks JCM, Kremer JAM . Karyotyping, congenital anomalies and follow-up of children after intracytoplasmic sperm injection with non-ejaculated sperm: a systematic review. Hum Reprod Update 2010;16:12-19.
17. Fedder J, Loft A, Parner ET, Rasmussen S, Pinborg A. Neonatal outcome and congenital malformations in children born after ICSI with testicular or epididymal sperm: a controlled national cohort study. Hum Reprod. 2013; 28: 230-240.
18. Wennerholm UB, Soderstrom-Anttila V, Bergh C, Aittoma¨ki K, Hazekamp J, Nygren K-G, Selbing A, Loft A Children born after cryopreservation of embryos or oocytes: a systematic review of outcome data. Hum Reprod 2009; 24: 2158-2172.

19. Desmyttere S, De Rycke M, Staessen C, Liebaers I, De Schrijver F, Verpoest W, Haentjens P, Bonduelle M. Neonatal follow-up of 995 consecutively born children after embryo biopsy for PGD Hum. Reprod. 2012; 27: 288-293.
20. Beukers F, van der Heide M, Middelburg KJ, Cobben JM, Mastenbroek S, Breur R, van der Lee JH, Hadders-Algra M, Bos AF, Kok JH; PGS Study Group Morphologic abnormalities in 2-year-old children born after in vitro fertilization/intracytoplasmic sperm injection with preimplantation genetic screening: follow-up of a randomized controlled trial. Fertil Steril. 2013; 99:408-413.
21. Halliday J, Oke K, Breheny S, Algar E, Amor DJ. Beckwith–Wiedemann syndrome and IVF: a case-control study. Am J Hum Genet 2004; 75: 526–528.
22. Källén B, Finnström O, Lindam A, Nilsson E, Nygren K-G, Otterblad Olausson P. Cancer Risk in Children and Young Adults Conceived by In Vitro Fertilization Pediatrics 2010;126;270.
23. Tararbit K, Lelong N, Thieulin A-C, Houyel L, Bonnet D, Goffinet F, Khoshnood B, on Behalf of the EPICARD Study Group The risk for four specific congenital heart defects associated with assisted reproductive techniques: a population-based evaluation Hum Reprod. 2013; 28: 367-374.
24. Silver RI, Rodriguez R, Chang TSK, Gearhart JP. In vitro fertilization is associated with an increased risk of hypospadias. J Urol 1999;161:1954-1957.
25. van der Zanden LFM, van Rooij LALM, Feitz WFZ, Franke B, Knoers NVAM, Roeleveld N. Aetiology of hypospadias: a systematic review of genes and environment Hum. Reprod. Update. 2012; 18: 260-283.
26. Carson C, Sacker A, Kelly Y, Redshaw N, Kurinczuk JJ, Quigley MA. Asthma in children born after infertility treatment: findings from the UK Millennium Cohort Study Hum Reprod (2013) 28: 471-479.
27. Hediger ML, Bell EM, Druschel CM, Buck Louis GM. Assisted reproductive technologies and children's neurodevelopmental outcomes. Fertil Steril. 2013; 99:311-317.

Trilogy 13. Toxicants and reproduction

The ovary: The impact of environmental toxicants on ovarian function

Robert F. Casper

University of Toronto, Toronto, Canada

Introduction

In North America, the main exposure to environmental toxicants is through inhalation or ingestion of air pollution or cigarette smoke. Polycyclic aromatic hydrocarbons (PAHs) are major toxicants resulting from the incomplete combustion of any type of fuel. Benzo[*a*]pyrene (BaP) and Dimethylbenz(a)anthracene (DMBA) are the two prevalent PAHs and everyone on the planet is exposed to these toxicants through car exhaust, furnace gases, and especially through cigarette smoking.

Smoking is a serious health concern with about half a million Americans and about 50,000 Canadians dying yearly from cigarette-related diseases. Smoking-related diseases and loss of productivity from smoking cost over 100 billion dollars annually. On average, cigarette smokers die about 10 years before nonsmokers. In Canada, it has been reported that about 30% of teenage girls smoke, and thus smoking may have a major impact on reproductive function in the future. It has been estimated that women who smoke undergo menopause 1-4 years earlier than nonsmokers and mathematical modeling suggests that destruction of about 25% of oocytes at birth is required to see a 2-year advance in age of menopause.

Diseases linked to smoking include several types of cancer including bladder, esophagus, larynx, mouth and throat, and especially lung, as well as chronic obstructive pulmonary disease and chronic heart and cardiovascular disease. A recent US Surgeon General report added a number of diseases that had previously not been attributed to tobacco use to this list including acute myeloid leukemia, cancer of the cervix and stomach, cataracts, periodontitis, and abdominal aortic aneurysms.

Aryl hydrocarbon receptor agonists

PAHs are responsible for epigenetic changes through binding to the aryl hydrocarbon receptor (AhR), a ubiquitous cytoplasmic protein, which is a member of the beta helix-loop-helix/PAS family. The AhR is considered an orphan receptor since an endogenous ligand has not been identified. When aryl hydrocarbons bind to AhR, the receptor forms a heterodimer with ARNT, which then binds to a dioxin response element on DNA and induces gene transcription, specifically induction of CYP1A1, CYP1B1, and aryl hydrocarbon hydroxylase (AHH). Expression of these genes leads to an increase in reactive oxygen species (ROS) production, which may cause cell membrane damage, lipid peroxidation, and DNA damage. The metabolism of BaP and DMBA to diol-epoxides by CYP1A1 and CYP1B1 also leads to the formation of DNA adducts, bulky molecules that bind to DNA and either cause mutations or prevent repair of mutations in DNA. We, therefore, hypothesized that environmental PAHs can cause cancer, or lead to reproductive problems, through the formation of DNA adducts or ROS or a combination of both.

Identification of resveratrol, an AhR antagonist

While on sabbatical in the laboratory of Dr. Edwin Milgrim in Paris in the late 1990s, I worked with a young French Ph.D., Jean Francois Savouret, and we became interested in finding an AhR antagonist that might prevent some of the problems related to environmental pollution. We were intrigued by the so-called "French Paradox," which refers to the low rate of coronary heart disease in France compared to other Western countries at the time despite similar risk factors such as high animal fat intake, low exercise levels, and, in particular, a very high rate of smoking. What differentiated France from most of the other developed countries at the time, however, was a very high consumption of wine, in particular red wine. We speculated that red wine may contain a substance that might antagonize the adverse effects of cigarette smoke and we developed a bioassay to identify ligands to the AhR by stably transfecting a breast cancer cell line with DNA containing a dioxin response element coupled to the thymidine kinase promoter and a chloramphenicol acetyltransferase (CAT) reporter gene. We then reviewed the literature to identify polyphenolic chemicals present in red wine and compared their chemical structure with that of dioxin or PAHs. We tested many of these chemicals in the bioassay to see if they could inhibit dioxin response element activation by dioxin (TCDD), the cognate aryl hydrocarbon receptor ligand.

Using the bioassay, we determined that trans-resveratrol, a trihydroxystilbene, was able to inhibit activation of the AhR with half maximal inhibition between the micromolar and nanomolar range. We went on to show specific binding to the AhR by displacement of radiolabeled TCDD and by translocation of the AhR from the cytoplasm into the nucleus cells in vitro. Finally, in vivo studies in rats were able to demonstrate that the induction of CYP1A1 and CYP1B1 by benzo[*a*]pyrene and dimethylbenz(a)anthracene could be completely inhibited by co-administration of resveratrol. These experiments, therefore, confirmed for the first time that resveratrol was a pure aryl hydrocarbon receptor antagonist with no apparent agonistic activity at all and appeared to be unique as a naturally occurring plant-based ligand (1).

Resveratrol is produced by grapes and is found in the skins and seeds. Resveratrol is also produced in large quantities in the root of a weed called polygonum cuspidatum, which is found growing wild in the Far East. Resveratrol concentrations are measureable in red wine since it is a lipid-soluble chemical that is extracted from the skin of the grape when in contact with alcohol. It is not present in white wine since juice is squeezed from the grapes and fermented separately from the skins. Since resveratrol is a phytoalexin and is used by plants to protect against mold and mildew, it is found in the highest concentrations in wines from countries with a temperate climate where the vines are exposed to some fungal pressure. This observation is consistent with the hypothesis that resveratrol may be a protective agent in French red wine that accounts for the low rate of heart disease.

Effects of PAH on reproduction

One of the negative health effects of environmental pollution is in the area of reproduction. Our group in Toronto has had a longstanding interest in examining the effects of cigarette smoking on both sperm and oocyte function. Almost 20 years ago, Maria Teresa Zenses in our laboratory showed that women who smoked had an increase in oocyte meiotic dysfunction resulting in a high proportion of diploid oocytes collected at the time of in vitro fertilization (IVF) compared to nonsmokers. She also found that even women who didn't smoke but who were exposed to second-hand cigarette smoke from a partner had an increased incidence of diploid oocytes as well (2). These oocytes, when fertilized, resulted in triploid embryos. We also demonstrated that sperm obtained from men who smoked contained PAH DNA adducts, which were transmitted to the embryo at the time of fertilization, thereby establishing a plausible mechanism for epigenetic changes in the embryo and fetus as a result of paternal cigarette smoking (3).

Xenograft model of human ovary

We were interested in examining the potential mechanism of the adverse effect of cigarette smoking on reproductive function and on the age of menopause and utilized an in vivo xenograft model developed in the laboratory by Dr. Ariel Weissman when he was a research fellow (4). We determined that human ovarian cortex could be transplanted subcutaneously into the flanks of nonobese diabetic/severe combined immunodeficiency (NOD-SCID) mice where the ovarian tissue would engraft, develop a blood supply, and follicles could be stimulated to grow after a few months using gonadotropins. This model also provided us with a means to examine the effects of the environmental toxicants found in cigarette smoke. We demonstrated that after exposure to DMBA, about half of the secondary follicles became atretic within 24 hours, about half of the primary growing follicles were atretic by 48 hours, and about 10% of primordial follicles became atretic by 72 hours. We demonstrated that follicle and oocyte death was likely related to Bax and p53 up-regulation in the ovaries after PAH exposure (5), and that Bax knockout mice had granulosa cells that seem to be resistant to apoptosis induced by PAHs (6). Finally, we demonstrated that co-treatment of these mice with resveratrol and DMBA prevented the upregulation of Bax and oocyte atresia. This work was published in collaboration with Jon Tilly's laboratory at Harvard.

Transgenerational effects of PAH

Dr. Jurisicova in our group went on to study the transplacental and lactational transfer of PAHs in a mouse model. Our goal was to investigate the possible adverse effects of maternal PAH exposure on the gonads of the offspring. To mimic smoking in humans, we administered a mixture of BaP and DMBA at a relatively low dose for 3 weeks before pregnancy and then again after delivery during lactation. We used a cross-fostering design with the pups divided at birth between lactating mothers given PAH or oil injections. As a result of this design, some of the pups were exposed to PAH during pregnancy only, some were exposed during lactation only, and some were exposed to PAHs both during pregnancy as well as during lactation. We were able to demonstrate that the aryl hydrocarbons administered triggered transcription of CYP1A1 in the lungs of the mothers and in the lungs of 3-week-old F-1 females, demonstrating that transplacental exposure of the offspring did occur. We also demonstrated significant atresia of the follicles in both groups of offspring with the highest level of atresia in the group that received PAH exposure both transplacentally and during lactation. Of major interest to us, in view of our previous work, pretreatment of the mice with resveratrol prevented the loss of ovarian follicles in the offspring. Mechanistically, we examined Bax immunostaining in the ovaries of 3-week-old mice that had been exposed to PAH or to oil injections to the mothers and found that Bax immunostaining was up-regulated following transplacental or lactational exposure to PAHs. Resveratrol pretreatment of the mothers inhibited Bax protein expression. We demonstrated that expression of a binding partner of Bax called Harikari (Hrk) was also increased after PAH exposure and could be inhibited by resveratrol pretreatment or by AhR knockout (7). In summary, we demonstrated that exposure of adult mice to PAH either preconceptionally or lactationally resulted in decreased primordial and primary follicle counts in F-1 offspring at the age of 3 weeks and at the age of 8 weeks. We were able to demonstrate increased cell death gene expression in the oocytes and granulosa cells of the offspring of PAH-exposed animals and we found that resveratrol, a naturally occurring stilbene produced by spermatocyte plants, was able to reverse the adverse effects of PAH exposure on the offspring. The findings of this study raised concerns clinically that women who smoke may transfer PAHs to their offspring, especially during breastfeeding since PAHs are present in the lipid portion of breast milk. However, we more recently identified an endogenous AhR modulator, 7-keto-cholesterol, that appears to be able to compete with PAH for binding to the DRE on DNA and to block gene expression induced by PAH in vitro (8). 7-keto-cholesterol is present in breast milk at concentrations greater than in serum and may play a protective role by blocking any adverse effects of breast milk PAH in the infants.

Effects of PAH on the male

We have previously shown that PAHs caused DNA damage and apoptosis of spermatozoa in BalbC mice and that these adverse effects could be prevented by resveratrol (9). Therefore, we also examined the testes of male offspring of the animals in the transgenerational experiment and found that there were many empty seminiferous tubules as a result of germ cell apoptosis in the mice at 3 weeks of age. Interestingly, and in contrast to the female offspring, the seminiferous tubules were repopulated with cells by 8 weeks of postnatal life. This finding suggests that the testes were able to regenerate their spermatogenic activity, likely as a result of germ line stem cells that are not completely destroyed by PAH exposure, whereas this phenomenon was not observed in the female offspring. This observation may be of interest in light of the recent data from the Tilly laboratory suggesting that oocyte stem cells exist. These oocyte stem cells may not be functional in replacing oocytes postnatally since neither mice nor humans seem to be able to regenerate oocytes from damaged ovaries.

Conclusion

Cigarette smoke and other sources of polycyclic aromatic hydrocarbons in environmental pollution have a negative effect on reproductive function. PAHs increase expression of cell death genes in the ovary and stimulate the formation of DNA adducts and ROS in all tissues. We have demonstrated that there may also be transgenerational effects of PAHs in an animal model with adverse effects on both male and female gametes. Resveratrol, a naturally occurring trihydroxystilbene, produced by spermatocyte plants, is an AhR antagonist that appears to be unique in that it has no AhR agonist activity and no observed toxicity. Resveratrol, in an appropriate delivery vehicle (it is highly lipophilic) might prove to be a valuable dietary supplement to prevent AhR-mediated toxicity clinically. More research is needed in this interesting area.

References

1. Casper RF, Quesne M, Rogers I, Shirota T, Jolivet A, Milgrom E, Savouret J-F. Resveratrol has antagonist activity on the aryl hydrocarbon receptor: Implications for prevention of dioxin toxicity. Molecular Pharmacology, 1999;56:784-790.
2. Zenzes MT, Wang P, Casper RF. Cigarette smoking may affect meiotic maturation of human oocytes. Human Reprod. 1995;10:3213-17.
3. Zenzes MT, Puy LA, Bielecki R, Reed TE. Detection of benzo[a]pyrene diol epoxide-DNA adducts in embryos from smoking couples: evidence for transmission by spermatozoa. Mol Hum Reprod. 1999;5:125-31.
4. Weissman A, Gotlieb L, Colgan T, Jurisicova A, Greenblatt EM, Casper RF. Preliminary Experience with Subcutaneous Human Ovarian Cortex Transplantation in the NOD-SCID Mouse Model. Biol Reprod, 1999;60:1462-1467.
5. Detmar J, Rabaglino T, Taniuchi Y, Oh J, Acton BM, Benito A, Nunez G, Jurisicova A. Embryonic loss due to exposure to polycyclic aromatic hydrocarbons is mediated by Bax. Apoptosis. 2006;11:1413-25.
6. Matikainen T, Perez G, Jurisicova A, Schlezinger JJ, Ryu, H-Y, Sakai T, Korsmeyer SJ, Casper RF, Sherr DH, Tilly JL. Aromatic hydrocarbon receptor-dependent bax gene expression is required for ovarian failure caused by biohazardous environmental chemicals. Nature Genetics, 2001;28:355-360.
7. Jurisicova A, Taniuchi A, Li H, Shang Y, Antenos M, Detmar J, Xu J, Matikainen T, Hernandez AB, Nunez G, Casper RF. Maternal exposure to polycyclic aromatic hydrocarbons diminishes murine ovarian reserve via induction of Harakiri. J Clin Invest. 2007;117:3971-8.
8. Savouret JF, Antenos M, Quesne M, Xu J, Milgrom E, Casper RF. 7-ketocholesterol is an endogenous modulator for the Aryl hydrocarbon Receptor. J Biol Chem 2001;276:3054-3-59.
9. Revel A, Raanani H, Younglai E, Xu J, Rogers I, Han R, Savouret J-F, Casper RF. Resveratrol, a natural aryl hydrocarbon receptor antagonist, protects sperm from DNA damage and apoptosis caused by Benzo(a)pyrene. Reproductive Toxicology. 2001;15:479-486.

Toxicants in pregnancy and neonatal outcome

Tracey Woodruff and Dylan Atchley

University of California, San Francisco, United States

Reproductive environmental health

A substantial body of knowledge has demonstrated that preconception and prenatal environmental exposures can adversely impact reproductive health throughout the life course (1-3). Furthermore, given the ubiquity of environmental exposures, they have been implicated in increases in adverse reproductive health outcomes such as autism (4), childhood cancer (5), preterm birth (6), and obesity in women (7). These increases have occurred relatively rapidly during various time periods starting after World War II, and they cannot be explained by genetics, which is a slower, more gradual process.

The environmental drivers of reproductive health are many and varied. Of critical concern for reproductive health professionals is the ubiquity of patient exposure to manufactured chemicals and metals (8). In the past 70 years, the manufacture and use of industrial chemicals has increased more than 15-fold (9). Currently in the United States, approximately 700 new chemicals are introduced into commerce each year and more than 84,000 chemical substances are listed by the US Environmental Protection Agency (EPA) for manufacturing, processing, or importation (10, 11); overall about 3,000 of these chemicals are used or imported in high volumes (greater than 1 million pounds) (10). But due to the current regulatory structure, unlike pharmaceuticals, the vast majority of environmental chemicals in commerce have entered the marketplace without comprehensive and standardized information on their reproductive or other chronic toxicities (12, 13).

Maternal exposure

Environmental chemicals are pervasive in all aspects of peoples' lives, including in air, water, soil, food, and consumer products. As a result, among pregnant women, daily exposure to many and varied toxic chemicals is now the norm. An analysis of National Health and Nutrition Examination Survey (NHANES) data from 2003-2004 found that virtually every pregnant woman in the United States was exposed to at least 43 different chemicals (14). Furthermore, occupational exposures (15) and other factors such as geography (16), race, and socioeconomic class (17) make certain populations of women particularly vulnerable to environmental chemical exposures. For example, in the United States, minority populations are more likely to live in the counties with the highest levels of outdoor air pollution (18) and to be exposed to a variety of indoor pollutants, including lead, allergens, and pesticides (19).

Many of the chemicals found in virtually all pregnant women are persistent organic pollutants (POPs), chemicals that are resistant to environmental degradation and remain in the environment for long periods of time. For example, the organochlorine pesticide DDT and several polychlorinated biphenyls (PCBs) were recently detected in nearly 100% of pregnant women sampled in the United States despite being banned in the United States for over 30 years, as well as in many other parts of the world (20). Other frequently detected compounds include persistent and bioaccumulative chemicals that have been more recently phased out such as several perfluorochemicals (PFCs) and polybrominated diphenylethers (PBDEs) (20). Furthermore, the persistent nature of these chemicals allows them to circulate throughout the global environment; studies have measured POPs and heavy metals in pregnant women in remote populations in the

Arctic, indicating a global incidence of pollution exposure (21).

Fetal exposure

Maternal body burden of chemicals during pregnancy can lead to fetal exposure, as chemicals can transfer across the placenta and into the fetus. In 2010, the National Cancer Institute's President's Report on Cancer observed that "to a disturbing extent babies are born 'pre-polluted'" (22). A wide range of chemicals have been detected in various fetal matrices, including pharmaceuticals, illicit drugs, alcohol, tobacco, metals, pesticides, PCBs, PBDEs, and phytoestrogens (23). Persistent chemicals (e.g., PBDEs, PFCs) are typically lipophilic or bind to proteins that enter the hepatic bloodstream circulation and can expose the fetus directly. Studies at birth of these classes of chemicals are a more reasonable proxy for early and mid-gestation exposures because of their long half-life. On the other hand, the transfer of non-lipophilic compounds that are rapidly metabolized (e.g., bisphenol A) is more difficult to predict as research suggests several possible metabolic determinants for fetal exposure.

The specific structure, chemical composition, and relative persistence of xenobiotic chemicals determine the pattern of placental transfer. Some xenobiotic chemicals are capable of bioaccumulating in the fetus resulting in greater exposure during this very sensitive period of development, while others are transferred in equal proportion. For example, fetal methyl mercury levels have been shown to be about 1.7 times greater than maternal levels (24). Maternal health conditions can also influence the extent to which chemicals can cross the placenta. For example, high blood pressure and maternal alcohol use during the second and third trimesters have been associated with relatively greater fetal blood lead concentration compared to maternal concentrations, while other factors appear to reduce the degree of transfer (25).

Critical and sensitive windows of development

Timing of exposure

The human reproductive system is particularly vulnerable to environmental chemicals when the exposure occurs during "critical" or "sensitive" windows of development (1, 26-28). This is because these are times of extensive developmental changes, such as cellular proliferation and rapidly changing and/or undeveloped metabolic, hormonal, and immunologic capabilities (29). Even very small amounts of chemical exposures during windows of vulnerability can either increase risk of or lead to adverse birth outcomes, as well as risks of disease and disability across the lifespan (30, 31). The link between fetal and other developmental exposures and increased risk of disease later in life is known as "developmental programming," or "the developmental origins of adult health and disease" and has been substantiated and refined by a large body of experimental and epidemiologic data (3, 29, 32).

Mechanisms of action

Three important mechanisms related to environmental chemical exposures during critical and sensitive windows of development are mutagenesis and the inter-related mechanisms of epigenetics and hormone disruption. Mutagens impact DNA directly. For example, ionizing radiation-induced cancer results from complex forms of DNA double-strand breaks (33). In contrast, "epigenetic" mechanisms disrupt gene expression integral to orchestrating healthy human development without changing DNA (34). Finally, "endocrine disrupting chemicals" (EDCs) act by "interfering with the synthesis, secretion, transport, binding, action, or elimination of natural hormones in the body that are responsible for the maintenance of homeostasis (normal cell metabolism), reproduction, development, and/or behavior" (35). Because hormonal regulation is critical to human reproduction, chemicals that perturb the endocrine system may cause permanent effects (1, 30, 36-38).

Neonatal health outcomes

Prenatal exposure to certain environmental chemicals is linked to a wide range of health consequences that can manifest across the lifetime of individuals and potentially be transmitted to the next generation (39). The dangers of prenatal exposure to cigarette smoke and alcohol have been well-established. Now, there is a growing body of evidence that environmental chemicals can have similar deleterious effects on reproduction and development. For example, pesticides are applied in large quantities in agricultural, community, and household settings and humans are exposed through a myriad of sources including food, water, and air. An analysis of NHANES data from 2003-2004 found that every pregnant women tested was exposed to at least one pesticide (14). Exposure to pesticides has been linked to impaired neurodevelopment (40, 41), impaired fetal growth (42), increased susceptibility to testicular cancer (43), and several childhood cancers (44).

Similarly, phthalates are a class of synthetically derived chemicals used in a variety of consumer goods such as medical devices, cleaning and building materials, personal care products, cosmetics, pharmaceuticals, food processing, and toys. Exposure occurs through ingestion, inhalation, and dermal absorption, and as with pesticides, NHANES data from 2003-2004 showed that every pregnant women tested was exposed to at least one phthalate (45). A number of phthalates have been shown to be anti-androgenic and exposure to phthalates has been linked to reduced masculine play in boys (46), reduced anogenital distance (47), shortened gestational age (48), and impaired neurodevelopment in girls (49).

For a more comprehensive list of examples of reproductive health impacts of prenatal exposure to environmental contaminants refer to Sutton et al., 2012 (50).

Evidence available for decision-making in environmental health

The type of scientific evidence available for clinical decision-making differs in character from the evidence used in environmental health science. The "gold-standard" for informing clinical risk-benefit decisions about medical interventions is a well-conducted, randomized controlled trial (RCT). However, in environmental health science, ethics virtually precludes RCTs to discover adverse impacts of environmental chemicals on health, and there is no comprehensive comparable weighing of health benefits and risks in the environmental arena (51) because chemicals are not designed to have a direct health benefit.

Therefore, clinicians must rely on animal and other non-human experimental data and human observational studies to shape patient recommendations and prevention strategies in environmental health. Studies have established the concordance of developmental and reproductive effects between in vitro animal and human studies and concluded that humans are as sensitive or more sensitive than even the most sensitive animal species (52, 53). Experimental animal studies are most appropriate for prevention of harmful chemical exposures as observational human studies can require many years and adverse effects in humans.

To bridge the gap between evidence streams in clinical and environmental health sciences, a methodology called the Navigation Guide has been developed to evaluate the quality of evidence and strength of recommendations about the relationship between the environment and reproductive health in uniform, simple, and transparent summaries that integrate best practices of evaluation in environmental and clinical health sciences (54).

Recommendations for prevention

The evidence linking environmental exposures to adverse reproductive and developmental health outcomes is sufficiently robust that leading scientists, reproductive health clinicians, and other clinical practitioners are calling for timely action to prevent harm (1, 22, 26, 31, 39). Reproductive health care providers can be extremely effective in preventing prenatal exposure to environmental threats to health because they are uniquely poised to intervene during pregnancy—and thus impact exposures during a critical window of human development. An important outcome of pregnancy is no longer just a healthy newborn but a human being optimally programmed for health from infancy through old age (3, 29, 55, 56). By taking steps to address the environmental drivers of health, reproductive health professionals can have a large and enduring beneficial impact on patient health.

Provide anticipatory guidance

Clinicians should intervene as early as possible during pregnancy to alert patients on how to avoid toxic, and ensure beneficial, environmental exposures. By the first prenatal care visit, exposure to environmental toxicants and disruptions of organogenesis may have already occurred. Reproductive health providers' patient interactions occur at an opportune time for affecting change. Individuals hoping to bear children are intensely interested in the impact of the environment on their pregnancies and the health of their future children, and they look to their health care providers for guidance on how to avoid potentially harmful exposures. Health providers can serve a critical role as a science-based source of guidance on how to avoid potentially adverse exposures (57, 58).

Reproductive health professionals do not need to be experts in environmental health to provide useful information to patients, take an exposure history, and make referrals when hazardous exposures are identified. Existing clinical experience and expertise in communicating risks of treatment are also largely transferable to environmental health. Physician contact time with a patient does not need to be the primary point of intervention; information and resources about environmental hazards can be successfully incorporated into childbirth class curriculum to help women and men make optimal choices for themselves and their children (59).
Resources for clinicians who want to learn more about reproductive environmental health and a set of low-literacy patient brochures on ways to avoid harmful chemical exposures can be found at http://prhe.ucsf.edu/prhe/.

Advance prevention-oriented policy

Evidence-based recommendations for preventing harmful environmental exposures must ultimately involve policy change (60). While action at the individual level can reduce exposure to some toxic chemicals (61-63), and while informed consumer-purchasing patterns can send a signal to the marketplace to help drive societal change (64, 65), individuals alone can do little to impact many harmful environmental exposures, such as from air and water pollution and those exacerbated by poverty. Thus, the role of clinicians extends well beyond the clinic (45, 66). The incorporation of the authoritative voice of health professionals in policy arenas is critical to translating emerging scientific findings into prevention-oriented action on a larger scale (50), and accordingly, many medical associations have taken steps in that direction (67).

References

1. Diamanti-Kandarakis E, Bourguignon JP, Giudice LC, Hauser R, Prins GS, Soto AM, et al. Endocrine-disrupting chemicals: an Endocrine Society scientific statement. Endocr Rev 2009;30:293-342.
2. Woodruff TJ, Janssen SJ, Guillette LJ, Jr., Giudice LC. Environmental impacts on reproductive health and fertility. 2010, New York, NY: Cambridge University Press.
3. Boekelheide K, Blumberg B, Chapin RE, Cote I, Graziano JH, Janesick A, et al. Predicting later-life outcomes of early-life exposures. Environ Health Perspect 2012;120:1353-61.
4. Rice C. Prevalence of autism spectrum disorders - Autism and Developmental Disabilities Monitoring Network, United States, 2006. MMWR Surveill Summ 2009;58:1-20.
5. U.S. Environmental Protection Agency. America's Children and the Environment. 2010 [cited 2010; Available from: http://www.epa.gov/envirohealth/children/child_illness/d6-graph.html].
6. Martin JA, Hamilton BE, Ventura SJ, Osterman MJK, Wilson EC, Mathews TJ, et al. Births: Final Data for 2010. in National Vital Statistics Reports. N.V.S. Service, Editor 2012, Centers for Disease Control and Prevention: Atlanta.
7. Fryar CD, Carroll MD, Ogden CL. Prevalence of Overweight, Obesity, and Extreme Obesity Among Adults: United States, Trends 1960–1962 Through 2009–2010. in Health E-Stat. N.C.f.H. Statistics, Editor 2012, U.S. Centers for Disease Control and Prevention,: Atlanta
8. American Congress of Obstetricians and Gynecologists. Environmental Exposures. Committee Opinion. . Obstet Gynecol In Review.
9. Federal Reserve Board. G.17 - Industrial Production and Capacity Utilization, Industrial Production for Chemicals (NAICS=325). 2008 August 14, 2009 [cited 2008 August 18, 2008];http://www.federalreserve.gov/datadownload/Download.aspx?rel=G17&series=4374e8caec6beeaa874d28776fa68c1e&filetype=spreadsheetml&label=include&layout=seriescolumn&from=01/01/1919&to=12/31/2009].
10. U.S. Environmental Protection Agency. Office of Pollution Prevention and Toxics Programs. 2007 January 2007 [cited 2011 May 3]; Available from: http://www.epa.gov/oppt/pubs/oppt101c2.pdf].
11. U.S. Environmental Protection Agency. TSCA Chemical Substance Inventory. 2012 [cited 2012 September 12]; Available from: http://www.epa.gov/oppt/existingchemicals/pubs/tscainventory/basic.html].
12. Vogel SA,Roberts JA. Why The Toxic Substances Control Act Needs An Overhaul, And How To Strengthen Oversight Of Chemicals In The Interim. Health Aff (Millwood) 2011;30:898-905.
13. Wilson MP,Schwarzman MR. Toward a new US chemicals policy: Rebuilding the foundation to advance new science, green chemistry, and environmental health. Environ Health Perspect 2009;117:1202.
14. Woodruff TJ, Zota AR, Schwartz JM. Environmental chemicals in pregnant women in the US: NHANES 2003-2004. Environ Health Perspect 2011;119:878-85.
15. Figa-Talamanca I. Occupational risk factors and reproductive health of women. Occup Med (Lond) 2006;56:521-31.
16. Zota AR, Park JS, Wang Y, Petreas M, Zoeller RT, Woodruff TJ. Polybrominated diphenyl ethers, hydroxylated polybrominated diphenyl ethers, and measures of thyroid function in second trimester pregnant women in California. Environ Sci Technol 2011;45:7896-905.
17. Morello-Frosch R, Zuk M, Jerrett M, Shamasunder B, Kyle AD. Understanding the cumulative impacts of inequalities in environmental health: implications for policy. Health Aff (Millwood) 2011;30:879-87.

18. Woodruff TJ, Parker JD, Kyle AD, Schoendorf KC. Disparities in exposure to air pollution during pregnancy. Environ Health Perspect 2003;111:942-6.
19. Adamkiewicz G, Zota AR, Fabian MP, Chahine T, Julien R, Spengler JD, et al. Moving Environmental Justice Indoors: Understanding Structural Influences on Residential Exposure Patterns in Low-Income Communities. Am J Public Health 2011.
20. Centers for Disease Control and Prevention. Fourth National Report on Human Exposure to Environmental Chemicals, Updated Tables. 2012: Atlanta, GA.
21. Artic Monitoring and Assessment Programme (AMAP). AMAP Assessment 2009: Human Health in the Arctic. 2009: Oslo.
22. Reuben SH,President's Cancer Panel. Reducing Environmental Cancer Risk: What We Can Do Now. 2010, National Cancer Institute: Bethesda.
23. Barr DB, Bishop A, Needham LL. Concentrations of xenobiotic chemicals in the maternal-fetal unit. Reproductive toxicology 2007;23:260-6.
24. Stern AH,Smith AE. An assessment of the cord blood: maternal blood methylmercury ratio: implications for risk assessment. Environ Health Perspect 2003;111:1465.
25. Harville E, Hertz-Picciotto I, Schramm M, Watt-Morse M, Chantala K, Osterloh J, et al. Factors influencing the difference between maternal and cord blood lead. Occup Environ Med 2005;62:263-269.
26. Grandjean P, Bellinger D, Bergman A, Cordier S, Davey-Smith G, Eskenazi B, et al. The faroes statement: human health effects of developmental exposure to chemicals in our environment. Basic & clinical pharmacology & toxicology 2008;102:73-5.
27. Crain DA, Janssen SJ, Edwards TM, Heindel J, Ho SM, Hunt P, et al. Female reproductive disorders: the roles of endocrine-disrupting compounds and developmental timing. Fertil Steril 2008;90:911-940.
28. Barker DJ. Fetal origins of coronary heart disease. Bmj 1995;311:171-4.
29. Newbold R,Heindel J. Developmental exposures and implications for early and latent disease. in Environmental Impacts on Reproductive Health and Fertility, G.J.L. Woodruff TJ JS, Giudice LC, Editor 2010, Cambridge University Press: Cambridge, UK. p. 92-102.
30. Vandenberg LN, Colborn T, Hayes TB, Heindel JJ, Jacobs Jr DR, Lee DH, et al. Hormones and Endocrine-Disrupting Chemicals: Low-Dose Effects and Nonmonotonic Dose Responses. Endocr Rev 2012;33:378-455.
31. Zoeller RT, Brown TR, Doan LL, Gore AC, Skakkebaek NE, Soto AM, et al. Endocrine-disrupting chemicals and public health protection: a statement of principles from the endocrine society. Endocrinology 2012;153:4097-110.
32. Warner MJ,Ozanne SE. Mechanisms involved in the developmental programming of adulthood disease. The Biochemical journal 2010;427:333-47.
33. National Research Council. Health risks from exposure to low levels of ionizing radiation: BEIR VII Phase 2. 2006, Washington, D.C.: National Academies Press. xvi, 406 p.
34. Olden K, Freudenberg N, Dowd J, Shields AE. Discovering how environmental exposures alter genes could lead to new treatments for chronic illnesses. Health Aff (Millwood) 2011;30:833-41.
35. Kavlock RJ, Daston GP, DeRosa C, Fenner-Crisp P, Gray LE, Kaattari S, et al. Research needs for the risk assessment of health and environmental effects of endocrine disruptors: a report of the US EPA-sponsored workshop. Environ Health Perspect 1996;104:715.
36. Colborn T, vom Saal FS, Soto AM. Developmental effects of endocrine-disrupting chemicals in wildlife and humans. Environ Health Perspect 1993;101:378-84.
37. Miller MD,Marty MA. Impact of Environmental Chemicals on Lung Development. Environ Health Perspect 2010;118.
38. Miller MD, Crofton KM, Rice DC, Zoeller RT. Thyroid-disrupting chemicals: interpreting upstream biomarkers of adverse outcomes. Environ Health Perspect 2009;117:1033-41.

39. Woodruff TJ, Carlson A, Schwartz JM, Giudice LC. Proceedings of the summit on environmental challenges to reproductive health and fertility: executive summary. Fertil Steril 2008;89:e1-e20.
40. Rauh VA, Garfinkel R, Perera FP, Andrews HF, Hoepner L, Barr DB, et al. Impact of prenatal chlorpyrifos exposure on neurodevelopment in the first 3 years of life among inner-city children. Pediatrics 2006;118:e1845-59.
41. Rauh V, Arunajadai S, Horton M, Perera F, Hoepner L, Barr DB, et al. 7-Year Neurodevelopmental Scores and Prenatal Exposure to Chlorpyrifos, a Common Agricultural Pesticide. Environ Health Perspect 2011.
42. Whyatt RM, Rauh V, Barr DB, Camann DE, Andrews HF, Garfinkel R, et al. Prenatal insecticide exposures and birth weight and length among an urban minority cohort. Environ Health Perspect 2004;112:1125.
43. Cohn BA, Cirillo PM, Christianson RE. Prenatal DDT Exposure and Testicular Cancer: A Nested Case-Control Study. Arch Environ Occup Health 2010;65:127-34.
44. Wigle DT, Arbuckle TE, Turner MC, Berube A, Yang Q, Liu S, et al. Epidemiologic evidence of relationships between reproductive and child health outcomes and environmental chemical contaminants. Journal of Toxicology and Environmental Health, Part B: Critical Reviews 2008;11:373-517.
45. Parker CL. Slowing global warming: benefits for patients and the planet. Am Fam Physician 2011;84:271.
46. Swan SH, Liu F, Hines M, Kruse RL, Wang C, Redmon JB, et al. Prenatal phthalate exposure and reduced masculine play in boys. Int J Androl 2010;33:259-69.
47. Swan SH, Main KM, Liu F, Stewart SL, Kruse RL, Calafat AM, et al. Decrease in anogenital distance among male infants with prenatal phthalate exposure. Environ Health Perspect 2005;113:1056.
48. Latini G, De Felice C, Presta G, Del Vecchio A, Paris I, Ruggieri F, et al. In utero exposure to di-(2-ethylhexyl) phthalate and duration of human pregnancy. Environ Health Perspect 2003;111:1783.
49. Engel SM, Zhu C, Berkowitz GS, Calafat AM, Silva MJ, Miodovnik A, et al. Prenatal phthalate exposure and performance on the Neonatal Behavioral Assessment Scale in a multiethnic birth cohort. Neurotoxicology 2009;30:522-8.
50. Sutton P, Woodruff TJ, Perron J, Stotland N, Conry JA, Miller MD, et al. Toxic environmental chemicals: the role of reproductive health professionals in preventing harmful exposures. Am J Obstet Gynecol 2012.
51. Raffensperger C,Tickner J, eds. Protecting Public Health and the Environment: Implementing the Precautionary Principle. 1999, Island Press: Washington, DC.
52. National Research Council (U.S.) Committee on Developmental Toxicology,National Research Council (U.S.) Commission on Life Sciences. Scientific frontiers in developmental toxicology and risk assessment. 2000, Washington, DC: National Academy Press. xviii, 327 p.
53. Kimmel CA, Holson JF, Hogue CJ, Carlo G. Reliability of Experimental Studies for Predicting Hazards to Human Development. in NCTR Technical Report for Experiment No. 60151984: Jefferson, AR.
54. Woodruff TJ, Sutton P, The Navigation Guide Work Group. An Evidence-Based Medicine Methodology To Bridge The Gap Between Clinical And Environmental Health Sciences. Health Aff (Millwood) 2011;30:931-937.
55. Lu MC. We can do better: improving perinatal health in America. J Womens Health (Larchmt) 2010;19:569-74.
56. Barker DJP. The developmental origins of adult disease. J Am Coll Nutr 2004;23:588S-595S.

57. Solomon G, Janssen S. Communicating with patients and the public about environmental exposures and reproductive risk. in Environmental Impacts on Reproductive Health and Fertility, T.J. Woodruff, et al., Editors. 2001, Cambridge University Press: Cambridge.
58. Solomon G,Janssen S. Talking with Patients and the Public about Endocrine-Disrupting Chemicals. in Endocrine-Disrupting Chemicals: From Basic Research to Clinical Practice, A. Gore, Editor 2007, Humana Press Totowa.
59. Ondeck M,Focareta J. Environmental Hazards Education for Childbirth Educators. The Journal of Perinatal Education 2009;18:31.
60. Lubick N. Advising Parents in the Face of Scientific Uncertainty: An Environmental Health Dilemma. Environ Health Perspect 2011;119.
61. Lu C, Toepel K, Irish R, Fenske RA, Barr DB, Bravo R. Organic diets significantly lower children's dietary exposure to organophosphorus pesticides. Environ Health Perspect 2006;114:260.
62. Rudel RA, Gray JM, Engel CL, Rawsthorne TW, Dodson RE, Ackerman JM, et al. Food Packaging and Bisphenol A and Bis(2-Ethylhexyl) Phthalate Exposure: Findings from a Dietary Intervention. Environ Health Perspect 2011.
63. Ji K, Lim Kho Y, Park Y, Choi K. Influence of a five-day vegetarian diet on urinary levels of antibiotics and phthalate metabolites: A pilot study with "Temple Stay" participants. Environ Res 2010;110:375-382.
64. Bailin PS, Byrne M, Lewis S, Liroff R. Public Awareness Drives Market for Safer Alternatives: Bisphenol A Market Analysis Report. 2008, Investor Environmental Health Network: Falls Church, VA.
65. Layton L. Wal-Mart bypasses federal regulators to ban controversial flame retardant. in The Washington Post2011: Washington, D.C.
66. Gould R,Russell C. Taking action to prevent harm. San Francisco Medicine 2010;83:27-29.
67. UCSF Program on Reproductive Health and the Environment. Professional Statements Database. 2012 [cited 2012; Available from: http://prhe.ucsf.edu/prhe/clinical/index.html#ps].

Trilogy 14. Contemporary approaches to polycystic ovary syndrome management (PCOS update)

Genetics of polycystic ovary syndrome

Zi-Jiang Chen

Shandong University, Jinan, China

Summary

Polycystic ovary syndrome (PCOS) can be viewed as a heterogeneous and complex disorder trigged by androgen excess, along with varying degrees of gonadotropic and metabolic abnormalities. It is the most common cause of female anovulatory infertility, with a prevalence of 6%-8% among women of reproductive age (1-3). PCOS was first described by Stein and Leventhal in 1935, but still remains controversial in diagnosis and unclear in its etiology.

As a complex disorder, PCOS is present with heterogeneous characteristics originating from the combined effect of both environmental and genetic factors. On the genetic aspects, a series of family and twin studies have demonstrated the heritable nature of PCOS. Meanwhile, several researchers have focused their attention on genetic association studies and tried to find the link between certain genes and PCOS.

A number of candidate-gene studies in PCOS have been conducted and are still under continuous and intense investigation (4). Major candidate genes can be categorized as: I) genes involved in the biosynthesis and the action of androgens; II) genes affecting insulin resistance; III) genes correlated with inflammatory cytokines; and IV) other candidate genes.

Hyperandrogenism is one of the fundamental characteristics and clinical manifestations of PCOS; thus, genes involved in steroidogenesis (e.g., *CYP11A, CYP17A, CYP21, EPHX1*, and *HSD17B6*) are the essential candidates. *CYP11A1* is a rate-limiting enzyme, and polymorphism D15S520 in *CYP11A1* is associated with PCOS susceptibility in Caucasians and Chinese (5-8). *CYP21* mutations in PCOS women were also found in some studies (9, 10). But for other candidates, very few consistent significant associations have been confirmed in PCOS.

Sex hormones and hormone receptors are the key regulators during folliculogenesis. *FSH, FSHR, LHCGR, AR,* and *SHBG* are all compelling candidate genes for PCOS. The SNP rs6166 (p.N680S) in exon 10 of *FSHR* has been reported to be associated with PCOS in Dutch and Japanese women (11, 12), but not in Chinese women with PCOS (13, 14). Inactivating mutations of *LHCGR* in females are associated with PCOS-like phenotypes such as increased luteinizing hormone (LH), enlarged ovaries, oligomenorrhea, resistance to LH or human chorionic gonadotropin (hCG), and infertility (15, 16). In gene *AR*, a repeat polymorphism of CAG showed a link with PCOS in an Australian study but was not considered a major determining factor in the development of PCOS (17, 18). Hogenveen et al. identified a missense mutation (P156L) within *SHBG* in 4 of 482 women with PCOS, hirsutism, or ovarian dysfunction (19). Xita et al. also confirmed that higher frequency of longer VNTR (variable number tandem repeats) exists in *SHBG* amongst Greek women with PCOS (20).

Insulin resistance is considered an important component of the PCOS pathogenesis. Genes such as *INS, INSR, IRS-1, IRS-1,* and *IGF* are all plausible candidates for PCOS. Several studies on these genes have yielded statistically significant associations, but most are still under debate; whereas, a body mass-related gene, *FTO*, has interesting functions in PCOS with obesity. A meta-analysis of 8 studies showed that the *FTO*-carrying risk allele of rs9939609 could amplify the effect more than 2 times on body mass index (BMI) and weight in PCOS (21).

To date, nearly 100 genes have been listed as PCOS candidates; however, very few correlate consistently with PCOS. New approaches based on whole genome open new and promising perspectives in the investigation of the genetic basis of this complex disorder. In PCOS genetic studies, the first genome-wide association study (GWAS) was "a major milestone" (22). It was conducted in Chinese with 744 women with PCOS and 895 unaffected controls from the same population as discovery set using the Affymetrix SNP 6.0 array. Three loci (2p16.3, 2p21, and 9q33.3) were detected to be associated with PCOS, as well as multiple SNPs in the genes *LHCGR, THADA,* and *DENND1A* (23). The *LHCGR* gene (on 2p16.3), which has been a fundamental candidate for PCOS, was confirmed again by this GWAS. The thyroid adenoma-associated gene, *THADA*, mapping to chromosome 2p21, was first identified as a target gene in thyroid benign tumors (24). Recent GWAS of T2D also reported that *THADA* is an associated gene that might affect pancreatic beta-cell function (25). *DENND1A* is located on chromosome 9q33.3 and encodes a domain of DENN (differentially expressed in normal and neoplastic cells), functioning as a guanine nucleotide exchange factor for the early endosomal small GTPase Rab35 (26).

More remarkably, these findings are replicated in a series of subsequent studies. First, a family-based transmission disequilibrium test (TDT) analysis followed up the GWAS findings and confirmed association and linkage of the *THADA* variants in Chinese PCOS trios (27). Then Goodarzi et al. (1,474 cases vs. 1,802 controls) and Welt et al. (1,131 cases vs. 17,607 controls) confirmed the association between *DENND1A* and PCOS in US and Icelandic European populations (28-29). Due to the differences existing in the linkage disequilibrium (LD) and minor allele frequencies of SNPs between European and Chinese, SNPs associated with Chinese (*THADA*: rs13429458 and rs12478601; *LHCGR*: rs13405728) are not well-replicated in Europeans. However, Goodarzi et al. replicated that other SNP rs12468394 in *THADA* has a risk to PCOS and Mutharasan et al. found strong evidence for association of PCOS with rs7562215 and rs10495960 in *LHCGR* (30). For some studies that cannot replicate the GWAS SNPs, please carefully consider LD pattern between different populations.

Considering that PCOS is a complicated endocrine-metabolic disorder, 3 loci found in the first GWAS (PCOS GWAS-I) are not sufficient, and a second GWAS (PCOS GWAS-II) was conducted again in Chinese with an enlarged sample size of 10,480 PCOS cases and 10,489 controls (31). In PCOS GWAS-II, another 8 new loci were identified, including SNPs in the plausible genes *FSHR* and *INSR*. A total of 11 loci related to PCOS have been uncovered by GWAS. Among them are a number of candidate genes within the susceptibility loci related to hormone and organ growth and in common with T2D: *FSHR* and *LHCGR* are plausible candidates related to folliculogenesis and ovulation; *INSR, HMGA2*, and *THADA* were also identified as candidate genes for T2D in recent GWAS (32, 33); 12q13.2 also confers risk to type 1 diabetes (34-39); and *YAP* and *HMGA2* ("pygmy" gene) may correlate with enlarged size of polycystic ovary. On the other hand, these genes also are involved in several pathways: INSR and *ERBB3* are implicated in the processes of female gamete generation; *LHCGR* and *FSHR* both encode hormone ligand-binding receptors; *FBP1* and *INSR* are related through the insulin signaling pathway; *YAP1* and *ERBB3* are both involved in the ERBB signaling pathway (40, 41); *LHCGR* and *ERBB3* are involved in the calcium signaling pathway (42); and *RAB5B* and *ERBB3* play roles in endocytosis (42). Those susceptibility loci provide clues into PCOS etiology researches. Recently, a third GWAS on PCOS was conducted in a Korean population, but it identified the gene *GYS2* that is specifically associated with BMI rather than PCOS per se (43). So far, efforts to identify PCOS susceptibility loci have focused on Asian populations; GWAS of other ethnic groups are in request.

In summary, among these candidate-gene studies, a number have yielded statistically significant associations; however, few with results are robustly reproducible. Whole-genome association studies otherwise provide more reliable and unbiased results, representing a new breakthrough in genetic study of female reproduction. Future association studies still need world-wide collaborations, expanding sample size to identify more susceptibility loci, and, based on these results, to specify subtypes of disease and explore subtype-related markers. Besides the pursuit of understanding the genetic mechanisms, the need also arises for establishing risk prediction models, developing less invasive methods of diagnosis, and creating more effective targeted treatments.

References

1. Carmina E, Lobo RA: Polycystic ovary syndrome (PCOS): arguably the most common endocrinopathy is associated with significant morbidity in women. The Journal of clinical endocrinology and metabolism 1999, 84(6):1897-1899.
2. Goodarzi MO, Azziz R: Diagnosis, epidemiology, and genetics of the polycystic ovary syndrome. Best practice & research Clinical endocrinology & metabolism 2006, 20(2):193-205.
3. Ehrmann DA, Barnes RB, Rosenfield RL, Cavaghan MK, Imperial J: Prevalence of impaired glucose tolerance and diabetes in women with polycystic ovary syndrome. Diabetes care 1999, 22(1):141-146.
4. Deligeoroglou E, Kouskouti C, Christopoulos P: The role of genes in the polycystic ovary syndrome: predisposition and mechanisms. Gynecological endocrinology : the official journal of the International Society of Gynecological Endocrinology 2009, 25(9):603-609.
5. Zhang CW, Zhang XL, Xia YJ, Cao YX, Wang WJ, Xu P, Che YN, Wu XK, Yi L, Gao Q et al: Association between polymorphisms of the CYP11A1 gene and polycystic ovary syndrome in Chinese women. Molecular biology reports 2012, 39(8):8379-8385.
6. Liu Y, Jiang H, He LY, Huang WJ, He XY, Xing FQ: Abnormal expression of uncoupling protein-2 correlates with CYP11A1 expression in polycystic ovary syndrome. Reproduction, fertility, and development 2011, 23(4):520-526.
7. Prazakova S, Vankova M, Bradnova O, Lukasova P, Vcelak J, Dvorakova K, Vondra K, Vrbikova J, Bendlova B: ((TTTTA), polymorphism in the promoter of the CYP11A1 gene in the pathogenesis of polycystic ovary syndrome). Casopis lekaru ceskych 2010, 149(11):520-525.
8. Pusalkar M, Meherji P, Gokral J, Chinnaraj S, Maitra A: CYP11A1 and CYP17 promoter polymorphisms associate with hyperandrogenemia in polycystic ovary syndrome. Fertility and sterility 2009, 92(2):653-659.
9. Witchel SF, Aston CE: The role of heterozygosity for CYP21 in the polycystic ovary syndrome. Journal of pediatric endocrinology & metabolism : JPEM 2000, 13 Suppl 5:1315-1317.
10. Escobar-Morreale HF, San Millan JL, Smith RR, Sancho J, Witchel SF: The presence of the 21-hydroxylase deficiency carrier status in hirsute women: phenotype-genotype correlations. Fertility and sterility 1999, 72(4):629-638.
11. Sudo S, Kudo M, Wada S, Sato O, Hsueh AJ, Fujimoto S: Genetic and functional analyses of polymorphisms in the human FSH receptor gene. Molecular human reproduction 2002, 8(10):893-899.
12. Valkenburg O, Uitterlinden AG, Piersma D, Hofman A, Themmen AP, de Jong FH, Fauser BC, Laven JS: Genetic polymorphisms of GnRH and gonadotrophic hormone receptors affect the phenotype of polycystic ovary syndrome. Hum Reprod 2009, 24(8):2014-2022.

13. Du J, Zhang W, Guo L, Zhang Z, Shi H, Wang J, Zhang H, Gao L, Feng G, He L: Two FSHR variants, haplotypes and meta-analysis in Chinese women with premature ovarian failure and polycystic ovary syndrome. Molecular genetics and metabolism 2010, 100(3):292-295.
14. Tong Y, Liao WX, Roy AC, Ng SC: Absence of mutations in the coding regions of follicle-stimulating hormone receptor gene in Singapore Chinese women with premature ovarian failure and polycystic ovary syndrome. Hormone and metabolic research = Hormon- und Stoffwechselforschung = Hormones et metabolisme 2001, 33(4):221-226.
15. Latronico AC, Chai Y, Arnhold IJ, Liu X, Mendonca BB, Segaloff DL: A homozygous microdeletion in helix 7 of the luteinizing hormone receptor associated with familial testicular and ovarian resistance is due to both decreased cell surface expression and impaired effector activation by the cell surface receptor. Mol Endocrinol 1998, 12(3):442-450.
16. Toledo SP, Brunner HG, Kraaij R, Post M, Dahia PL, Hayashida CY, Kremer HTAP: An inactivating mutation of the luteinizing hormone receptor causes amenorrhea in a 46,XX female. The Journal of clinical endocrinology and metabolism 1996, 81(11):3850-3854.
17. Hickey T, Chandy A, Norman RJ: The androgen receptor CAG repeat polymorphism and X-chromosome inactivation in Australian Caucasian women with infertility related to polycystic ovary syndrome. The Journal of clinical endocrinology and metabolism 2002, 87(1):161-165.
18. Wang R, Goodarzi MO, Xiong T, Wang D, Azziz R, Zhang H: Negative association between androgen receptor gene CAG repeat polymorphism and polycystic ovary syndrome? A systematic review and meta-analysis. Molecular human reproduction 2012, 18(10):498-509.
19. Hogeveen KN, Cousin P, Pugeat M, Dewailly D, Soudan B, Hammond GL: Human sex hormone-binding globulin variants associated with hyperandrogenism and ovarian dysfunction. The Journal of clinical investigation 2002, 109(7):973-981.
20. Xita N, Tsatsoulis A, Chatzikyriakidou A, Georgiou I: Association of the (TAAAA)n repeat polymorphism in the sex hormone-binding globulin (SHBG) gene with polycystic ovary syndrome and relation to SHBG serum levels. The Journal of clinical endocrinology and metabolism 2003, 88(12):5976-5980.
21. Wojciechowski P, Lipowska A, Rys P, Ewens KG, Franks S, Tan S, Lerchbaum E, Vcelak J, Attaoua R, Straczkowski M et al: Impact of FTO genotypes on BMI and weight in polycystic ovary syndrome: a systematic review and meta-analysis. Diabetologia 2012, 55(10):2636-2645.
22. Strauss JF, 3rd, McAllister JM, Urbanek M: Persistence pays off for PCOS gene prospectors. The Journal of clinical endocrinology and metabolism 2012, 97(7):2286-2288.
23. Chen ZJ, Zhao H, He L, Shi Y, Qin Y, Li Z, You L, Zhao J, Liu J, Liang X et al: Genome-wide association study identifies susceptibility loci for polycystic ovary syndrome on chromosome 2p16.3, 2p21 and 9q33.3. Nature genetics 2011, 43(1):55-59.
24. Drieschner N, Belge G, Rippe V, Meiboom M, Loeschke S, Bullerdiek J: Evidence for a 3p25 breakpoint hot spot region in thyroid tumors of follicular origin. Thyroid : official journal of the American Thyroid Association 2006, 16(11):1091-1096.
25. Zeggini E, Scott LJ, Saxena R, Voight BF, Marchini JL, Hu T, de Bakker PI, Abecasis GR, Almgren P, Andersen G et al: Meta-analysis of genome-wide association data and large-scale replication identifies additional susceptibility loci for type 2 diabetes. Nature genetics 2008, 40(5):638-645.
26. Marat AL, McPherson PS: The connecdenn family, Rab35 guanine nucleotide exchange factors interfacing with the clathrin machinery. The Journal of biological chemistry 2010, 285(14):10627-10637.

27. Zhao H, Xu X, Xing X, Wang J, He L, Shi Y, Zhao Y, Chen ZJ: Family-based analysis of susceptibility loci for polycystic ovary syndrome on chromosome 2p16.3, 2p21 and 9q33.3. Hum Reprod 2012, 27(1):294-298.
28. Goodarzi MO, Jones MR, Li X, Chua AK, Garcia OA, Chen YD, Krauss RM, Rotter JI, Ankener W, Legro RS et al: Replication of association of DENND1A and THADA variants with polycystic ovary syndrome in European cohorts. Journal of medical genetics 2012, 49(2):90-95.
29. Welt CK, Styrkarsdottir U, Ehrmann DA, Thorleifsson G, Arason G, Gudmundsson JA, Ober C, Rosenfield RL, Saxena R, Thorsteinsdottir U et al: Variants in DENND1A are associated with polycystic ovary syndrome in women of European ancestry. The Journal of clinical endocrinology and metabolism 2012, 97(7):E1342-1347.
30. Mutharasan P, Galdones E, Penalver Bernabe B, Garcia OA, Jafari N, Shea LD, Woodruff TK, Legro RS, Dunaif A, Urbanek M: Evidence for Chromosome 2p16.3 Polycystic Ovary Syndrome Susceptibility Locus in Affected Women of European Ancestry. The Journal of clinical endocrinology and metabolism 2012.
31. Shi Y, Zhao H, Cao Y, Yang D, Li Z, Zhang B, Liang X, Li T, Chen J, Shen J et al: Genome-wide association study identifies eight new risk loci for polycystic ovary syndrome. Nature genetics 2012, 44(9):1020-1025.
32. Voight BF, Scott LJ, Steinthorsdottir V, Morris AP, Dina C, Welch RP, Zeggini E, Huth C, Aulchenko YS, Thorleifsson G: Twelve type 2 diabetes susceptibility loci identified through large-scale association analysis. Nature genetics 2010, 42(7):579-589.
33. Zeggini E, Scott LJ, Saxena R, Voight BF, Marchini JL, Hu T, de Bakker PIW, Abecasis GR, Almgren P, Andersen G: Meta-analysis of genome-wide association data and large-scale replication identifies additional susceptibility loci for type 2 diabetes. Nature genetics 2008, 40(5):638-645.
34. Hakonarson H, Qu HQ, Bradfield JP, Marchand L, Kim CE, Glessner JT, Grabs R, Casalunovo T, Taback SP, Frackelton EC et al: A novel susceptibility locus for type 1 diabetes on Chr12q13 identified by a genome-wide association study. Diabetes 2008, 57(4):1143-1146.
35. Plagnol V, Howson JMM, Smyth DJ, Walker N, Hafler JP, Wallace C, Stevens H, Jackson L, Simmonds MJ, Bingley PJ: Genome-Wide Association Analysis of Autoantibody Positivity in Type 1 Diabetes Cases. PLoS genetics 2011, 7(8):e1002216.
36. Cooper JD, Walker NM, Healy BC, Smyth DJ, Downes K, Todd JA: Analysis of 55 autoimmune disease and type II diabetes loci: further confirmation of chromosomes 4q27, 12q13.2 and 12q24.13 as type I diabetes loci, and support for a new locus, 12q13.3-q14.1Analysis of 55 autoimmune disease and type II diabetes loci in T1D. Genes and immunity 2009, 10:S95-S120.
37. Barrett JC, Clayton DG, Concannon P, Akolkar B, Cooper JD, Erlich HA, Julier C, Morahan G, Nerup J, Nierras C: Genome-wide association study and meta-analysis find that over 40 loci affect risk of type 1 diabetes. Nature genetics 2009, 41(6):703-707.
38. Burton PR, Clayton DG, Cardon LR, Craddock N, Deloukas P, Duncanson A, Kwiatkowski DP, McCarthy MI, Ouwehand WH, Samani NJ: Genome-wide association study of 14,000 cases of seven common diseases and 3,000 shared controls. Nature 2007, 447(7145):661-678.
39. Todd JA, Walker NM, Cooper JD, Smyth DJ, Downes K, Plagnol V, Bailey R, Nejentsev S, Sarah F, Payne F: Robust associations of four new chromosome regions from genome-wide analyses of type 1 diabetes. Nature genetics 2007, 39(7):857-864.
40. Joshi-Tope G, Gillespie M, Vastrik I, D'Eustachio P, Schmidt E, de Bono B, Jassal B, Gopinath GR, Wu GR, Matthews L: Reactome: a knowledgebase of biological pathways. Nucleic acids research 2005, 33(suppl 1):D428-D432.

41. Matthews L, Gopinath G, Gillespie M, Caudy M, Croft D, De Bono B, Garapati P, Hemish J, Hermjakob H, Jassal B: Reactome knowledgebase of human biological pathways and processes. Nucleic acids research 2009, 37(suppl 1):D619-D622.
42. Ogata H, Goto S, Sato K, Fujibuchi W, Bono H, Kanehisa M: KEGG: Kyoto encyclopedia of genes and genomes. Nucleic acids research 1999, 27(1):29-34.
43. Hwang JY, Lee EJ, Jin Go M, Sung YA, Lee HJ, Heon Kwak S, Jang HC, Soo Park K, Lee HJ, Byul Jang H et al: Genome-wide association study identifies GYS2 as a novel genetic factor for polycystic ovary syndrome through obesity-related condition. Journal of human genetics 2012, 57(10):660-664.

Global differences in presentation of polycystic ovary syndrome

Fahrettin Kele timur

Erciyes University, Kayseri, Turkey

PCOS is one of the most common public health problems seen in women of reproductive age. Male phenotype has not been clearly defined. Despite changes in diagnostic criteria over decades, some of the manifestations are essential to the diagnosis of PCOS. Among these are the clinical signs and symptoms of hyperandrogenemia including hirsutism, acne, and alopecia; hormonal findings including increased levels of testosterone, androstenedione, and dehydroepiandrosterone sulfate (DHEAS); and menstrual or fertility problems, which include oligomenorrhea/amenorrhea, anovulation, and infertility.

A number of recent studies have revealed that PCOS is associated with metabolic abnormalities due to insulin resistance that also lead to carbohydrate intolerance, increased risk for type 2 diabetes, dyslipidemia characterized by low levels of high-density lipoprotein (HDL)-cholesterol, increased levels of triglycerides and low-density lipoprotein (LDL)-cholesterol, acanthosis nigricans (AN), and increased cardiovascular morbidity (1, 2, 3). Obese PCOS women are more insulin resistant and are at higher risk for cardiovascular disease when compared to non-obese PCOS women. Insulin sensitizers, especially metformin, may have some beneficial effects on insulin resistance, resumption of menses, and atherogenic dyslipidemia in obese PCOS women. There are some discrepancies in the literature regarding the effectiveness of metformin in the treatment of non-obese PCOS women. Interestingly, the effectiveness of metformin in non-obese PCOS women may vary among populations (2).

Although insulin resistance has not been included in the diagnostic criteria for PCOS, it may account for some clinical or biochemical abnormalities (4, 5). The degree of insulin resistance, and therefore the frequency of insulin resistance-related manifestations, differs among populations. It was demonstrated that Mexican-American women with PCOS are more insulin resistant than a comparable group of white women. However, DHEAS (the production level of which is more than 95%, is adrenal in origin, and is accepted as a useful marker for adrenal androgen production) was found to be significantly lower in Mexican-American women compared to their white counterparts. In that study, no association was found between circulating insulin and serum DHEAS levels. Therefore, the differences in DHEAS production and insulin sensitivity between Mexican-American population and age- and weight-matched white women with PCOS are consistent with genetic heterogeneity (6). Women of Middle Eastern origin with PCOS are referred at a younger age and are characterized by decreased body mass index (BMI) and increased insulin resistance when compared to Caucasian women with PCOS (7). In another study reported 20 years ago, PCOS and ethnicity were suggested independent risk factors for insulin sensitivity in Caribbean-Hispanic women (8).

Hirsutism, which is defined as the presence of excess terminal hair in androgen-sensitive areas of the female body, is seen in approximately 10% of the population. PCOS, idiopathic hirsutism, and idiopathic hyperandrogenemia are functional causes of hirsutism. Nonclassical congenital adrenal hyperplasia, hyperprolactinemia, androgen-secreting adrenal or ovarian tumors, acromegaly, and Cushing syndrome are rare causes of hirsutism. The most common cause of hirsutism is PCOS. Consequently, a great number of patients with PCOS seek medical advice due to hirsutism, the frequency of which differs among the various populations. Mechanisms underlying hirsutism also may be different among varying ethnicities. Asian women are rarely hirsute while Mediterranean women, including Turkish and Greek populations, are more hirsute (9). On the other hand, Caucasian women were found to be less hirsute but paradoxically more hyperandrogenemic (7). The enzyme 5α-reductase converts testosterone to the more potent androgen dihydrotestosterone. The activity of this enzyme varies among different populations, and differences in its activity may explain why the prevalence of hirsutism is not equal in different populations. A detailed medical history and physical examination are essential in the investigation of hyperandrogenism, and specific variations due to the differences in genetic background of hirsutism patients should be considered. Additionally, cut-off values for the most commonly used hair scoring system, the Ferriman-Gallwey scoring system, depend on racial and ethnic variability. Population-based cut-off values for Ferriman-Gallwey would probably be more beneficial in the investigation of hirsutism (10). In a study performed in Sri Lanka, young indigenous South Asians with PCOS were found to have greater odds of being centrally obese with a third having the metabolic syndrome. Of the PCOS patients, 79.7% had hirsutism and 74.6% had significant hirsutism. On the other hand, acanthosis nigricans, which is accepted as a clinical sign of insulin resistance, was significantly common in PCOS women in this population (11).

Recent data suggest that the Chinese population with PCOS has remarkably different phenotypes. Chinese women with PCOS have been found to have increased risk of impaired glucose tolerance (IGT) and noninsulin-dependent diabetes mellitus (NIDDM) in a study including 102 PCOS patients (12). Zhang et al. divided PCOS patients into 4 subgroups including oligo and/or anovulation plus hyperandrogenism plus polycystic ovarian morphology; oligo and/or anovulation plus hyperandrogenism; hyperandrogenism plus polycystic ovarian morphology; and oligo and/or anovulation plus polycystic ovarian morphology. They found that the most common PCOS phenotype was the group with oligo and/or anovulation plus polycystic ovarian changes, which was named as a nonhyperandrogenic phenotype. The classic phenotype (oligo and/or anovulation plus hyperandrogenism) was the rarest phenotype (13). In an Australian study, both women with polycystic ovarian changes and PCOS with cycle irregularity had significantly higher concentrations of serum fasting and stimulated insulin independent of androgens and body mass index than those with normal cycles. According to that study, ultrasound evidence predicts similar metabolic sequelae to PCOS and can therefore be used for studies of genetics and long-term risks for this condition (14).

The major androgens in the circulation of normal premenopausal women include testosterone, androstenedione, and DHEAS. The least required initial tests for the differential diagnosis of hyperandrogenism are total testosterone measured by high-quality RIA or free androgen index, which is calculated by the measurement of total testosterone and sex hormone-binding globulin (SHBG). Studies comparing the importance of androgens in the diagnosis of PCOS in different populations are very rare. Interestingly, from a hormonal point of view, androstenedione has been suggested as the hormone that should be measured for the documentation of hyperandrogenism in Icelandic women. In the same study, polycystic ovarian morphology by ultrasound has been found to be a universal finding in PCOS women (15). Cytochrome P450c17α is an enzyme that binds progesterone and converts it to 17-OH progesterone by 17α-hydroxylase activity and 17-OH progesterone to androstenedione by 17,20-lyase activity. This enzyme is active in both the ovaries and adrenal glands. Dysregulation of cytochrome P450c17α enzyme may cause the exaggerated secretion of adrenal and ovarian androgens in PCOS. Adrenocorticotropic hormone (ACTH)-stimulated and gonadotropin-releasing hormone (GnRH) agonist-stimulated 17-OH progesterone levels in PCOS women were found to be different in various populations (16, 17, 18).

The current data suggest that there are significant regional, ethnic, racial, and social variations in PCOS women in terms of clinical presentation, hormonal abnormalities, reproductive disorders, and metabolic problems. Existence of different phenotypes in women with PCOS should be kept in mind during assessment. Medical history should include the features of the population in which the patient is living given that ethnic origin is affected by both genetic and environmental changes and that the PCOS woman may present a variety of complaints based on these. Therefore, an approach to a woman with PCOS depends on the characteristics of the relevant population. Not only are clinical and laboratory features important in the diagnosis of PCOS, but a response to treatment may also be affected by ethnic background. More long-term prospective studies including molecular genetic analysis in various populations are needed to understand the relation between ethnicity and phenotype of women with PCOS.

References

1. Azziz R, Carmina E, Dewailly D, Diamanti-Kandarakis E, Escobar-Morreale HF, Futterweit W, Janssen OE, Legro RS, Norman RJ, Taylor AE et al. The Androgen Excess and PCOS Society criteria for the polycystic ovary syndrome: the complete task force report. Fertil Steril 2009; 91:456-488.
2. Sahin Y, Unluhizarci K, Yilmazsoy A, Yikilmaz A, Aygen E, Kelestimur F. The effects of metformin on metabolic and cardiovascular risk factors in nonobese women with polycystic ovary syndrome. Clin Endocrinol 2007; 67:904-908.
3. Kaya MG, Calapkorur B, Karaca Z, Yildirim S, Celik A, Akpek M, Unluhizarci K, Kelestimur F. The effects of treatment with drospirenone/ethinyl oestradiol alone or in combination with metformin on elastic properties of aorta in women with polycystic ovary syndrome. Clin Endocrinol 2012; 77:885-892.
4. Unluhizarci K, Karababa Y, Bayram F, Kelestimur F. The investigation of insulin resistance in patients with idiopathic hirsutism. J Clin Endocrinol Metab 2004; 89:2741-2744.
5. Unluhizarci K, Ozocak M, Tanriverdi F, Atmaca H, Kelestimur F. Investigation of hypothalamo-pituitary-gonadal axis and glucose intolerance among the first-degree female relatives of women with polycystic ovary syndrome. Fertil Steril 2007; 87:1377-82.
6. Kauffman RP, Baker VM, DiMarino P, Castracane VD. Hyperinsulinemia and circulating dehydroepiandrosterone sulfate in white and Mexica-American women with polycystic ovary syndrome. Fertil Steril 2006; 85:1010-1016.
7. Glintborg D, Mumm H, Hougaard D, Ravn P, Andersen M. Ethnic differences in Rotterdam criteria and metabolic risk factors in a multiethnic group of women with PCOS studied in Denmark. Clin Endocrinol 2010; 73:732-738.
8. Dunaif A, Sorbara L, Delson R, Green G. Ethnicity and Polycystic Ovary Syndrome are associated with independent and additive decreases in insulin action in Caribbean-Hispanic women. Diabetes 1993; 42: 1462-8.
9. Diamanti-Kandarakis E, Kouli CR, Bergiele AT, Filandra FA, Tsianateli TC, Spina GG, Zapanti ED, Bartzis MI. A survey of the polycystic ovary syndrome in the Grek island of lesbos: hormonal and metabolic profile. J Clin Endocrinol Metab 1999; 84:4006-4011.
10. Escobar-Morreale H, Carmina E, Dewailly D, Gambineri A, Kelestimur F, Moghetti P, Pugeat M, Wijeyaratne CN, Witchel S, Norman RJ. Epidemiology, diagnosis and management of hirsutism: a consensus statement by the Androgen Excess and Polycystic Ovary Syndrome (AE-PCOS) Society. Hum Reprod Update 2012; 18:146-70.
11. Wijeyaratne CN, Seneviratne Ruwanthi de A, Dahanayake S, Kumarapeli V, Palipane E, Kuruppu N, Yapa C, Seneviratne Rohini A, Balen AH. Phenotype and metabolic profile of South Asian women with polycystic ovary syndrome (PCOS): results of a large database from a specialist Endocrine Clinic. Hum Reprod 2011; 26: 202-13.
12. Chen X, Yang D, Lin L, Feng S, Wang L. Abnormal glucose tolerance in Chinese women with polycystic ovary syndrome. Hum Reprod 2006;21:2027-2032.

13. Zhang HY, Zhu FF, Xiong J, Shi XB, Fu SX. Characteristics of different phenotypes of polycystic ovary syndrome based on the Rotterdam criteria in a large-scale Chinese population. BJOG 2009; 116:1633-9.
14. Norman RJ, Hague WM, Masters SC, Wang XJ. Subjects with polycystic ovaries without hyperandrogenemia exhibit similar disturbances in insülin and lipid profiles as those with polycystic ovary syndrome. Hum Reprod 1995;10:2258-2261
15. Welt CK, Arason G, Gudmundsson JA, Adams J, Palsdottir H, Gudlaugsdottir G, Ingadottir G, Crowley WF. Defining constant versus variable phenotypic features of women with polycystic ovary syndrome using different Ethnic groups and populations. J Clin Endocrinol Metab 2006; 91:4361-8. 14
16. ahin Y, Kele timur F. 17-Hydroxyprogesterone response to buserelin testing in polycystic ovary syndrome. Clin Endocrinol 1993; 39: 151-155.
17. ahin Y, Kele timur F. 17-Hydroxyprogesterone response to gonadotrophin-releasing hormone agonist buserelin and adrenocorticotrophin in polycystic ovary syndrome : investigation of adrenal and ovarian cytochrome P 450 c17- dysregulation. Hum Reprod 1997; 12: 910-913.
18. Pasquali R, Patton L, Cognigni GE, Gambineri A. 17-Hydroxyprogesterone responses to gonadotrophin-releasing hormone disclose distinct phenotypes of functional ovarian hyperandrogenism and polycystic ovary syndrome. J Clin Endocrinol Metab 2007; 92:4208-4217.

Management of polycystic ovary syndrome: a patient-centered approach

Basil C. Tarlatzis, Gesthimani Mintziori, Dimitrios G. Goulis

Aristotle University of Thessaloniki, Thessaloniki, Greece

Introduction

Polycystic ovary syndrome (PCOS) is the most common endocrine disorder of women, with an incidence between 6% and 10% based on the National Institutes of Health (NIH) criteria and as high as 20% to 22% based on American Society of Reproductive Medicine/European Society of Human Reproduction and Embryology (ASRM/ESHRE) criteria (1, 2). Its clinically variable phenotype includes oligo- or anovulation, hyperandrogenism (either clinical or biochemical), and the presence of polycystic ovaries, with two of the three being necessary to establish the diagnosis (1, 2).

Patient-centered PCOS management

If the primary concern is skin problems

Hirsutism is present in about 70% of women with PCOS and should be evaluated biochemically. On the other hand, acne and alopecia are not commonly associated with hyperandrogenemia and, therefore, should not be regarded as evidence of hyperandrogenemia. The main aims should be the reduction of androgen production, decreasing the fraction of circulating free testosterone, and limiting androgen bioactivity at the hair follicle. The slow turnover of the terminal hair should be considered in managing hirsutism.

1. **Oral contraceptive pills (OCPs).** The first-line therapy for treatment of hirsutism in women with PCOS is an estrogen-progestin contraceptive. OCPs suppress the secretion of luteinizing hormone (LH) and lead to a decrease in ovarian androgen production. The estrogenic fraction increases the levels of sex hormone-binding globulin (SHBG), which, in turn, results in a decrease in free testosterone concentrations. The progestin in the pill can compete for 5α-reductase and the androgen receptor. The OCPs also decrease adrenal androgen production by a mechanism yet unclear, possibly due to a decrease in adrenocorticotropic hormone (ACTH) concentrations. An estrogen-progestin contraceptive is suggested as first-line pharmacologic therapy for most women (3).
2. **Anti-androgens (spironolactone, flutamide, and finasteride).** Anti-androgens may be prescribed in combination with OCPs to block androgen action at the hair follicles. An anti-androgen is suggested to be added after 6 months of OCP use, if the cosmetic response is suboptimal (3).
3. **Insulin-sensitizing agents (metformin, pioglitazone)** have little effect on hirsutism and acne (4). Endocrine Society (ES) Clinical Practice Guidelines suggest against their routine use as they are associated with minimal or no benefit and are less effective than treatment with OCPs and/or antiandrogens (3).
4. **Isotretinoin** is not effective in hirsutism but can be beneficial in severe cases of acne.
5. **Eflornithine hydrochloride,** as topical treatment, may be helpful in hair removal.

6. **Physical approaches** may be helpful in hair removal. These approaches involve removal of hair by mechanical means such as shaving, waxing, depilatories, electrolysis, or laser treatment.

If the primary concern is menstrual irregularity/endometrial protection

1. **Lifestyle modifications (diet, exercise, behavioral modification) and pharmacological treatment or bariatric surgery.** Weight management is recommended as first-line management for women with PCOS. As little as a 5% to 10% weight loss can help restore menstrual function (5). Weight management is defined as prevention of excess weight gain or achieving and maintaining reduced weight in those who are already overweight. Weight management requires a multidisciplinary approach that involves dietary and behavioral interventions as well as interventions to increase physical activity. Reproductive, metabolic, and psychological features of PCOS can be increased by weight loss only (6).
2. **OCPs.** They have been recommended for over 30 years to treat women with PCOS, as they restore menstrual cyclicity and can be used to protect endometrium from hyperplasia, dysfunctional uterine bleeding, and possibly endometrial cancer (7). Due to possible long-term metabolic outcomes, it has been suggested that OCPs could be combined with insulin sensitizers, anti-androgens, or both in an attempt to positively address metabolic abnormalities, especially in young women with the syndrome (8).
3. **Insulin-sensitizing agents.** Insulin-sensitizing agents may reduce ovarian androgen production and restore normal menstrual cyclicity. After initiating metformin therapy, it may take up to 6 months for ovulatory cycles to ensue. Intermittent progestin therapy could be used in combination with metformin during the initial anovulatory period.
4. **Intermittent progestin therapy.** In anovulatory women with PCOS the continued exposure of endometrium to estrogens unopposed by progesterone results in hyperplasia. This could be restored in most women by the administration of progesterone or by inducing ovulation. Medroxyprogesterone acetate (10 mg) can be used for 7 to 10 days every 1 to 2 months. Intermittent progestin therapy has no effect on contraception or other symptoms of PCOS, like acne or hirsutism.

If the primary concern is infertility

The recognition of the controversies surrounding the treatment of PCOS led to a second international workshop endorsed by ESHRE and ASRM, held in Thessaloniki, Greece in 2007, to address the therapeutic challenges raised in women with infertility and PCOS (9). According to the Thessaloniki Consensus, the following therapeutic interventions have been proposed to address infertility in women with PCOS.

1. **Lifestyle modifications (diet, exercise, behavioral modification) and pharmacological treatment or bariatric surgery**. Interventions in subfertile women with PCOS should start from preconception period with counseling in an attempt to identify and address all potential risk factors. Obesity is a risk factor that is related to anovulation, pregnancy loss, and late pregnancy complications as well as to failure or delayed response to other treatments proposed (clomiphene citrate, gonadotropins). Weight loss is recommended as first-line therapy in obese women with PCOS seeking pregnancy (9).
2. **Insulin-sensitizing agents.** The effectiveness of insulin-sensitizing drugs in improving reproductive outcomes and metabolic parameters for women with PCOS has been assessed in a recent Cochrane review (10). The study involved 44 trials (3,992 women) and showed that clinical pregnancy rates were improved for metformin versus placebo and for met-

formin and clomiphene versus clomiphene alone. Metformin was also associated with a significantly higher incidence of gastrointestinal disturbances than placebo, but no serious adverse effects were reported. In the studies that compared metformin and clomiphene alone, there was evidence of an improved live birth rate and clinical pregnancy rate in the group of obese women who took clomiphene. When metformin was administered in infertile patients with PCOS, who receive gonadotropins for in vitro fertilization (IVF) and intracytoplasmic sperm injection (ICSI) cycles, there was no clinical effect on rates of pregnancy or live birth, but it reduces the risk of ovarian hyperstimulation syndrome (OHSS) and improved the rates of miscarriage and implantation (11).

3. **Clomiphene citrate.** Clomiphene citrate (CC) is a selective estrogen receptor modulator (SERM) that increases production of gonadotropins by inhibiting negative feedback on the hypothalamus. CC, the dihydrogen citrate salt of clomiphene, has been the most widely used treatment for fertility enhancement for the past 40 years. Its primary indication is infertility secondary to oligo-ovulation or anovulation in normogonadotropic, normoprolactinemic, euthyroid women (WHO class 2), like women with PCOS. It is a drug of low cost that does not require close monitoring, is taken orally, and has relatively few adverse effects. The main factors that predict outcome of treatment are obesity, hyperandrogenemia, and age (12). Approximately 75%–80% of patients with PCOS will ovulate after CC and the conception rate of those women ovulating on CC has been calculated up to 22% per cycle (9).
4. **Gonadotropins and gonadotropin-releasing hormone (GnRH)-analogues.** The main indication of gonadotropins is ovulation induction in normogonadotropic (WHO class 2) anovulatory women who have not ovulated or conceived with CC treatment and/or insulin-sensitizing agents. Women with PCOS and anovulatory infertility treated with gonadotropins are at high risk for OHSS. That is why, in women with PCOS, a low-dose, step-up protocol has been suggested (13). Currently, the regimens utilized are: Step-up regimens (stepwise follicle-stimulating hormone [FSH] increase), step-down regimen (loading dose of FSH with a subsequent stepwise reduction), and combination approaches (9). The duration of gonadotropin therapy generally should not exceed 6 ovulatory cycles. The routine use of GnRH-agonists during ovulation induction with gonadotropins in women with PCOS is not justified according to the Thessaloniki Consensus due to the significantly higher hyperstimulation rate, the associated risk of multiple pregnancies, and the additional inconvenience and cost of concomitant GnRH-agonist administration. There is also limited evidence for increases in pregnancy success with the concomitant GnRH-agonist administration (9).
5. **Aromatase inhibitors.** Aromatase inhibitors (including letrozole and anastrozole) have been proposed as an alternative treatment to CC therapy in infertile women with PCOS (14). Currently, there is insufficient evidence to recommend letrozole over that of CC in infertile anovulatory women with PCOS (15).
6. **Laparoscopic ovarian diathermy/surgical ovulation induction.** According to a recent Cochrane review, there was no evidence of a significant difference in rates of clinical pregnancy, live birth, or miscarriage in women with CC-resistant PCOS undergoing laparoscopic ovarian diathermy (LOD) compared to other medical treatments. However, a reduction in multiple pregnancy rates was reported in women undergoing LOD (16). The main concerns of using LOD in everyday practice are related to long-term effects on intra-abdominal adhesions and ovarian function (17).
7. **Assisted reproduction techniques.** It is generally estimated that around 20% of all IVF patients are diagnosed with PCOS. However, PCOS women are difficult to hyperstimulate in a controlled manner. In vitro fertilization treatment should be reserved for those who have not managed to conceive with other medical treatments. At the time, there is no con-

sensus regarding the preferred ovarian hyperstimulation protocol (including type and dose of gonadotropin, GnRH agonist or antagonist co-treatment) (17). However, the GnRH antagonist protocol could significantly reduce the risk of OHSS (18). In vitro maturation (IVM) of oocytes collected from unstimulated (or minimally stimulated) polycystic ovaries could be an alternative option for women with PCOS (19).

If the primary concern is long-term outcomes and quality of life

The Amsterdam ESHRE/ASRM-Sponsored third PCOS Consensus Workshop Group addressed the various women's health aspects of PCOS (20). The latter has a significant detrimental effect on quality of life compared to controls, with weight issues being most probable to affect quality of life (21).

Weight loss can have influential effects on metabolic and psychological features of PCOS (6). Five percent to 10% weight loss can lead to increased glucose tolerance and better body composition (5). Lifestyle management that results in weight loss can improve surrogate markers of metabolic disease/syndrome (evidence Level A) (20). Lifestyle management can also have an influential effect on the prevention of diabetes (Level B) (20). Metformin may be used for impaired glucose tolerance and type 2 diabetes (Level A) (20). However, there is concern for the use of other insulin-sensitizing agents, such as thiazolidinediones and glucagon-like peptide-1 (GLP-1) drugs (20, 22).

It has been suggested that women with PCOS should undergo psychological screening to improve long-term prognosis. Until it is possible to disentangle potential features of the disorder from reactions to it, specific psychological screening cannot be recommended. However, based on the consultation and the patient's perception of her problems, appropriate counseling and intervention should be offered (Level C) (20).

Conclusions

The management of PCOS should be tailored to the individual's risk profile, needs, concerns, and treatment goals. It may require interdisciplinary approach and long-term care. Current symptoms should be addressed according to patient's concerns, such as hirsutism, fertility, or psychosocial issues. Interventions to prevent related future health problems, including diabetes, should also be considered.

References

1. Revised 2003 consensus on diagnostic criteria and long-term health risks related to polycystic ovary syndrome. Fertil Steril 2004;81:19-25.
2. Revised 2003 consensus on diagnostic criteria and long-term health risks related to polycystic ovary syndrome (PCOS). Hum Reprod 2004;19:41-7.
3. Martin KA, Chang RJ, Ehrmann DA, Ibanez L, Lobo RA, Rosenfield RL, Shapiro J, Montori VM, Swiglo BA. Evaluation and treatment of hirsutism in premenopausal women: an endocrine society clinical practice guideline. J Clin Endocrinol Metab 2008;93:1105-20.
4. Harborne L, Fleming R, Lyall H, Sattar N, Norman J. Metformin or antiandrogen in the treatment of hirsutism in polycystic ovary syndrome. J Clin Endocrinol Metab 2003;88:4116-23.
5. Vause TD, Cheung AP, Sierra S, Claman P, Graham J, Guillemin JA, Lapensee L, Stewart S, Wong BC. Ovulation induction in polycystic ovary syndrome. J Obstet Gynaecol Can 2010;32:495-502.

6. Moran LJ, Hutchison SK, Norman RJ, Teede HJ. Lifestyle changes in women with polycystic ovary syndrome. Cochrane Database Syst Rev 2011;CD007506.
7. Ehrmann DA. Polycystic ovary syndrome. N Engl J Med 2005;352:1223-36.
8. Ibanez L, de ZF. Low-dose flutamide-metformin therapy for hyperinsulinemic hyperandrogenism in non-obese adolescents and women. Hum Reprod Update 2006;12:243-52.
9. Consensus on infertility treatment related to polycystic ovary syndrome. Fertil Steril 2008;89:505-22.
10. Tang T, Lord JM, Norman RJ, Yasmin E, Balen AH. Insulin-sensitising drugs (metformin, rosiglitazone, pioglitazone, D-chiro-inositol) for women with polycystic ovary syndrome, oligo amenorrhoea and subfertility. Cochrane Database Syst Rev 2012;5:CD003053.
11. Palomba S, Falbo A, La Sala GB. Effects of metformin in women with polycystic ovary syndrome treated with gonadotrophins for in vitro fertilisation and intracytoplasmic sperm injection cycles: a systematic review and meta-analysis of randomised controlled trials. BJOG 2013;120:267-76.
12. Imani B, Eijkemans MJ, te Velde ER, Habbema JD, Fauser BC. A nomogram to predict the probability of live birth after clomiphene citrate induction of ovulation in normogonadotropic oligoamenorrheic infertility. Fertil Steril 2002;77:91-7.
13. White DM, Polson DW, Kiddy D, Sagle P, Watson H, Gilling-Smith C, Hamilton-Fairley D, Franks S. Induction of ovulation with low-dose gonadotropins in polycystic ovary syndrome: an analysis of 109 pregnancies in 225 women. J Clin Endocrinol Metab 1996;81:3821-4.
14. Mitwally MF, Casper RF. Use of an aromatase inhibitor for induction of ovulation in patients with an inadequate response to clomiphene citrate. Fertil Steril 2001;75:305-309.
15. Costello MF, Misso ML, Wong J, Hart R, Rombauts L, Melder A, Norman RJ, Teede HJ. The treatment of infertility in polycystic ovary syndrome: a brief update. Aust N Z J Obstet Gynaecol 2012;52:400-3.
16. Farquhar C, Brown J, Marjoribanks J. Laparoscopic drilling by diathermy or laser for ovulation induction in anovulatory polycystic ovary syndrome. Cochrane Database Syst Rev 2012;6:CD001122.
17. Health and fertility in World Health Organization group 2 anovulatory women. Hum Reprod Update 2012;18:586-99.
18. Xiao J, Chen S, Zhang C, Chang S. Effectiveness of GnRH antagonist in the treatment of patients with polycystic ovary syndrome undergoing IVF: a systematic review and meta analysis. Gynecol Endocrinol 2013;29:187-91.
19. Siristatidis CS, Maheshwari A, Bhattacharya S. In vitro maturation in sub fertile women with polycystic ovarian syndrome undergoing assisted reproduction. Cochrane Database Syst Rev 2009;CD006606.
20. Fauser BC, Tarlatzis BC, Rebar RW, Legro RS, Balen AH, Lobo R, Carmina E, Chang J, Yildiz BO, Laven JS, Boivin J, Petraglia F, Wijeyeratne CN, Norman RJ, Dunaif A, Franks S, Wild RA, Dumesic D, Barnhart K. Consensus on women's health aspects of polycystic ovary syndrome (PCOS): the Amsterdam ESHRE/ASRM-Sponsored 3rd PCOS Consensus Workshop Group. Fertil Steril 2012;97:28-38.
21. Jones GL, Hall JM, Balen AH, Ledger WL. Health-related quality of life measurement in women with polycystic ovary syndrome: a systematic review. Hum Reprod Update 2008;14:15-25.
22. Franks S. When should an insulin sensitizing agent be used in the treatment of polycystic ovary syndrome? Clin Endocrinol (Oxf) 2011;74:148-51.

Trilogy 15. Optimizing assisted reproductive technology outcomes/evidence-based medicine

Chasing the holy grail of pregnancy rates – at the expense of safety?

Paul Devroey

Centre for Reproductive Medicine, Brussels, Belgium

Are pregnancies that occur after infertility treatment at high risk? Several negative events have been mentioned, such as premature deliveries and intrauterine growth restriction. What are the obvious causes for these events? One could question that in vitro fertilization (IVF) as such does play an important role. Moreover, these women are in general older and on certain occasions more obese. Apparently, the risk factor is closely related to the occurrence of multiple pregnancies. These multiple pregnancies induce premature deliveries, intrauterine growth retardation, and increased rates of mortality of the offspring.

Also, from the assisted reproductive technology surveillance of 2009 from the United States, it is apparent that multiple births are a substantial risk for the outcome of IVF. In 2009 a total of 146,244 procedures were performed. The multiple birth rates ranged in some states from 35% to 60.8%. Most of these children were twins. Promotion of single-embryo transfers is mandatory to reduce these multiple births.

In a recent publication the International Committee for Monitoring Assisted Reproductive Technologies (ICMART) published the data of 2004. 954,743 cycles resulting in 237,809 babies were born. Also in this report the proportion of twin deliveries was 25.1%.

One can question if single-embryo transfer imposed by legislation will be a valuable approach. In Turkey by law, mandatory single-embryo transfer has been regulated. The results of this new rule favored the new policy: a significant reduction of multiple pregnancies has been obtained and no differences were observed in clinical pregnancy rates and live birth rates.

It is quite surprising to observe that still today ovarian hyperstimulation syndrome (OHSS) is present in many clinics worldwide. This syndrome is for sure the most important complication. It occurs in about 5% of stimulated cycles. In recent publications it has been highlighted that this complication can potentially be fatal. In the Netherlands out of 100,000 stimulated cycles, 3 deaths induced by OHSS have been reported. Also some fatalities due to ovarian stimulation complicated by fatal adult respiratory distress syndrome have been observed. Many causative measures have been proposed as a therapeutic armamentarium: vaginal ascites punctures, heparin administration, and dopamine to improve diuresis.

As a preventive measure, coasting has been proposed. However, it has been demonstrated in a retrospective study, comprising 2,948 patients, that 327 required coasting (11%). In this particular study, a long gonadotropin-releasing hormone (GnRH) agonist protocol was used. OHSS occurred in 32 of the coasted women (10%).

Limited attention has been given to the obstetrical outcome of IVF pregnancies in OHSS. It has been demonstrated that in 40 women with OHSS, 22.5% suffered from early OHSS and 75.5% from late OHSS. It should be noted that thromboembolic complications occurred in 10%, pregnancy induced hypertension in 21%, and preterm labor in 36%.

The main question relates to the following: Is iatrogenic OHSS avoidable and erasable? Can we use the drugs differently and can we opt for different treatment strategies? Apparently, the way to avoid OHSS is to change down-regulation strategies from GnRH agonist to GnRH antagonist protocols. If GnRH antagonists are used, there is no need to trigger final egg maturation with human chorionic gonadotropin (hCG). HCG can be routinely replaced by GnRH agonist.

It has been demonstrated that in oocyte donor programs the occurrence of OHSS can be eliminated. This observation implies that also for regular IVF, if no fresh embryos are replaced, we can obtain the status of an OHSS-free clinic.

The important option has to be taken if, in patients at risk, a fresh embryo replacement will be performed. The ultimate debate is related to the patients at risk of OHSS. It has been demonstrated that patients who develop $\geq$ 18 oocytes at the end of the follicular phase are at risk for OHSS. If it has been decided to replace a fresh embryo, the following strategy has been proposed: administration of GnRH agonist to trigger ovulation and the administration of 1,500 IU of hCG after egg retrieval. In this condition ongoing pregnancy rates are normalized. However, this approach has to be taken with great caution since it is predictable that some cases of OHSS will still occur. One could propose that a strict number of retrieved oocytes could be the momentum to decide on fresh transfer or a freeze-all policy.

To avoid any occurrence of OHSS there is only one option: the freeze-all strategy. In this option either oocytes or embryos can be vitrified. For sure, this strategy implies a well-developed vitrification program. Also, it has to be noticed that in case of the replacement of vitrified oocytes or embryos, the transfer can be performed in ideal conditions. Needless to say a natural endometrium or an artificial cycle is more receptive than a stimulated one. In several centers worldwide, the implantation rates after the transfer of cryopreserved embryos are significantly increased compared with the fresh group.

In conclusion, a policy of single embryo replacement should be implemented worldwide. Also related to the progress in vitrification programs, the strategy of freeze-all oocytes or embryos should be implemented in case of risk of OHSS. The long GnRH agonist approach for down-regulation should be replaced by GnRH antagonist in combination with GnRH agonist to trigger final egg maturation.

References

Aljawoan FY et al. Prediction of ovarian hyperstimulation syndrome in coasted patients in an IVF/ICSI program. J Hum Reprod Sci. 2012 Jan;5(1):32-6.

Braat DD et al. Maternal death related to IVF in the Netherlands 1984-2008. Hum Reprod. 2010 Jul;25(7):1782-6.

Courbiere B et al. Obstetric outcome of women with in vitro fertilization pregnancies hospitalized for ovarian hyperstimulation syndrome: a case-control study. Fertil Steril 2011 Apr;95(5):1629-32.

Devroey P et al. An OHSS-Free Clinic by segmentation of IVF treatment. Hum Reprod. 2011 Oct;26(10):2593-7.

Fineschi V et al. An immunohistochemical study in a fatality due to ovarian hyperstimulation syndrome. Int J Legal Med. 2006 Sep;120(5):293-9.

Humaidan P. Luteal phase rescue in high-risk OHSS patients by GnRHa triggering in combination with low-dose HCG: a pilot study. Reprod Biomed Online. 2009 may;18(5):630-4

Kol S, Itskovitz-Eldor J. Gonadotropin-releasing hormone agonist trigger: the way to eliminate ovarian hyperstimulation syndrome--a 20-year experience. Semin Reprod Med. 2010 Nov;28(6):500-5.

Melo M et al. GnRH agonist versus recombinant hCG in an oocyte donation programme: a randomized, prospective, controlled, assessor-blind study. Repord Biomed Online. 2009 Oct;19(4):486-92.
Papanikolaou EG et al. Early and late ovarian hyperstimulation syndrome: early pregnancy outcome and profile. Hum Reprod 2005 Mar;20(3):636-41.
Seyhan A et al. Severe early ovarian hyperstimulation syndrome following GnRH agonist triggering with the addition of 1500 IU hCG. Hum Reprod. 2013 Apr 30.(Epub ahead of print).
Shapiro BS et al. Evidence of impaired endometrial receptivity after ovarian stimulation for in vitro fertilization: a prospective randomized trial comparing fresh and frozen-thawed embryo transfer in normal responders. Fertil Steril.2011 Aug;96(2):344-8.
Sullivan EA et al. Internation Committee for Monitoring Assisted Reproductive Technologies (ICMART) world report: assisted reproductive technology 2004. Hum Reprod. 2013 May;28(5):1375-90.
Sunderam S et al. Assisted reproductive technology surveillance-United states, 2009. MMWR Surveillance Summ. 2012 Nov 2;61(7):1-23.
Yilmaz N et al. The impact of single embryo transfer policy on pregnancy outcomes after legislation change. Gynecol Endocrinol. 2013 June; 29(6):600-2.
Zollner U, Dietl J. Perinatal risks after IVF and ICSI. J Perinat Med. 2013 Jan; 41(1):17-22.

Systematic reviews: Building blocks for the best practice of assisted reproductive technology

Cindy Farquhar

University of Auckland, Auckland, New Zealand

Introduction

Over the past 50 years there has been an exponential growth in clinical research. This growth has mirrored the technological advances in the field of reproductive medicine, such as assisted reproduction and ovulation induction. While such growth is welcome, it has also presented clinicians with some challenges. The busy clinician who needs to be well informed and up to date struggles with the volume and complexity of research papers. The approach of simply reading a single study is no longer considered sufficient to be up to date as that single paper probably does not represent the body of all the available evidence. The overwhelming number of studies available and the need to appraise the studies means that important findings may be overlooked.

The response to this problem has been the development of systematic reviews that summarize the studies on a particular topic. Over the past 20 years systematic reviews have become a useful and important tool for clinicians. They can enable clinicians and patients to make health care decisions based on evidence from all the available high-quality studies. The reason they are called systematic is that they systematically and explicitly describe their methods so that bias can be limited (Liberati 2009). They particularly seek to minimize bias by having pre-specified criteria for including, appraising, and summarizing the studies. The use of meta-analysis, a statistical method that combines the results of primary studies, allows for the calculation of more precise estimates of the effects of health care than those from the primary studies.

The move towards publishing systematic reviews has been led by the Cochrane Collaboration, which is focused on identifying reliable evidence and preparing systematic reviews of therapeutic interventions using randomized controlled trials (RCTs). The Collaboration has invested heavily in developing and improving the methodology of systematic reviews over the past two decades (Higgins 2011). Collaborative review groups have evolved within the Cochrane Collaboration, which now cover most areas of health care. There are currently 53 Cochrane Review Groups internationally and eight of these deal directly with the field of obstetrics and gynecology and women's health. These are the Cochrane Pregnancy and Childbirth Group, Cochrane Menstrual Disorders and Subfertility Group, Cochrane Incontinence Group, Cochrane Gynaecological Cancer Group, Cochrane Fertility Regulation Group, Cochrane Neonatal Group, Cochrane Sexually Transmitted Infections Group, and the Cochrane Breast Cancer Group.

The Cochrane Subfertility Group was one of the earliest Cochrane groups and commenced in 1992 at the University of Leeds. The Cochrane Menstrual Disorders Group commenced in 1996 at the University of Auckland. At the end of 1997 the two groups were merged and became the Cochrane Menstrual Disorders and Subfertility Group (CMDSG). Since that time the CMDSG has become the third most productive group in the Cochrane Collaboration. To date (March 2013) 166 full Cochrane reviews have been published, covering most topics within the scope. In addition, 53 protocols have been published and are currently being converted into full reviews. The CMDSG includes 800 authors from around the world who have now been trained in the preparation of systematic reviews. There is a board of 21 editors based in 7 counties with an editorial office based at the University of Auckland, New Zealand. The Collaboration provides a range of training resources including workshops in different Cochrane Centres around the world, online training, and individual assistance in preparing reviews. The Collaboration has invested considerable resources in improving the methodology of Cochrane Reviews (CRs) and in the software used to write CRs.

Why systematic reviews?

Systematic reviews summarize the results of randomized controlled trials in a broad range of topics. Instead of conducting your own search for studies and then sifting them for quality and applicability, a systematic review has already undertaken these steps for the reader. Each of these reviews has identified the clinical question, prepared a protocol that is then published, searched for the RCTs from usually 4-8 databases (with no language restriction), appraised the risk of bias within the studies, extracted the data independently, and summarized the data using meta-analysis. Perhaps the most challenging part of writing reviews is keeping them up to date – the Cochrane collaboration gold standard is to update reviews every two years. About 30% of our reviews have been updated in the past 2 years, 40% in the past 3 years, and 71% in the past 5 years.

There are almost 50 systematic reviews on the different steps that make up an assisted reproduction cycle (Farquhar 2013) and there are 34 other reviews on fertility interventions such as intrauterine insemination and ovulation induction. In the field of menstrual disorders there are 34 reviews on pelvic pain conditions including endometriosis; 11 on disorders of menstrual cycling such as polycystic ovarian syndrome, premenstrual syndrome, and hirsutism; 10 on heavy menstrual bleeding; 18 on gynecological surgery for non-malignant conditions; and 10 on management of menopausal symptoms.

Systematic reviews - building block for guidelines?

Systematic reviews are particularly useful to develop guidance for clinicians. A range of guidelines have used Cochrane reviews as an important source of evidence. For example, the ESHRE Guidelines for the Management of Women with Endometriosis (which has recently been sent out for comment) cites 15 Cochrane reviews (ESHRE 2013). This will be made easier in the future as all of the Cochrane reviews on endometriosis will be summarized in an overview (Brown 2013). The National Institute for Health and Clinical Excellence (NICE) guideline Fertility: Assessment and Treatment for People with Fertility Problems has been published in 2013, and 58 Cochrane reviews have been referenced (NICE 2013). Other examples of guidelines that have used Cochrane reviews are the Heavy Menstrual Bleeding published by NICE in 2007, which cited 14 Cochrane reviews (NICE 2007), and the committee opinions of the American Society for Reproductive Medicine, which also cite Cochrane reviews such as blastocyst transfers, preimplantation genetic screening, and single embryo transfer.

Some changes in policy have resulted from systematic reviews, although not always Cochrane reviews. A major focus of the past decade in reproductive medicine has been to reduce the harms associated with multiple pregnancy. The focus on pregnancy rates has come with the cost of increasing multiple pregnancies. The observation that the rate of pregnancy increased dramatically from 7.4% when only one embryo was transferred to over 20% when two or more embryos were transferred (Wood 1984) failed to appreciate that poor pregnancy rates when one embryo was transferred largely reflected the circumstance that only one embryo was available (Brinsden 2003). As a result multiple births have risen in most countries that offer assisted reproduction. There were some early calls to restrict the number of embryos transferred to two in recognition of the increased rate of perinatal mortality and morbidity associated with multiples, and the adverse consequences for families (Kerin 1983). A worldwide shift to double embryo transfer (DET) occurred after Templeton and Morris (1998) showed that DET had similar pregnancy rates, but far fewer higher-order multiples, than transfers of three or more embryos.

The first Cochrane review considering the number of embryos that should be transferred after in vitro fertilization (IVF) and intracytoplasmic sperm injection (ICSI) was published in 2004 (Pandian 2004). The authors found that "three small, poorly reported trials compared transfer of two versus one embryo in a single cycle, and one small, poorly reported trial compared transfer of two versus four embryos in a single cycle." They considered it "unlikely that the conclusions are robust enough to catalyse a change in clinical practice." The updated Cochrane Review published in 2009 included a further three trials. Notably, there were now two trials comparing DET to serial SET (with the second transfer either a fresh or frozen embryo). A much stronger conclusion was reached: "although the use of SET in a fresh IVF cycle results in lower livebirth rates, subsequent transfer of a frozen embryo can provide outcomes that are not significantly different to one fresh cycle of DET. The results have been clearly demonstrated in younger women. Single embryo transfer has a major impact in reducing twins in IVF."

Clinical practice with regard to the number of embryos being transferred is changing, albeit slowly. In Sweden (Ferraretti 2012), Australia, and New Zealand (Farquhar 2010), SET accounts for 70% of embryo transfers. Change has been slow in the United Kingdom (Templeton 2010) and in the United States (Fell 2012), despite the American Society for Reproductive Medicine's guidelines on the number of embryos transferred (ASRM & SART 2009), which cite the 2009 Cochrane Review and recommend that "for patients under the age of 35 who have a more favourable prognosis, consideration should be given to transferring only a single embryo."

Another example of a Cochrane Review highlighting harms is the review of preimplantation genetic screening (PGS) (Twist 2010). PGS was hailed in the early 2000s as a breakthrough for women of advanced maternal age. The hope was that pregnancy outcomes would be improved by identifying and transferring only euploid embryos. The review was first published in 2006 and updated in 2010. The first version of the review had only one RCT but the update had 9 RCTs including 1,589 women who underwent PGS with fluorescence in situ hybridization technique (FISH) for three different indications: advanced maternal age (5 RCTs), repeated failed implantation, and recurrent miscarriage. The results showed a 40% decrease in live births for women of advanced maternal age and a 60% decrease in repeated implantation failures. The authors recommended that newer techniques currently being developed, such as comparative genome hybridization (CGH), should be properly evaluated before routine clinical application is recommended. The ESHRE PGD Consortium published a position statement in 2010 stating, "The only effective way to resolve the debate is to perform more well-designed and well-executed clinical trials" (ESHRE PGD 2010).

Other contributions of systematic reviews

Systematic reviews have led to improved reporting of important outcomes. The editors of the Cochrane Menstrual Disorders and Subfertility Group have been able to highlight the deficiencies in clinical trial design in infertility interventions and the failure to report live birth outcomes. We have called for reporting of live birth as the most important outcome in fertility trials and also highlighted the need to report adverse events including ovarian hyperstimulation syndrome (OHSS) and multiple pregnancy (Clarke 2010, Vail 2003, Farquhar, and Vail 2006).

Systematic reviews have identified gaps in the evidence. These gaps have also been identified in a range of publications including editorials and also in lists generated by the NICE Fertility Guidelines in 2013 (NICE Fertility Guidelines 2013, Farquhar and Johnson 2004). There have been more than 2,000 new RCTs in reproductive medicine published over the past decade (Figure 1). Many of those new RCTs have been in the initiated following the publication of an analysis of Cochrane reviews highlighting the gap in evidence. Once the RCTs are published then the new data can be included in new and updated reviews. Some examples include laparoscopic ovarian drilling, studies of methotrexate for ectopic pregnancy, fallopian sperm perfusion, studies of the levonorgestrel intrauterine system for heavy menstrual bleeding, hysterectomy techniques, and laparoscopic uterine nerve ablation for dysmenorrhea.

Conclusion

In conclusion, the Cochrane Collaboration over the past 20 years has pioneered critical thinking about clinical research and synthesis. Developments in the field of reproductive medicine have allowed for 165 reviews to be published on a wide range of topics of interest to clinicians and their patients. With the continuing expansion of interventions in reproductive medicine there will be an ongoing need for such reviews. The development of clinical practice guidelines is the obvious place for systematic reviews to make an impact.

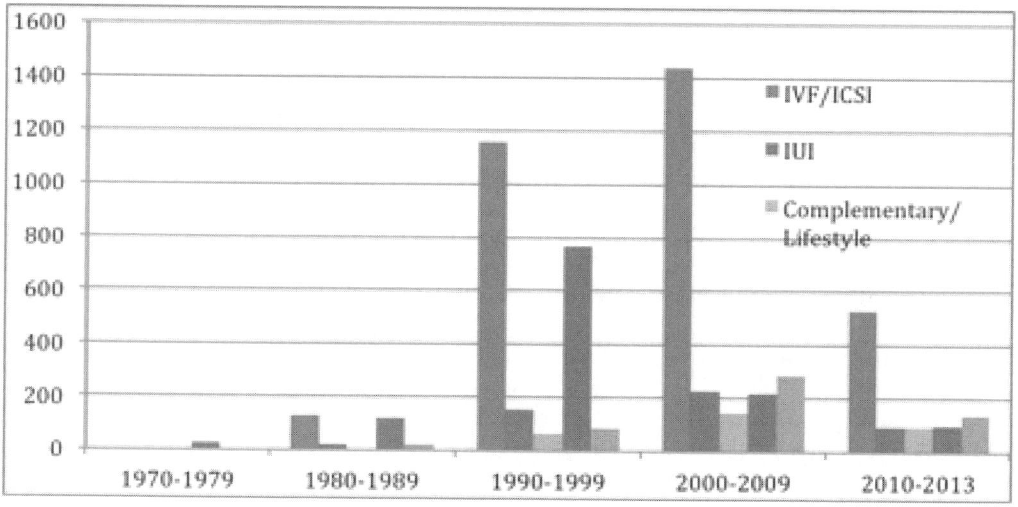

Figure 1. Number of randomized controlled trials published on fertility treatments 1970- 2013. (Source Cochrane Menstrual Disorders and Subfertility Group Register of Studies)

References

Brinsden P. Controlling the high order multiple birth rate: the European perspective. Reprod Biomed Online 2003;6(3):339-344.

Brown J, Farquhar C, Dias S. Endometriosis: an overview of Cochrane Reviews (Protocol). Cochrane Database of Systematic Reviews 2012, Issue 1. Art. No.: CD009590. DOI: 10.1002/14651858.CD009590.

Clarke J, van Rumste MME, Faruqhar CM, Johnson NP, Mol BWJ, Herbison P. Measuring outcomes in fertility trials: can we rely on clinical pregnancy rates? Fertility and sterility 2010; 94(5):1647-51.

ESHRE Endometriosis Guideline Development Group 2013 . Management of Women with Endometriosis (draft guideline) http://www.eshre.eu/binarydata.aspx?type=doc&sessionId=dhxqnrv5jhqpiw45ttwpuxup/ESHRE_ENDOMETRIOSIS_GUIDELINE_Draft_version_for_review.pdf

Farquhar CM, Johnson N P. The Evidence base for current treatments in infertility. Brit J Obstet & Gynae 2004; 111: 1-2.

Farquhar CM, Rishworth JR, Brown J, , Nelen WLDM. Assisted reproductive technology: an overview of Cochrane Reviews [Protocol]. Cochrane Database of Systematic Reviews [2013], In press.

Farquhar CM, Vail A. Pitfalls in Systematic Reviews. Current opinion in Obstetrics and Gynaecology 2006. 18:433-439.

Farquhar CM, Wang YA, Sullivan EA. A comparative analysis of assisted reproductive in Australia and New Zealand 2004-2007. Human Reproduction 2010. Electronic publication 22/07/2010.

Fell DB, Joseph K. Temporal trends in the frequency of twins and higher-order multiple births in Canada and the United States. BMC Pregnancy Childbirth 2012;12(1):103-109.

Ferraretti AP, Goossens V, de Mouzon J, Bhattacharya S, Castilla JA, Korsak V, et al. Assisted reproductive technology in Europe, 2008: results generated from European registers by ESHRE. Hum Reprod 2012;27(9):2571-84.

Harper JC, E. Coonen, M. De Rycke, G. Harton, C. Moutou, T. Pehlivan, J. Traeger-Synodinos, M.C. Van Rij, V. Goossens. ESHRE PGD consortium data collection X: cycles from January to December 2007 with pregnancy follow-up to October 2008. Hum. Reprod. (2010) 25 (11): 2685-2707.

Higgins JPT, Green S (editors). Cochrane Handbook for Systematic Reviews of Interventions Version 5.1.0 [updated March 2011]. The Cochrane Collaboration, 2011. Available from www.cochrane-handbook.org.

Kerin JF, Warnes GM, Quinn PJ, Jeffrey R, Kirby C, Matthews CD, et al. Incidence of multiple pregnancy after in-vitro fertilisation and embryo transfer. Lancet 1983;2(8349):537-40.

Liberati A, Altman DG, Tetzlaff J, Mulrow C, Gøtzsche PC, et al. (2009) The PRISMA statement for reporting systematic reviews and meta-analyses of studies that evaluate health care interventions: Explanation and elaboration. PLoS Med 6: e1000100.

Maheshwari A, Griffiths S, Bhattacharya S. Global variations in the uptake of single embryo transfer. Hum Reprod Update 2011;17(1):107-20.

NICE 2007: National Collaborating Centre for Women's and Children's Health. Heavy Menstrual Bleeding. Commissioned by the National Institute for Clinical Excellence. London: RCOG Press, 2007.

NICE 2013: National Collaborating Centre for Women's and Children's Health. Fertility: Assessment and Treatment for People with Fertility Problems. Commissioned by the National Institute for Clinical Excellence. London: RCOG Press, 2nd edition 2013.

Pandian Z, Bhattacharya S, Ozturk O, Serour G, Templeton A. Number of embryos for transfer following in-vitro fertilisation or intra-cytoplasmic sperm injection. Cochrane Database Syst Rev. 2009;(2):CD003416

Pandian Z, Templeton A, Serour G, Bhattacharya S. Number of embryos for transfer after IVF and ICSI: a Cochrane review. Hum Reprod 2005;20(10):2681-7.

Practice Committee of the American Society for Reproductive Medicine (ASRM); Practice Committee of the Society for Assisted Reproductive Technology (SART). Guidelines on number of embryos transferred. Fertil Steril 2009;92(5):1518-9.

Templeton A. Elective single versus double embryo transfer. BMJ 2010;341:c7083.

Tiitinen A, Halttunen M, Härkki P, Vuoristo P, Hyden-Granskog C. Elective single embryo transfer: the value of cryopreservation. Hum Reprod 2001;16(6):1140-4.

Templeton A, Morris JK. Reducing the risk of multiple births by transfer of two embryos after in vitro fertilization. N Engl J Med 1998;339(9):573-7.ional Collaborating Centre for

Twisk M, Mastenbroek S, van Wely M, Heineman MJ, Van der Veen F, Repping S. Preimplantation genetic screening for abnormal number of chromosomes (aneuploidies) in in vitro fertilization or intracytoplasmic sperm injection (Review).
Vail A, Gardener E. Common statistical errors in the design and analysis of subfertility trials. Hum Reprod. 2003 May;18(5):1000-4.
Wood C, Downing B, Trounson A, Rogers P. Clinical implications of developments in in vitro fertilisation. BMJ 1984;298(6450):978-80.

Translating evidence into practice

Siladitya Bhattacharya

University of Aberdeen, Aberdeen, United Kingdom

Summary

Evidence-based medicine requires the integration of research evidence, clinical expertise, and patient values and is believed to represent the best quality of clinical care. Robust data on interventions are ideally derived from appropriately performed systematic reviews and meta-analyses of randomized trials. In their absence, other sources of evidence include individual trials, controlled observational studies, case series, case studies, and expert opinion. Recommendations based on research evidence have been historically graded in a number of different ways. *The Grading of Recommendations Assessment, Development and Evaluation* or *GRADE* system, introduced in 2000, is thought to be superior to the earlier methods as it is able to capture not just the quality of the underlying data but also the consistency, clinical relevance, and external validity of the whole body of evidence (Guyatt et al, 2008).

Transfer of research knowledge to practitioners, managers, policy makers, and consumers is a complex process. It is becoming increasingly clear that individual studies are inappropriate as the unit for knowledge translation because they rarely provide definitive evidence to inform clinical practice. With the exception of some large trials, output from most individual studies can be unhelpful due to inherent bias or random variations in their results.

The currency of evidence translation: systematic reviews and guidelines

The sheer volume of research data and the requirement for appropriate skills and time to identify, read, and appraise relevant paper and electronic publications is such that individual papers are unsuitable as agents of evidence translation. The accepted currency of knowledge transfer is well-conducted, up-to-date systematic reviews and guidelines based on them. The Cochrane Collaboration has ensured the creation of a body of high-quality, peer-reviewed secondary research, which is updated on a regular basis. The paucity of randomized trials in some areas of reproductive medicine means that many of these Cochrane reviews are inconclusive due to lack of sufficient evidence. This can be frustrating to individual practitioners who are unable to make robust clinical decisions based on these published data alone. This is where a multidisciplinary guideline development group can use the GRADE system to assess the risks and benefits and interpret the relevance of the available evidence in the appropriate social, cultural, and economic context. The resulting guidelines aim to facilitate clinical decisions by making recommendations for clinicians, managers, patients, and policy makers. They involve an explicit process of evaluation of outcomes of alternative management strategies and clear criteria for downgrading and upgrading the quality of evidence. The process of moving from evidence to recommendations is transparent, acknowledging consumers' values and preferences.

The AGREE (Appraisal of Guidelines, Research, and Evaluation) instrument is a tool that assesses the methodological rigor and transparency of the methods by which a guideline is developed. The modified AGREE tool (AGREE II) comprises 23 items organized into the original six quality domains: i) scope and purpose; ii) stakeholder involvement; iii) rigor of development; iv) clarity of presentation; v) applicability; and vi) editorial independence (Bowers et al., 2010) and is used by most guideline development groups. Finally, for guidelines to remain contemporary, there is an obligation to update them on a regular basis (Shekelle et al., 2001).

Dissemination

Mere availability of secondary research and guidelines based on them is not sufficient to influence practice. There is a need for a policy of active dissemination among stakeholders. While it is acknowledged the target audience comprises health care providers, managers, policy makers, and consumers, it is less clear as to who should be primarily responsible for dissemination of evidence to these groups. This role is context related and could be an individual (clinician, researchers, or consumer), group, professional body, or health care organization (Grimshaw et al., 2012), depending on the target audience. The issue of credibility of the person or group responsible for dissemination is important, and authoritative endorsement from a professional organization, opinion leader, or government organizations can be a powerful lever for change.

Planned knowledge translation is more likely to be successful if the dissemination strategy is informed by a preliminary assessment of the likely barriers and facilitators.

Interventions used to improve dissemination of evidence include strategies for behavior change in professionals, printed educational materials, educational meetings, educational outreach visits by a trained person to meet with providers in their own setting, input from local opinion leaders, audit and feedback, reminders (patient or encounter-specific information designed to prompt a health professional to recall information), tailored interventions to overcome specific barriers, and multifaceted interventions. In addition to these, other interventions have targeted strategies to enhance information and communication among consumers (Grimshaw et al., 2012).

Distribution of printed guidelines alone has been shown to be ineffective in achieving changes in practice: guidelines are more likely to be effective if they are disseminated by an active educational intervention and implemented by patient-specific reminders relating directly to professional activity.

Other strategies focus on policy makers and senior health service managers. Formal and informal interactions between researchers and policy makers (policy networks and advisory committees) and research that is consistent with the values and beliefs of officials have been shown to increase use of research evidence in planning policy.

Factors responsible for gaps between evidence and practice

Social and personal factors

Acceptance of evidence-based care can only occur where the evidence is congruent with patients' beliefs and clinicians' preferences (Brozek et al., 2009). Failure to include patient-centered outcomes (e.g., disregarding quality of life or adverse effects) and placing excessive emphasis on surrogate outcomes of questionable importance to patients are common reasons for non-compliance with evidence-based treatment.

For service providers and consumers alike, it may be difficult to implement interventions that are counterintuitive or inconsistent with prevailing attitudes, cultural views, or personal and professional experience. An example is the case of elective single-embryo transfer in assisted reproduction in order to minimize the risk of iatrogenic multiple pregnancies. The effectiveness of this intervention in reducing the risk of multiples without compromising live birth rates in women with good prognosis is underpinned by robust data from randomized trials. These data show comparable success rates after either single-embryo transfer followed by replacement of a frozen single embryo and double-embryo transfer in a fresh in vitro fertilization treatment. Despite support from opinion leaders and regulatory authorities, this policy is yet to be implemented widely across the globe, mainly due to financial considerations, couples' and clinicians' strongly held beliefs about prejudicing success rates, and an active preference for twins.

Lack of resources

Barriers to the flow of evidence into practice can occur at an individual, group, or organizational (Brodribb et al., 2010) level. Despite practitioners' willingness to follow well-designed guidelines, resource constraints have been the major limiting factor in the implementation of elective single-embryo transfer, which has had a much higher uptake in countries where IVF is funded by the state as opposed to countries where couples have to pay - and, of course, where it is enforced by legislation (Maheshwari et al., 2011).

Interpretation of guidance: the role of education

While professional groups generally support evidence-based practice, there are clear differences in the way available research findings are interpreted. Differences amongst clinicians' understanding of research findings need to be acknowledged and the way they approach clinical uncertainty understood (O'Donell, 2004). This is particularly true in situations where often there are few data to support clinical decision-making. Examples in assisted reproduction include interventions to improve ovarian response in poor responders and to enhance embryo implantation following in vitro fertilization. Formal training in critical appraisal skills as well as a basic understanding of statistics as part of a clinical curriculum could foster an environment favorable to the practice of EBM (Mittal et al., 2010). Other barriers to widespread adoption of evidence-based practice include financial disincentives, lack of skill or equipment, local standards of care that are inconsistent with desired standards, and lack of appropriate knowledge and skills. Finally, a key element is appropriate professional–patient interaction in terms of communication and joint decision- making (Davies et al., 2007).

Measures of successful evidence translation

Views on appropriate endpoints of knowledge translation vary according to the perspective and background of stakeholders. There is debate about the influence of personal beliefs and preferences and policy context that can result in evidence-informed as opposed to evidence-based practice. Ultimately, the end point has to be changes in professional behavior and beyond that to improved health outcomes.

Conclusion

In recent years our focus has mainly been on evidence synthesis; it is time to concentrate on knowledge translation activities that can lead to better professional decision-making and improved clinical outcomes. The key challenge is to narrow the gap between the availability of evidence and its use in day-to-day practice. Guidelines sensitive to local sociocultural and economic factors are key tools for quality improvement in the presence of appropriate dissemination strategies.

References

Bowers MC, Kho ME, Browman GP, Burgers JS, Cluzeau F, Feder G, Fervers B, Graham ID, Grimshaw J, Hanna SE, Littlejohns P, Makarski j, Zitzelsberger L, For the AGREE Next Steps Consortium. AGREE II: Advancing guideline development, reporting and evaluation in health care. Preventive Medicine 2010;51:421-424.

Brodribb W. Barriers to translating evidence-based breastfeeding information into practice. Acta Paediatrics 2010 Dec 3. doi: 10.1111/j.1651-2227.2010.02108.x. [Epub ahead of print].

Brozek JL, Aki A, Coello A, Lang D, Jaeschke R, Williams JW, Phillips B, Lelgemann M, Lethaby A, Bousquet J, Guyatt GH, Schunemann HJ, For GRDAE working Group. Grading quality of evidence and strength of recommendations in clinical practice guidelines. Allergy 2009;64:669-677.

Grimshaw JM, Eccles MP, Lavis JN, Hill SJ, Squires JE. Knowledge translation of research findings Implementation Science 2012 7:50.

Guyatt GH Oxman AD, Vist GE, Kunz R, Falck-Ytter Y, Alonso-Coello P GRADE: an emerging consensus on rating quality of evidence and strength of recommendations. BMJ 2008;336:924–926.

Kulier R, Gee H, Khan K. Five steps from evidence to effect: exercising clinical freedom to implement research findings. British Journal of Obstetrics and Gynaecology 2008;115:1197-1202.

Maheshwari A, Griffiths S, Bhattacharya S. Global variations in the uptake of single embryo transfer. Hum Reprod Update. 2011 Jan-Feb;17(1):107-20.

Mittal R, Perakath B. Evidence-based surgery: knowledge, attitudes, and perceived barriers among surgical trainees. Journal of Surgical Education. 2010; 67:278-282.

O Donnell CA. Attitudes and Knowledge of primary care professionals towards evidence-based practice: a poster survey. Journal of Evaluation in Clinical Practice 2004;10:197-205.

Shekelle PG, Ortiz E, Rhodes S, Morton SC, Eccles MP, Grimshaw JM, Woolf SH. Validity of the agency for Healthcare Research and Quality Clinical Practice Guidelines. How quickly do guidelines become outdated? JAMA 2001;286:1461-1467.